COMMUNICATION DISORDERS OF THE AGED

COMMUNICATION DISORDERS OF THE AGED
A Guide for Health Professionals

by

Ronald L. Schow, Ph.D.,
John M. Christensen, Ph.D.,
John M. Hutchinson, Ph.D., and
Michael A. Nerbonne, Ph.D.

Department of Speech Pathology and Audiology
Idaho State University

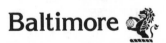

UNIVERSITY PARK PRESS
Baltimore

UNIVERSITY PARK PRESS
International Publishers in Science and Medicine
233 East Redwood Street
Baltimore, Maryland 21202

Typeset by Action Comp. Co., Inc.
Manufactured in the United States of America by The Maple Press Company

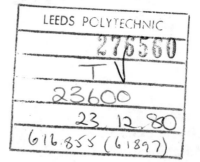

Library of Congress Cataloging in Publication Data

Main entry under title:

Communication disorders of the aged.

Bibliography: p.
Includes index.
1. Geriatrics. 2. Speech, Disorders of.
3. Hearing disorders. 4. Communicative disorders.
I. Schow, Ronald L.
RC952.5.C63 618.9′768′55 78-2596
ISBN 0-8391-1237-8

Dedicated to
the older generation—
especially some favorites,
our parents

Contents

Foreword

Given the rapidly developing interest in the topic of aging, the publication *Communication Disorders of the Aged: A Guide for Health Professionals* by Schow, Christensen, Hutchinson, and Nerbonne is a welcome event. The book adds substance to the set of concerns that have been expressed by those who have written about the psychosocial adjustment of the elderly. The discussions it contains underscore the fact that for human beings of any age to live meaningful and happy lives they must continue to communicate with others.

When interaction with others is blunted by loss of hearing or by language fractionation, the effects can be dehumanizing. For it is through the language process that human beings share their needs, hopes, aspirations, and innermost thoughts. Surely nonverbal communication often partially supplements, or substitutes for, verbal communication; but it does not offer the possibilities for so comprehensive an exchange as does the verbal.

As people grow older and transcend the world of work for that of retirement, there is simply more time for enjoying the social relationships that are so important to a happy existence. Without the ability to hear, understand, and reply, the socialization process is thwarted and the older persons become isolated from those about them. And with this isolation comes the feeling of being apart from, as contrasted to that of being a part of, the world about them.

The authors of this book present in a most logical manner the case for assisting those older persons who sustain disorders of communication. Their broad-ranging and comprehensive discussions first deal with the dynamics of the normal communication process and then provide the reader with a view of those psychobiological changes that take place as the human organism ages. Against this backdrop the authors develop in detail their insights into the specific types of disorders of communication that are frequently observed in older people.

Although audiologists and speech/language pathologists have been serving the needs of older persons for years, the present work serves to highlight the growing importance of this age group. As their numbers increase, older people will draw much more heavily upon the skills of all those who serve them.

Since most older people continue to live in their own homes or those of relatives, the importance of the role of the family in the delivery of care to those who sustain disorders of communication cannot be overemphasized. It is the family which provides the principal source of support to the elderly, and there must be understanding of the behavior that can be expected from the older members of the family who sustain disorders of communication. Unless there is this understanding and unless coping strategies are adequately developed, life can become tedious and frustrating for all concerned. The timely chapter at the end of the book deals well with this important topic.

Health professionals will find the work of Schow, Christensen, Hutchinson, and Nerbonne very valuable as they encounter older persons with disorders of communication. The understanding on the part of the health professionals will be increased by the material presented in this book, and this increased understanding will have a telling effect upon the eventual adjustments that are made by, and for, those older persons who sustain communication disorders.

Herbert J. Oyer, Ph.D.
Professor, Audiology and Speech Sciences
Dean, The Graduate School
Michigan State University

Preface

There has been a growing national and international interest in gerontology and the problems of aging. This certainly has been true with the profession of speech/language pathology and audiology. However, to date, the literature concerning communicative disorders among the elderly has been rather scattered in professional journals and books. Furthermore, widespread misunderstanding and lack of information exist among nearly all health professionals regarding the nature and impact of speech, hearing, and language disorders among the elderly. This book represents an effort to collect, for perhaps the first time, the scattered literature and present it in a readable fashion to all health professionals regardless of academic and clinical training.

The idea for this book was generated when all four authors became involved in presenting a series of workshops for nursing homes in the state of Idaho under the auspices of Program IMPACT of the Higher Education Act of 1965, Title I: Community Service and Continuing Education, U.S. Office of Education and the Idaho State Commission for Higher Education Facilities. At these workshops, we became acutely aware of the need for greater professional understanding of the communication problems of the elderly. In subsequent conversations with our colleagues around the country, it became clear that this situation was not unique to Idaho; it was clearly a national problem. We hope this volume provides an educational tool for the health professional—including the speech/language pathologist and audiologist—as well as a means to better diagnosis and rehabilitation for our elderly handicapped who desperately need and deserve these services.

We are all indebted to our wives and families for assistance and encouragement. Special thanks are extended to Dean Paul Leiby of the College of Health Related Professions and other members of the administration who have supported this endeavor. Finally, our appreciation is tendered to Jacque Overton and Diane Hutchinson for their cheerful preparation of the manuscript in the face of some rather immediate deadlines as well as to Jeff Webster who helped design the jacket.

COMMUNICATION DISORDERS OF THE AGED

Section I
OVERVIEW

Chapter 1
Introduction

Discussion is presented pertaining to the current and future status of the elderly in this country. Statistics demonstrate the anticipated growth in the number of persons over 65 years of age, and the high incidence of speech, language, and hearing disorders in the age group is discussed. Emphasis is placed on the need for increased awareness on the part of all professions working with the elderly regarding all types of communication disorders.

A NEGLECT FOR GERONTOLOGY

It is a curious fact that until recently the entire area of gerontology has received relatively little attention by health-related professionals. Evidence of a general nature has existed for some time concerning the profound effects which the aging process can have on a man's physical, psychological, and social well-being that seemingly would have resulted in a strong effort to address ourselves to these issues. But it has only been in the past few years that aging has received the attention it so desperately needs. We Americans in particular seem to have been guilty of ignoring the entire issue of aging. A strong urge prevails in this country to remain young and continually appear youthful at all costs. Utility in our society seems at times to be almost totally linked with age, with the elderly often being perceived as noncontributors. The term "ageism" has been suggested by Butler and Lewis (1973) to indicate an automatic prejudice toward the elderly. Attitudes of this nature have, in part, been responsible for making the elderly one of the most neglected and misunderstood minorities in our society today.

Evidence of this absence of a strong commitment toward gerontology is especially apparent in certain areas of the health professions. A survey conducted by Senator Charles Percy with the 114 medical schools in the country is quite revealing in this regard. Of the 87 schools responding, only three indicated that geriatrics is taught as a specialty in their curricula (Kent, 1977). Senator Percy compared the results of this survey with those conducted in 1970 and 1974 and concluded that slow but increasing awareness of the needs of the elderly is occurring in schools of medicine. This information is somewhat alarming when data presented by Somers (1972) and Somers and Somers (1968) regarding health care of the elderly are considered. Somers (1972) noted that although the elderly comprise only a small percent of the current population, they are the major users of medications, professional time, and health dollars. Those above 65 years of age occupy 33% of the 1 million hospital beds and 95% of the 1.2 million long-term beds in the country. In addition, the aged account for more office calls for medical treatment by a physician than any other age group (Libow, 1977). The emphasis of the training that many physicians receive is clearly not consistent with the composition of the patients they serve.

Academic preparation in gerontology in the field of social work also appears less than adequate. The Council on Social Work Education (1975) reported that of the 84 schools of social work which are accredited in the United States, only 26 offer concentrations or special work with the aging.

The disciplines of speech pathology and audiology have likewise failed to some degree in responding to the needs of the elderly. Data from a Metropolitan Life Insurance report (1976), Schow and Nerbonne (1976), and Miller and Ort (1965) have indicated that the incidence of hearing loss in the elderly ranges from 20 to nearly 97%, depending upon the nature of the group evaluated. Statistics also indicate the presence of a high incidence of speech and/or language disorders in the aging, with an estimate of such cases approaching 1 million (Spahr, 1971). And yet few of the training programs in speech pathology or audiology currently offer specific coursework in gerontology. This fact was documented some time ago by Morley (1963) and appears not to have changed substantially since then. Only in recent years has the literature in speech and hearing contained any extensive work related to the communication problems associated with senescence.

A CHANGING ATTITUDE

Recent developments, however, suggest that the situation may be changing considerably. More and more attention is being focused on the gerontologic population by the general public, with increased involvement occurring within governmental agencies and scientific communities on matters associated with the elderly. Perhaps one of the major factors which serves to explain this accelerated interest is the realization that, like the inevitability of death and taxes, each of us will grow old at some point in the future, and the present circumstances associated with this condition are, in many instances, not good. Each of us simply wishes to improve the living conditions of the elderly because we anticipate becoming a member of this minority ourselves someday, and we wish to avoid many of the adverse conditions that currently exist for the aged.

Another probable explanation regarding the recent emphasis on aging is found in some of the statistical information available from the U.S. Bureau of Census (1977). The number of individuals in this country over 65 years of age has grown rapidly, with 23 million currently being included in this age group. This represents approximately one-tenth of the total U.S. population. It is projected that by the year 2040 this number will swell to a total of nearly 55 million with one out of every six persons being over 65. Figure 1-1 demonstrates the anticipated increase in the number of individuals over 65 years of age from the present until the year 2040. The increases observed will undoubtedly have a strong influence on society in the future.

COMMUNICATION AND THE ELDERLY

Out of the ever-increasing body of knowledge concerning gerontology, a number of areas of major need or concern have arisen. One of these

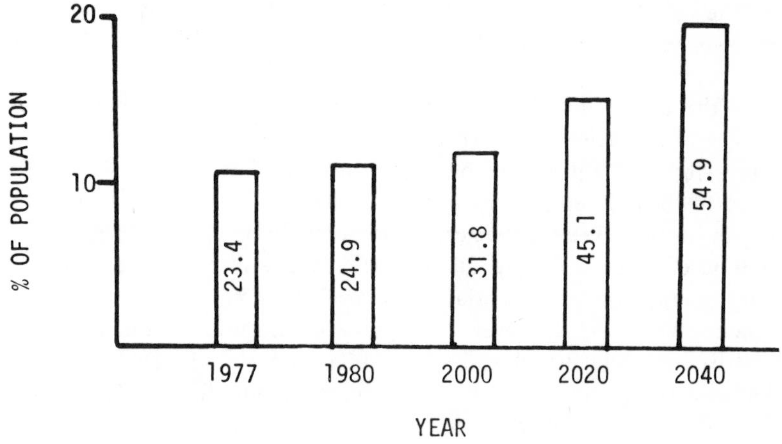

Figure 1-1. Projected percentage of the total population that is 65 years or older. Actual number (in millions) is noted in the bar. (Source: U.S. Bureau of Census, 1977.)

areas which has been recognized as being particularly crucial to the aged is that of communication. The importance of this process is pointed out in a recently published book entitled *Aging and Communication* (Oyer and Oyer, 1976), in which the various interrelationships that exist between these two important factors are explored in detail. Among other issues, the book considers the role of communication for the aging in such areas as mass media, interaction with older people, consumerism, organizations for the elderly, education, and religion. All of these areas are rich with needs for communication and involve special difficulties for the elderly. As Oyer and Oyer point out, at a time in life when communication is most important, the older individual experiences a diminished capacity to communicate that is usually the direct result of some type of physiologic deterioration associated with the process of aging. This is reflected outwardly in a diminished ability to hear and comprehend what is presented and/or to express oneself in a normal fashion.

It is this diminished ability on the part of the aged to communicate that is of utmost concern in this book. An attempt is made to present information that will create an increased awareness on the part of the reader about the various types of speech, language, and hearing disorders observed in the elderly. Material is presented regarding the diagnosis and remediation of communication disorders in this specific population, as is information concerning proper referral sources and procedures. Of particular interest is the discussion on the role of professionals other than speech pathologists and audiologists, such as nurses and family members, in dealing with the communication problems of the elderly. Because we anticipate that the book will be used by persons with a wide degree of variability in expertise in speech and hearing, we have included a list of suggested readings at the conclusion of each chapter to provide guidance to those interested in pursuing particular topics in a more in-depth fashion. We recognize that some of the material included may not be of direct value to all readers because of the quite divergent backgrounds of the potential audience for whom the material is intended. We hope, however, that much of the information presented will be beneficial to all and will serve to increase the awareness and knowledge of communication problems among the aged. Progress toward this end will make it possible for the elderly to compensate more readily for whatever speech, language, and/or hearing problems they may possess, a goal all of us share.

SUGGESTED READINGS

Cottrell, F. Aging and the Aged. Dubuque, Iowa: William C. Brown, 1974.
Mayer, A. The graying of America. Newsweek, 89, 50–64 (Feb., 1977).

REFERENCES

Butler, R., and Lewis, M. Aging and Mental Health. St. Louis: C. V. Mosby, 1973.

Council on Social Work Education. Summary of information on Master of Social Work programs, 1975.

Kent, S. Is training in geriatric medicine being neglected? Geriatrics, 32, 110–114 (1977).

Libow, L. The issues in geriatric medical education and postgraduate training: Old problems in a new field. Geriatrics, 32, 99–101 (1977).

Metropolitan Life Insurance Co. Hearing impairments in the United States. Metropolitan Life Insurance Statistics, 57, 7–9 (1976).

Miller, M., and Ort, R. Hearing problems in a home for the aged. Acta Otolaryngologica, 59, 33–44 (1965).

Morley, D. The training and experience of graduate students in communication problems of the aging. Asha, 5, 819–821 (1963).

Oyer, H., and Oyer, J. Communicating with older people: Basic considerations. In H. Oyer and J. Oyer (eds.), Aging and Communication. Baltimore: University Park Press, 1976.

Schow, R., and Nerbonne, M. Hearing levels in nursing home residents. Research Laboratory Report 1, pp. 1-10. Department of Speech Pathology and Audiology, Idaho State University, Pocatello, 1976.

Somers, A. The nation's health issues for the future. Annals of the American Academy of Political and Social Sciences, 399, 160 (1972).

Somers, H., and Somers, A. Medicare and the Hospitals. Washington, D.C.: The Brookings Institute, 1968.

Spahr, F. 1971 White House Conference on Aging. Asha, 13, 14–17 (1971).

U.S. Bureau of Census. Current Population Reports, Series P-25, No. 704. Projections of the population of the U.S.: 1977-2050. Washington, D.C.: U.S. Government Printing Office, July 1977.

Chapter 2
Anatomic and Physiologic Bases of the Communication Process

In this chapter a general overview is presented of the structures of importance in the process of communication, including speech, language, and hearing functions. The major divisions of the central nervous system are reviewed, with specific reference to their roles in communication. The intent is to provide a ready reference for other material associated with the aged that is presented in the remainder of the volume.

In identifying and discussing the anatomic structures involved in the total process of communication, it is desirable for the sake of presentation to segregate the related material into two major divisions: the auditory system; and the speech and language systems. The intent is to relate anatomic and physiologic information regarding these systems to the process of communication.

THE AUDITORY SYSTEM

Man's entire auditory system can be partitioned into two general subdivisions: the peripheral auditory mechanism and the central auditory mechanism. The peripheral portion of the ear traditionally has been considered to include three major sections: the outer ear, the middle ear, and the inner ear (see Figure 2-1). The peripheral auditory structures generally serve to receive auditory stimuli in the form of acoustic energy and to convert or transduce this initially into a suitable form of vibratory energy, followed by another conversion to electrochemical energy. It is this signal which is then transmitted to the other major portion of the auditory system, the central auditory mechanism. Within the central mechanism are the critical structures of the brain stem and higher cortical areas of the brain which are directly or indirectly involved in the process of

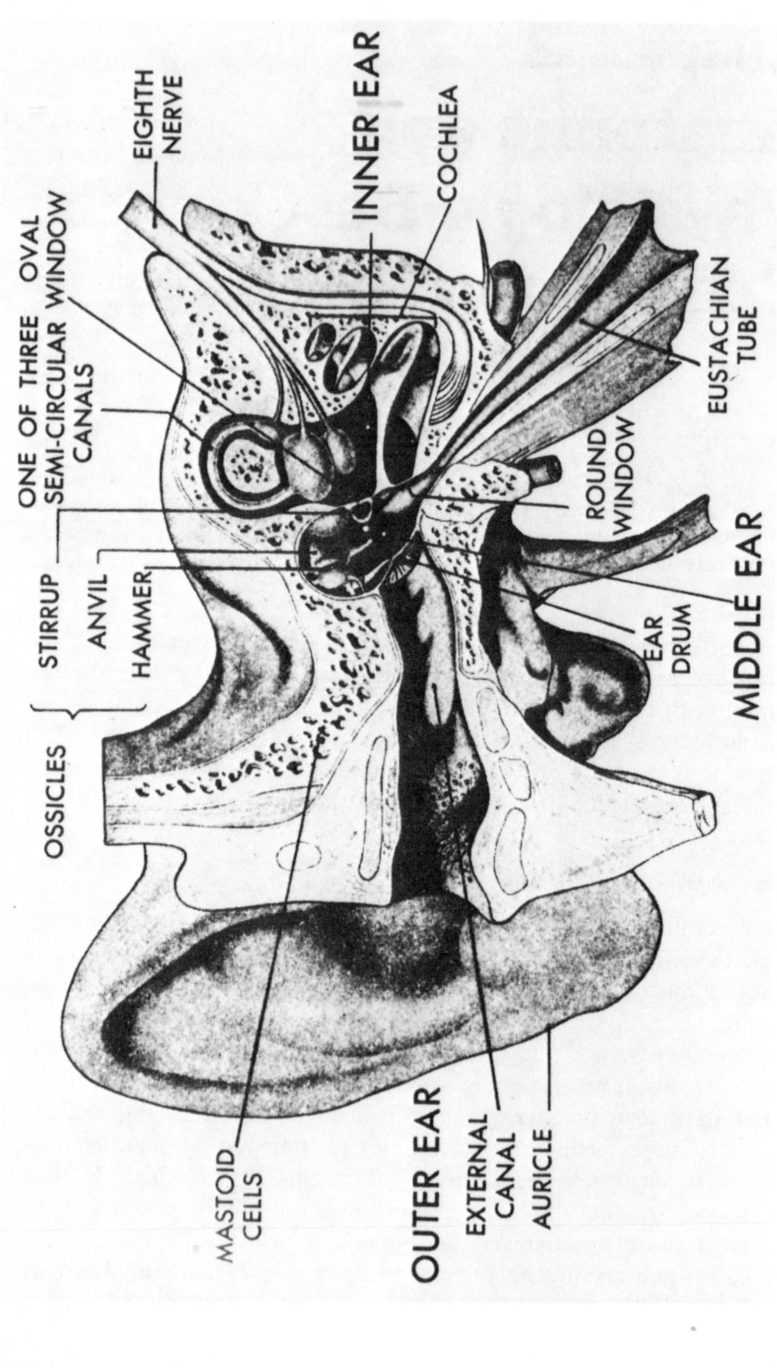

Figure 2-1. Sectional diagram of the human ear. (Source: Sonotone Corporation, Elmsford, N.Y.; reproduced by permission.)

hearing. It is here that much of the information received by the peripheral structures is decoded and processed for the purpose of perception.

The major anatomic and physiologic features of the structures within the auditory system are identified and discussed, beginning with the peripheral portion and concluding with the central auditory structures.

The Peripheral Auditory Mechanism

Outer Ear The outer or external ear is that portion of the auditory mechanism which, for the most part, is outwardly visible. Its chief function is to collect and direct sound waves to the structures of the middle ear. Two major structures are contained within this division of the ear: the auricle, or pinna, and the external auditory meatus.

Auricle The auricle or pinna is the most prominent structure of the hearing mechanism (see Figure 2-2); it is that part of the outer ear shaped vaguely in the form of a cup or funnel and is

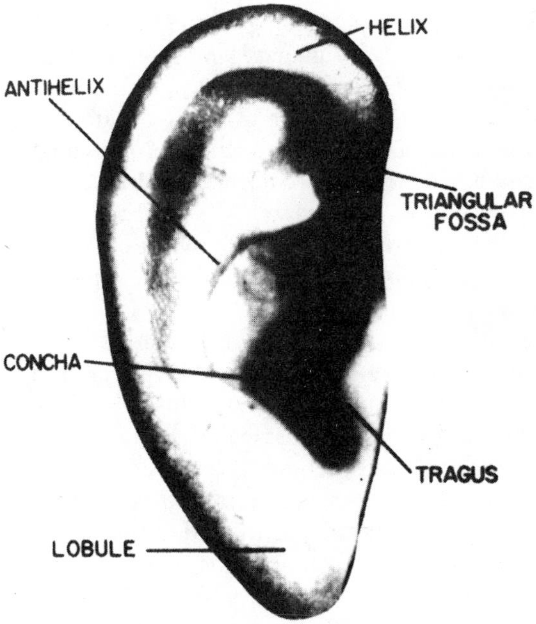

Figure 2-2. The human pinna (auricle). (Source: Durrant and Lovrinic, 1977.)

located on the side of the head. The pinna is composed entirely of cartilage which is covered with skin, and has a number of landmarks on its contoured surface. The outermost rim of the pinna if referred to as the helix. Another ridge on the pinna which runs inside of and parallels the helix is the antihelix. The extreme lower portion, which may extend downward to some degree in certain individuals, is called the lobule. Immediately above the lobule is the antitragus. Just anterior to the opening to the ear canal is a tiny protruding structure, the tragus. The depression in the pinna bounded by the tragus, antitragus, and antihelix is referred to as the concha. The concha serves as the opening into the external auditory meatus. The auricle's role in the hearing process is a minor one. It does serve to some extent to collect and direct sound waves into the ear canal, but its contribution is, at best, a slight one.

External auditory meatus This tube-like structure is continuous with the auricle and extends medially into an opening in the temporal bone of the skull. It is generally 26–30 mm long, with a width of approximately 7 mm. The canal is entirely lined with skin and is terminated medially by the tympanic membrane, or eardrum.

The outer one-third of the external canal traverses through cartilage. This portion of the lining of the canal contains tiny cilia, or hairs, and the subaceous glands, which secrete a waxy substance known as cerumen. The presence of the hair and cerumen serve somewhat to prevent the entrance of foreign material into the inner portion of the canal. The inner two-thirds of the canal pass through bone and contain none of the cilia or wax-producing glands found in the outer portion of the meatus. The external auditory meatus is tilted at a slight upward angle as it traverses into the skull. This, together with the action of the cilia and wax, serves to help protect the middle and inner ear structures.

Middle Ear Just behind the eardrum is a relatively small (2 cm^3) space known as the tympanic cavity or middle ear. This tiny area contains a number of structures critical for hearing, including the eardrum, the Eustachian tube, the ossicles, and a number of important muscles and ligaments. As a unit, the middle ear cavity transduces the acoustic energy it receives at the eardrum into vibratory or mechanical energy and transfers this to the next portion of the auditory system, the inner ear.

Tympanic membrane This structure, commonly referred to as the eardrum, serves as a partition between the outer and middle ear and is located at the end of the innermost portion of the ear canal.

It is an extremely thin and delicate structure and is circular in shape, as shown in Figure 2-3.

Most of the tympanic membrane is made up of three separate layers of tissue. The outer layer is made up of cutaneous tissue that is continuous with the tissue lining the ear canal. The inner layer is composed of mucousal tissue which lines the entire middle ear cavity, and the middle layer is composed of fibrous connective tissue. That portion of the eardrum having these three layers of tissue is termed the pars tensa. A small triangular portion of the drum, the pars flaccida, is located in the upper part of the membrane and does not have a middle or fibrous layer. This makes the pars flaccida more flexible than the pars tensa, allowing the tympanic membrane to be highly responsive and mobile as sound waves strike it. The eardrum is cone shaped, with its center, or umbo, protruding slightly into the middle ear cavity.

Ossicles The ossicles, a chain-like network made up of three tiny bones, bridge the middle ear cavity and connect the outer and inner ear portions of the hearing mechanism (see Figure 2-4). The first of these, the malleus, is attached to the middle tissue layer of the eardrum. Because of this, when sound waves create movement of the tympanic membrane the malleus is also set into motion. The second ossicle, the incus, is attached to the malleus and also joins

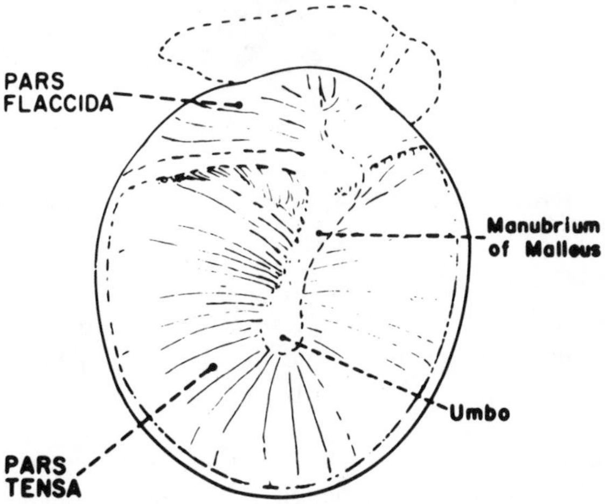

Figure 2-3. Lateral view of the right tympanic membrane. (Source: Anson and Donaldson, 1973.)

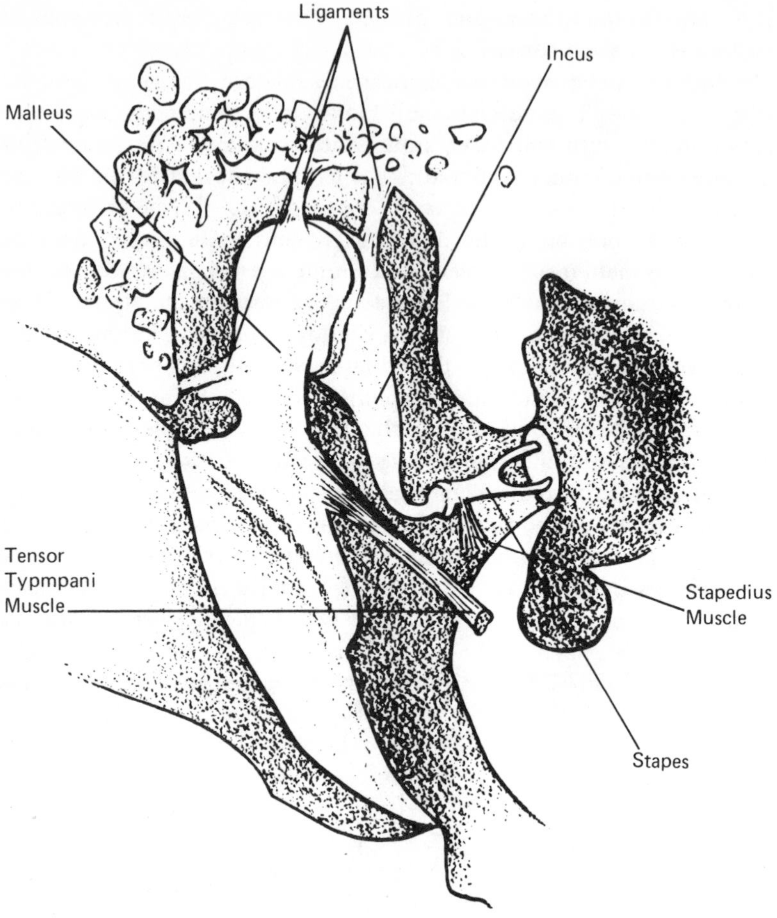

Figure 2-4. The ossicles together with their associated ligaments and muscles. (Source: Adapted from Palmer, 1972.)

with the last ossicle, the stapes, to form the entire ossicular chain. It is the stapes which fits into the oval window, an opening of the bony covering of the inner ear, and thereby initiates the stimulation of the sensory structures contained in that portion of the auditory system.

The ossicles therefore work as a unit, with the movement of the malleus triggering similar action in the remainder of the chain, first with the incus and then with the stapes. The lever action which results during the movement of the ossicles plays a critical role in explaining the acute hearing which man enjoys.

Muscles and ligaments The entire ossicular chain is suspended within the middle ear cavity by a series of ligaments which attach to numerous locations on the three bones. These ligaments generally function to hold the ossicles in place during their vibration and to assist in the termination of ossicular movement once a sound has ceased, minimizing the amount of distortion created in the auditory system.

Two muscles, the stapedius and the tensor tympani, are located within the middle ear. The stapedius muscle originates on the posterior wall of the middle ear cavity and attaches to the stapes. When this muscle contracts, the stapes is pulled somewhat from the oval window, altering its normal movement. The tensor tympani originates near the Eustachian tube and attaches to the malleus. Its contraction exerts a strong pull on the malleus medially and anteriorly within the middle ear. These two muscles have been shown to contract automatically when an individual is exposed to intense auditory stimulation. Contraction of these two muscles reduces the mobility of the ossicular chain and results in the transfer of less energy to the inner ear. Thus, these muscles play a minor role in the protection of the ear from damage resulting from exposure to intense sound.

Eustachian tube This very important structure is a canal which connects the middle ear cavity with the nasopharynx, near the back of the throat. The tube is normally closed and can be opened through muscular action associated with activities such as swallowing or yawning. The Eustachian tube allows for the exchange of air in and out of the middle ear cavity, a function vital to maintaining normal hearing. It is very important that the air pressure on both sides of the eardrum be equal so that the drum may move freely during stimulation; and since the tissues of the middle ear continually absorb air, the Eustachian tube must allow for the entrance of additional air into the middle ear. Failure to equalize the air pressure in the middle ear cavity with the outside pressure results in the eardrum being retracted into the middle ear cavity under pressure, making it less responsive to sound waves which reach it and creating a mild decrease in hearing acuity.

Inner Ear In addition to containing the end organ for hearing, the inner ear also holds the end organ for balance. Both are encased in the same bony capsule which is part of the temporal bone of the skull. The balance mechanism, sometimes termed the vestibular system, is composed of several critical structures, including the saccule and utricle and three fluid-filled semicircular canals. These components work together in a complex fashion to provide us with much needed information pertaining to equilibrium.

Our concern at this time, however, is with the end organ for hearing. This portion of the inner ear is termed the cochlea and contains a highly complex network of structures vital to the process of hearing.

The inner ear contains both a bony or osseous labyrinth and a membranous labyrinth. The osseous labyrinth is a series of cavities enclosed in the temporal bone, while the membranous labyrinth is a network of fluids and tissues found within the bony labyrinth. Both are shown in Figures 2-5 and 2-6.

The auditory portion of the inner ear, the cochlea, has a coiled shape somewhat like that of a snail. The footplate of the stapes fits into the oval window, which serves as an opening through the bony capsule into a space within the inner ear referred to as the vestibule. The vestibule is a common area within the inner ear for both the cochlear and vestibular systems and connects directly to the basal portion of the cochlea.

The cochlea contains three separate tube-like structures, the scala vestibuli, scala tympani, and scala media. The scala vestibuli

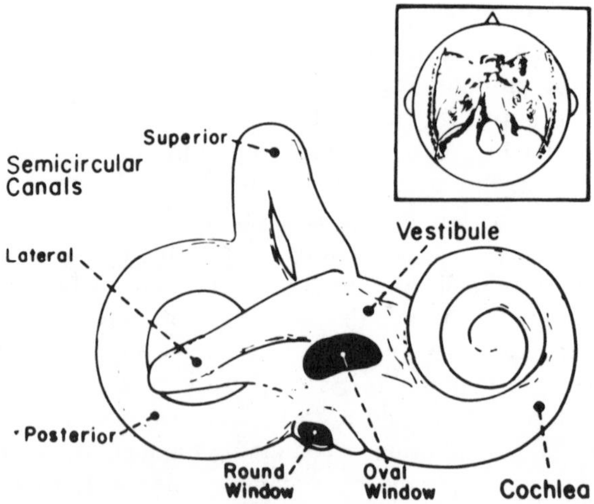

Figure 2-5. The osseous bony labyrinth (right ear) as viewed from a slightly lateral and slightly anterior (inset) perspective. (Source: Based on drawings of Sobatta, 1954; and after Schuknecht, 1974.)

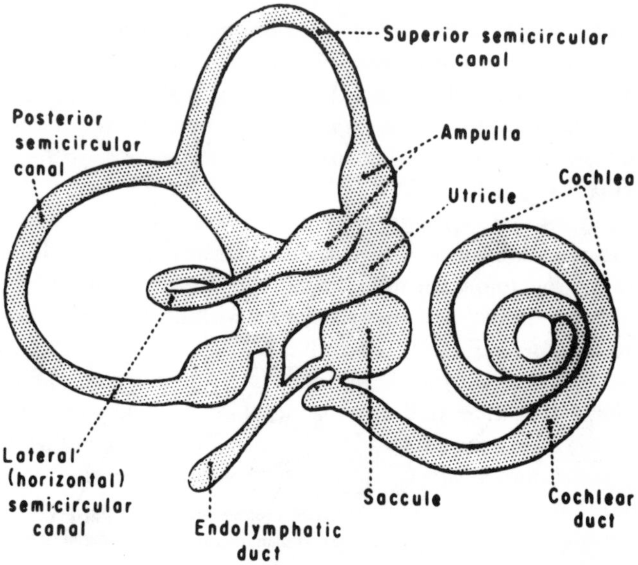

Figure 2-6. Partially schematic drawing representing the shape and parts of the right membranous labyrinth. (Source: DeWeese and Saunders, 1968.)

and scala tympani are located above and below the scala media and are filled with a fluid called perilymph, as is the vestibule. Though considered separate chambers, the scala vestibuli and scala tympani do join at a common point at the apex of the cochlea called the helicotrema. The scala tympani terminates with a structure similar to the oval window termed the round window, which is another opening through the bony labyrinth of the inner ear into the middle ear cavity (see Figure 2-7).

The scala media is located between these two chambers and is filled with another type of fluid called endolymph. Reissner's membrane separates it from the scala vestibuli, while the basilar membrane partitions it from the scala tympani.

Within the scala media is the organ of Corti. This end organ for hearing rests on the basilar membrane and the scala media, together with the scala vestibuli and scala tympani, wrap around the two and one-half turns of the snail-shaped cochlea.

The organ of Corti is made up of three to four rows of outer hair cells and a single row of inner hair cells, which have tiny cilia on their superior surface that are in contact with the tectorial membrane, a structure which hangs over them. Nerve fibers associated

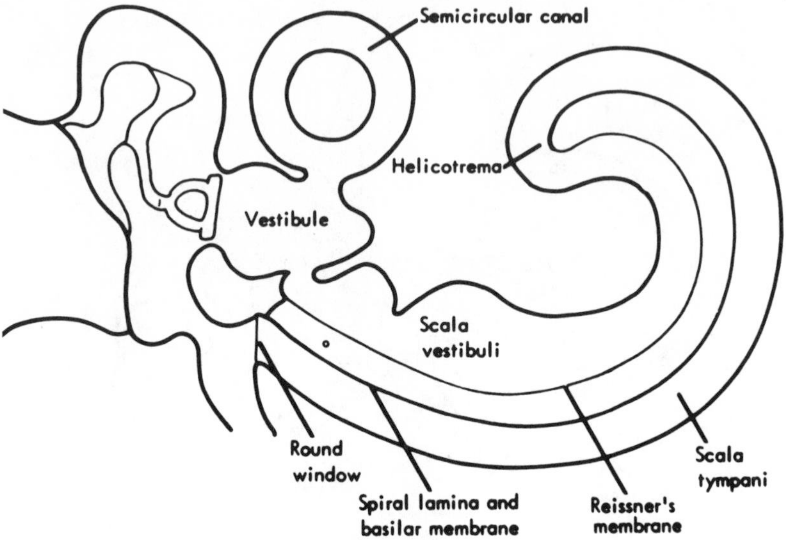

Figure 2-7. Schematic of the hearing mechanism, illustrating the relationship between the vestibule, scala vestibuli, scala tympani, and the cochlear duct. (Source: Zemlin, 1968, *Speech and Hearing Science,* © 1968. Reprinted by permission of Prentice-Hall, Inc., Englewood Cliffs, N.J.)

with the auditory nerve are embedded in the basilar membrane and innervate each of the more than 20,000 inner and outer hair cells in this very complex sensory structure. A cross-sectional view of these and other structures is shown in Figure 2-8.

Movement of the stapes in and out of the oval window creates displacement within the perilymph, causing the round window to bulge in and out in response to the action of the stapes. This fluid movement is also transmitted to the scala media and the sensory structures of the organ of Corti. Displacement of the endolymph and the basilar membrane occurs. Movement of the basilar membrane triggers the movement of the hair cell cilia through a shearing action which occurs between the basilar and tectorial membranes. The action of the cilia results in displacement of the hair cells, which in turn initiates electrochemical changes within the hair cells which trigger neural impulses within the nearby nerve fibers. These impulses are carried through the auditory nerve eventually to the next major division of the auditory system, the central auditory mechanism.

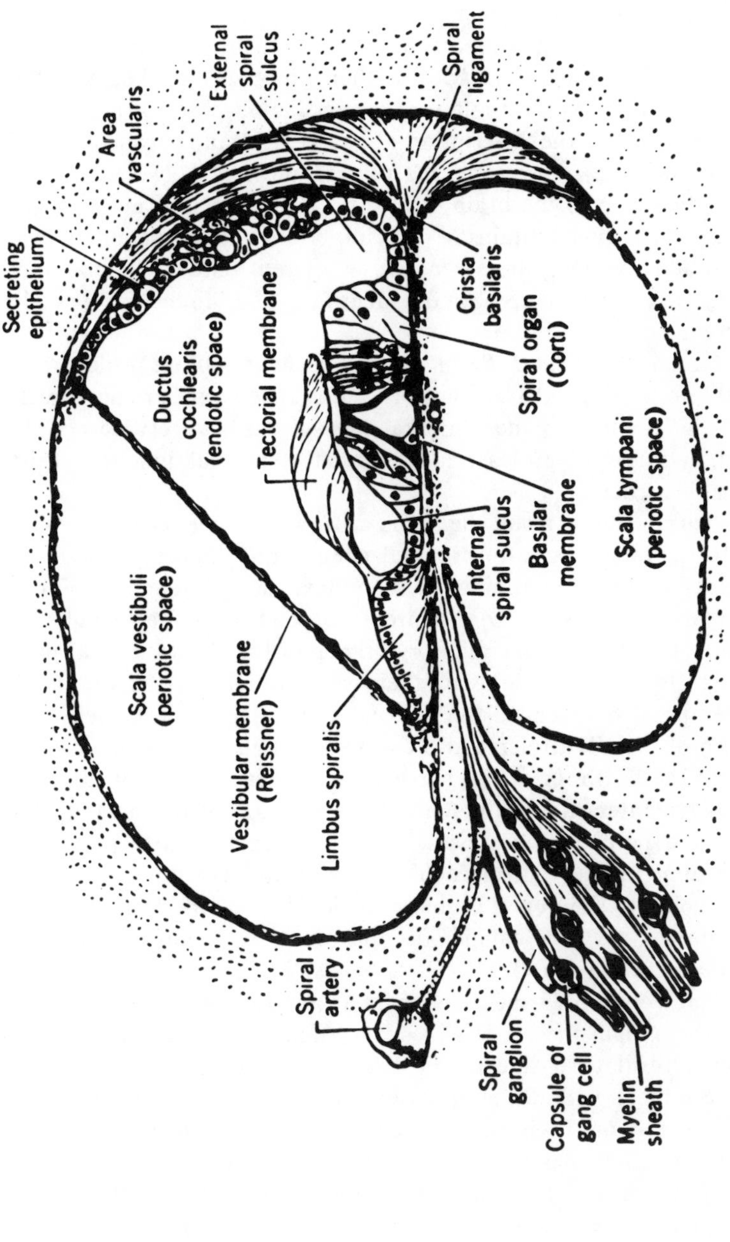

Figure 2-8. Illustration of the division of the cochlea into the scale vestibuli, scala media (cochlear duct), and scala tympani. (Source: Stevens, 1951.)

The Central Auditory Mechanism

Although basic intensity and frequency coding of auditory information occurs within the peripheral auditory system at the level of the cochlea, portions of the central auditory tract provide further coding as well. All of this information is then processed by the important structures of the central auditory system for purposes of perception.

To facilitate the description of the central auditory pathway, it is advantageous to separate the central auditory network into two major divisions: 1) the brain stem, and 2) the cerebral auditory cortex. Each division contains several important centers or junctions of neural activity along the ascending or afferent pathway of the auditory network which are briefly identified and discussed (see also Figure 2-9).

Eighth Nerve and Brain Stem The neural fibers which make up the ascending central auditory pathway do not extend directly from the cochlea to the temporal lobe of the auditory cortex. Instead, a series of at least four separate neuronal junctions exists along this tract.

Neural fibers from the hair cells within the cochlea collect within the modiolus to form spiral ganglia and then proceed to the cochlear nuclei, the first of the auditory neural junctions. These fibers are termed first-order neurons. Beyond the spiral ganglia the fibers collect to form the auditory branch of the VIIIth cranial nerve and exit from the modiolus on their way through a small channel in the temporal bone called the internal auditory canal. The vestibular branch of the VIIIth nerve also courses through this opening as well, as does the VIIth, or facial, nerve. The cochlear portion of the auditory nerve enters the brain stem at the junction of the medulla and pons, and here the fibers split into two branches, with one group proceeding to the ventral cochlear nuclei and the other branch of fibers going to the dorsal cochlear nuclei. It is at the location where the internal auditory canal joins the brain stem that VIIIth nerve tumors are often found.

The second-order neurons begin at the cochlear nuclei. Some of them then begin the process of decussation, in which neurons cross to the contralateral side of the brain stem via the trapezoid body and terminate within the superior olivary complex. The fact that nerve fibers from each ear do decussate here and at higher levels of the neural tract makes it less likely that neural destruction on one side of the central pathway will result in a total loss of hearing in that ear. Other second-order neurons emerge from the cochlear

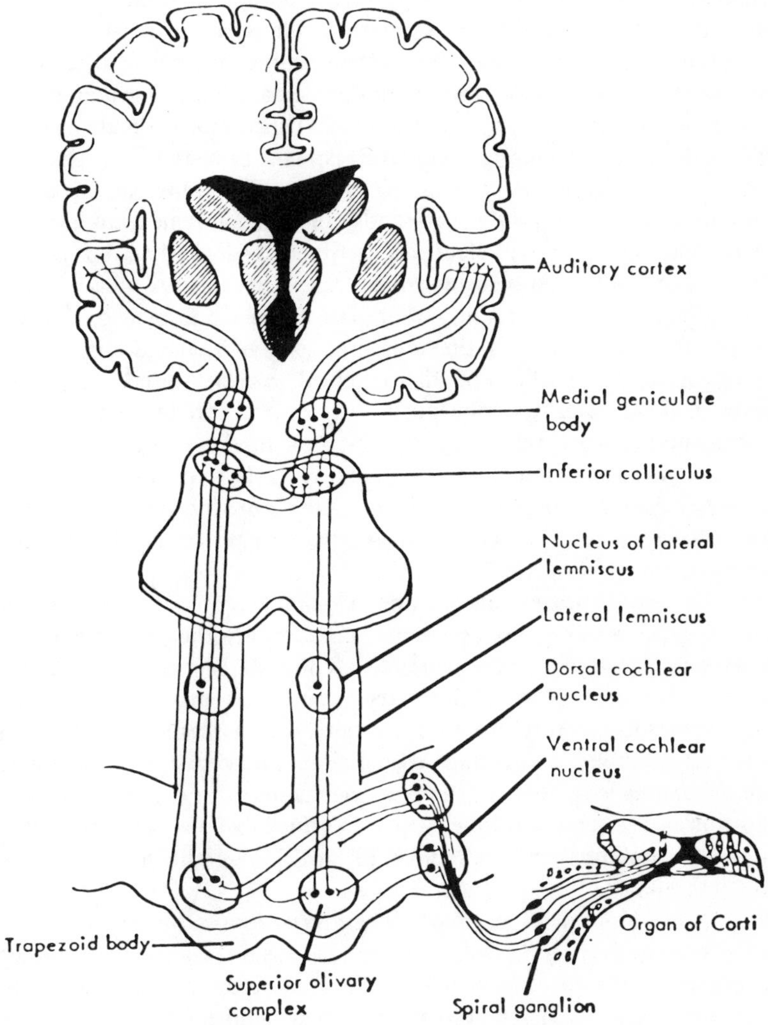

Figure 2-9. Ascending pathways of the cochlear branch of the VIIIth nerve. (Source: Zemlin, 1968, *Speech and Hearing Science,* © 1968. Reprinted by permission of Prentice-Hall, Inc., Englewood Cliffs, N.J.)

nuclei and remain on an ipsilateral (same side) ascending tract. Some of these fibers proceed to a second neural junction, the superior olivary complex, before ascending as third-order neurons through the lateral lemniscus. Others lead directly through the lateral lemniscus after leaving the cochlear nuclei. All fibers eventually reach the next neural junction, the inferior colliculus. A portion of the neurons may pass through the inferior colliculus, going directly to the next stopping point, the medial geniculate body. Further decussation of neurons occurs at the level of the inferior colliculus, which is felt to be the center for reflexive response to sound.

Cerebral Auditory Cortex Whatever the number and location of the synapses may be, apparently all ascending neurons synapse with neurons in the nucleus of the medial geniculate body. The fourth- or fifth-order neurons then travel through an area referred to as the auditory radiations, where the fibers are fanned out. These fibers then terminate in the temporal lobe of the auditory cortex. This particular portion of the cerebral cortex, found below the Sylvian fissure and bounded posteriorly by the parietal and occipital lobes, makes up a relatively large portion of the entire area of the cortex. Audition stands as the temporal lobe's primary function. According to Brodman's numbering system, this particular region of the cortex includes areas 41 and 42, considered to be the primary acoustic reception areas.

The entire process of audition, particularly for complex stimuli-like speech, requires the active participation of other portions of the cortex in addition to those already identified. Working in conjunction with the anterior auditory reception areas are more posterior and superior auditory areas of the cortex. It is here that functions such as auditory recognition, association, and recall are thought to be accomplished. This is felt to be particularly true of the superior portion of the temporal lobe, where Wernicke's area is located. This is elaborated further in Chapter 13, which contains material concerning aphasia.

The temporal lobes of both hemispheres of the brain appear to play very important roles in the process of audition. Although decussation of ascending neural fibers does occur to link each of the two peripheral auditory systems, the two hemispheres are believed not to duplicate all functions in the processing of auditory stimuli. Rather it is felt that there is some degree of cerebral dominance and specificity in audition. In most individuals the right ear appears to be able to retrieve more information than the left. The perception of speech, in particular, seems to be controlled for the most part by the left hemisphere, while the processing of nonverbal auditory stimuli is carried out predominantly by the right hemisphere. Thus, a lesion of the left temporal lobe would have more serious implications for the perception of speech than would a similar lesion of the right temporal lobe. Yet, even though a certain degree of specialization exists between the two auditory areas of the brain, a high degree of redundancy in the functions of the two lobes is present.

SPEECH AND LANGUAGE SYSTEMS

The speech process can be presented in terms of the three major functions of respiration, phonation, and articulation. Although the speech and language systems are considered here as separate entities, the reader should bear in mind that speech production and language use are actually complex and integrated processes. The speech process is based on an internalized language system which is stored, organized, and retrieved from the central nervous system. For this reason, the central nervous system is also discussed relative to language usage.

The Peripheral Speech Mechanism

Speech Respiration Speech respiration is a complex series of activities; a complete description of them exceeds the limits of this chapter. For this reason, only the key features of speech respiration are presented. Readers desiring more detailed information are referred to the works of Zemlin (1968) and Minifie, Hixon, and Williams (1973).

Merely defining respiration as a gas exchange process does not fully describe the respiratory activities required for speech. In English, only pulmonic egressive air flow is used to power the larynx and carry the generated speech signal through and out of the vocal tract. This outward air flow derives its power from the activities of the thoracic and abdominal muscular systems of the torso. Dividing the torso into two compartments, the thorax and abdomen, is a thin muscular septum known as the diaphragm. The diaphragm functions to draw air into the lungs when it contracts downward and thereby increases thoracic volume. The activities of the diaphragm are aided by the thoracic muscles, which enlarge the size of the rib cage when they contract. Although the dimensions of the torso may decrease as a result of abdominal muscle contractions, the size of the thorax is usually decreased by passive factors. These passive factors include rib torsion, gravity, and tissue elasticity, which are particularly effective during the initial stages of exhalation.

The solitary nucleus in the medulla controls normal respiration along with secondary expiratory-inspiratory centers in the medulla associated with the reticular formation. These centers coupled with a gamma-loop system at the spinal level help regulate speech respiration. The phrenic nerves, served by the solitary nucleus and the secondary respiration centers, exit from the cervical vertebrae (C-4 and C-5) and innervate the diaphragm. Thoracic cage movements are effected by the intercostal nerves (T-1 and T-2). Rapid thoracic volume changes during speech and resulting transient muscle loads are monitored by a spinal level gamma-loop system. This spinal level system acts as a servo-mechanism to automatically and subconsciously stabilize intercostal muscle length (Campbell, 1964).

The volume of air inhaled and exhaled by an adult during quiet respiration (tidal volume) depends to a large extend on age, size, and sex of the individual. For young adult men a tidal volume of 750 cc is average while 339 cc is typical for women (Zemlin, 1968). Respiratory volumes in the aged are significantly less and the reader is referred to Chapter 5 for details.

Investigations of speech respiration have revealed that this activity differs in several important ways from normal quiet respiration. For instance, it has been found that the external intercostal muscles of the thorax, which help expand the rib cage, are also active during speech exhalation. Apparently these muscles serve to check or regulate the collapse of the thorax as effected by passive exhalation forces (Draper, Ladefoged, and Whitteridge, 1959). The research of Hixon, Goldman, and Mead (1973) has shown that for speech purposes a slightly greater volume of air is used than for quiet respiration. These authors have also reported that there is an interactive relationship between respiratory phenomena and linguistic factors such as stress and phrase length. For example, expired air volumes in speech are governed by phrase length with few utterances in normal speech extending beyond the point of physiologic rest.

Phonation The process of oral communication depends on the transmission of sound waves through the air to the ears of the listener. When we talk to each other, the sound waves comprising the speech signal are, in part, generated by the larynx, which is situated at the upper end of the trachea. This sound generation process is referred to as phonation.

Air expired from the lungs is modified in the larynx by the vocal folds to produce phonation in the form of whispering or voicing. Whispering is produced by air-flow turbulence at the folds while voicing results from a cyclic opening and closing action. Voicing is the more important of these two forms of phonation since it it the primary sound used in speech. To produce voice the vocal folds are adducted (closed) and subglottic air pressure is increased from the lungs. This increase in pressure forces the vocal folds apart and permits a puff of air to escape. Myoelastic recoil forces bring the folds back together assisted by reduced air pressure on the walls of the folds (van den Berg, 1958). This process is repeated in a cyclic fashion to produce a quasi-periodic train of air puffs. These air puffs are the acoustic source of voicing and can be produced with varying intensities, qualities, and frequencies.

The larynx itself consists of nine cartilages and a complex system of intrinsic muscles (see Figures 2-10 and 2-11). This primary structure is supported and moved within the neck by muscle groups above (suprahyoids) and below (infrahyoids) the hyoid bone. Collectively these muscles are referred to as the extrinsic muscles of the larynx (Figure 2-12). The five major cartilages of the larynx are the paired arytenoids, a signet ring-shaped cricoid, the shield-like thyroid, and the epiglottis. The relationship of the five major cartilages to each other and to their articulatory movements is important for the functioning of the larynx as a valve and as a speech sound apparatus. The epiglottis moves in a posterior direction to help close off the larynx during swallowing. The cricoid cartilage tilts back and forth in an anteroposterior rocking motion relative to the thyroid and thus lengthens or shortens the vocal folds by its movements (Stone and Nuttall, 1974). As can be seen in Figure 2-13 posterior rocking movements of the cricoid cartilage carry the arytenoids backward and thus lengthen the vocal folds while anterior movements shorten the folds. The articulatory motions of the arytenoid cartilages are more complex and consist of rocking, gliding, and rotatory motions relative to the cricoid cartilage on which they are situated. The gliding motions of the arytenoids along the posterior edge of the cricoid cartilage effect either closure (adduction) or opening (abduction) of the vocal folds. Arytenoid rocking and rotary motions effect fine tension control in the vocal folds. Hence, the

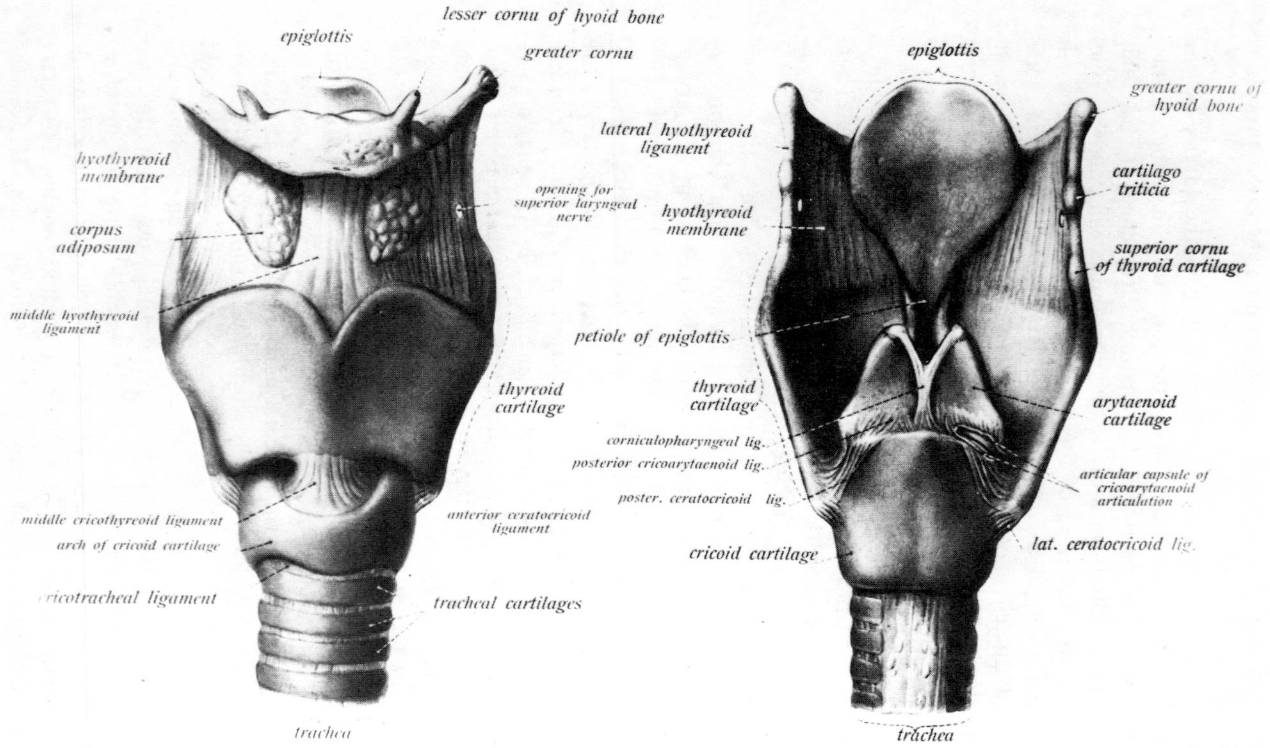

Figure 2-10. Cartilages and intrinsic muscles of the larynx. (Source: Sobotta and McMurrich, 1906.)

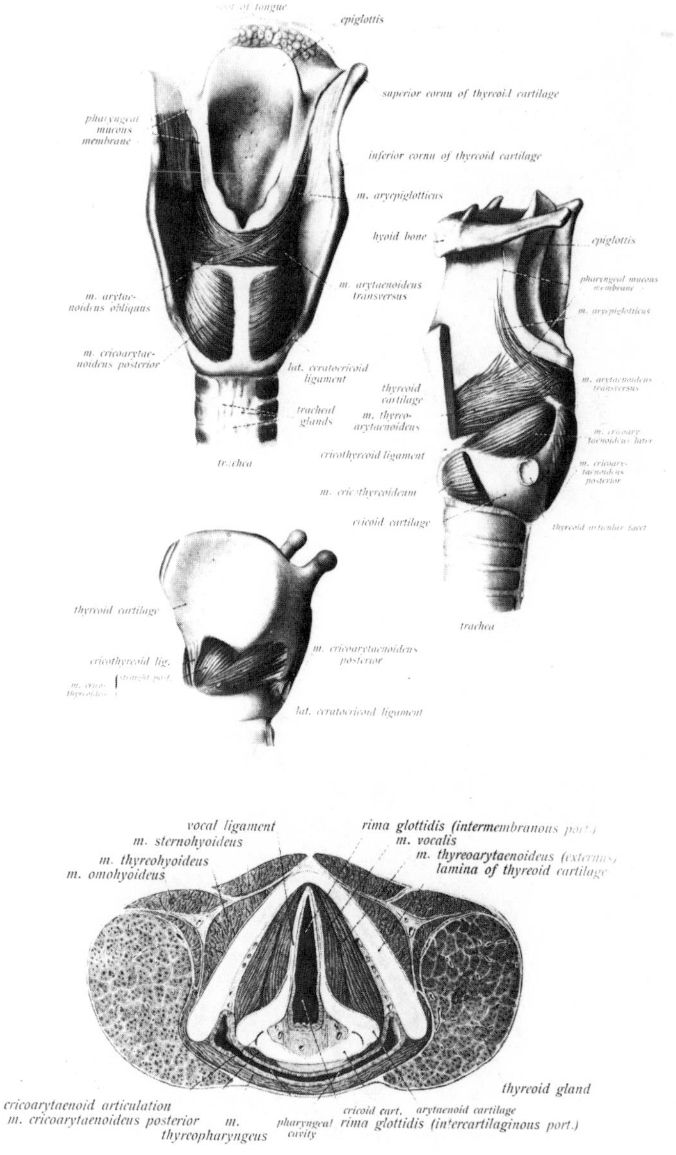

Figure 2-11. The intrinsic muscles of the larynx. (Source: Sobotta and McMurrich, 1906.)

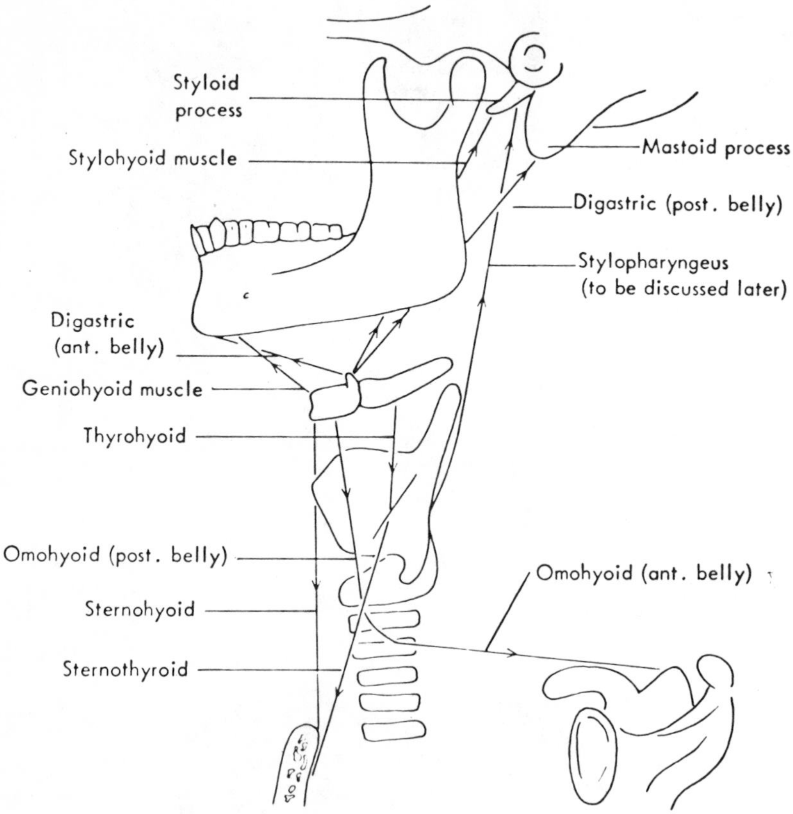

Figure 2-12. The extrinsic muscles of the larynx. (Source: Zemlin, 1968.)

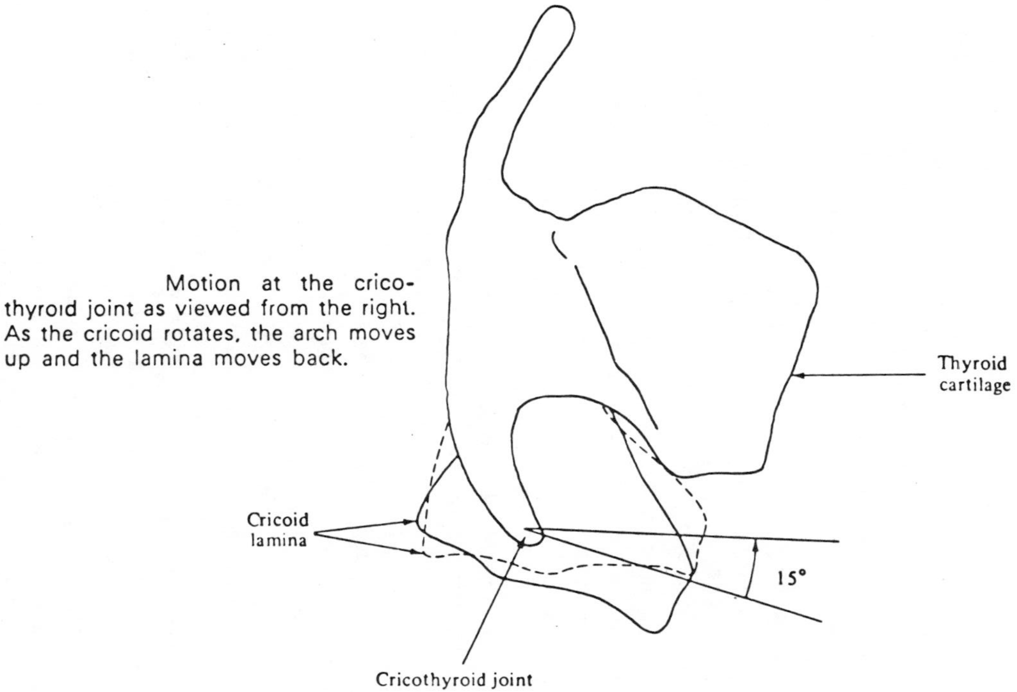
Motion at the crico-thyroid joint as viewed from the right. As the cricoid rotates, the arch moves up and the lamina moves back.
Thyroid cartilage
Cricoid lamina
15°
Cricothyroid joint

Figure 2-13. Action of the intrinsic muscles. (Source: Broad, 1973, in Minifie, Hixon, and Williams: *Normal Aspects of Speech, Hearing, and Language,* © 1973, p. 133. Reprinted by permission of Prentice-Hall, Inc., Englewood Cliffs, N.J.)

muscles of the larynx act on these major cartilages to change the configuration of the opening between the vocal folds (the glottis) and effect laryngeal valving. This valving action prohibits food and fluids from entering the trachea and regulates air flow from the lungs during exertion and speech phonation.

Neural control of the larynx is accomplished through the superior and recurrent laryngeal nerves which are branches of the vagus or *X*th cranial nerve. Neurologic research has also demonstrated that feedback-loops through these nerves from mechanoreceptors monitor laryngeal functions. These monitored functions include muscle tension and length, cartilage movements, and subglottic air pressure (Wyke, 1969).

Articulation The articulatory structures of speech are part of the vocal tract which consists of pharyngeal, nasal, and oral cavities (Figure 2-14). The pharyngeal cavity is a muscular tube which begins at the level of the glottal opening and extends upward to where it opens into the oral and nasal cavities. The nasal cavity consists of two narrow passages coursing in an anteroposterior direction separated by a medial septum. The oral cavity consists of the mouth extending back to the posterior faucial pillar. Most of this cavity is filled by the highly muscular tongue. Sounds generated by the larynx pass through the vocal tract and are further modified into speech. By altering the size and shape of the vocal tract in a coordinated series of rapid articulatory movements the various sounds of speech may be produced. These articulatory movements basically consist of valving actions by the larynx, soft palate (velum), tongue, and lips. Of these, the contacts and constrictions formed by the tongue are largely responsible for the various sounds produced during speech. Constrictions in the vocal tract are usually produced by the more mobile structures working against immovable portions of the tract such as the posterior pharyngeal wall, hard palate, and teeth. The size and shape of the vocal tract and the column of air within determine which portions of the sound spectrum produced at the larynx and other constrictions will escape from the lips. That is, as the vocal tract assumes various articulatory shapes the column of air within will be modulated in unique patterns producing the characteristic sounds of speech.

Peripherally, the articulatory mechanism is served by the Vth (trigeminal), VIIth (facial), IXth (glossopharyngeal), Xth (vagus), and XIIth (hypoglossal) cranial nerves. The nuclei of these nerves are located in the brain stem and are discussed further in the section

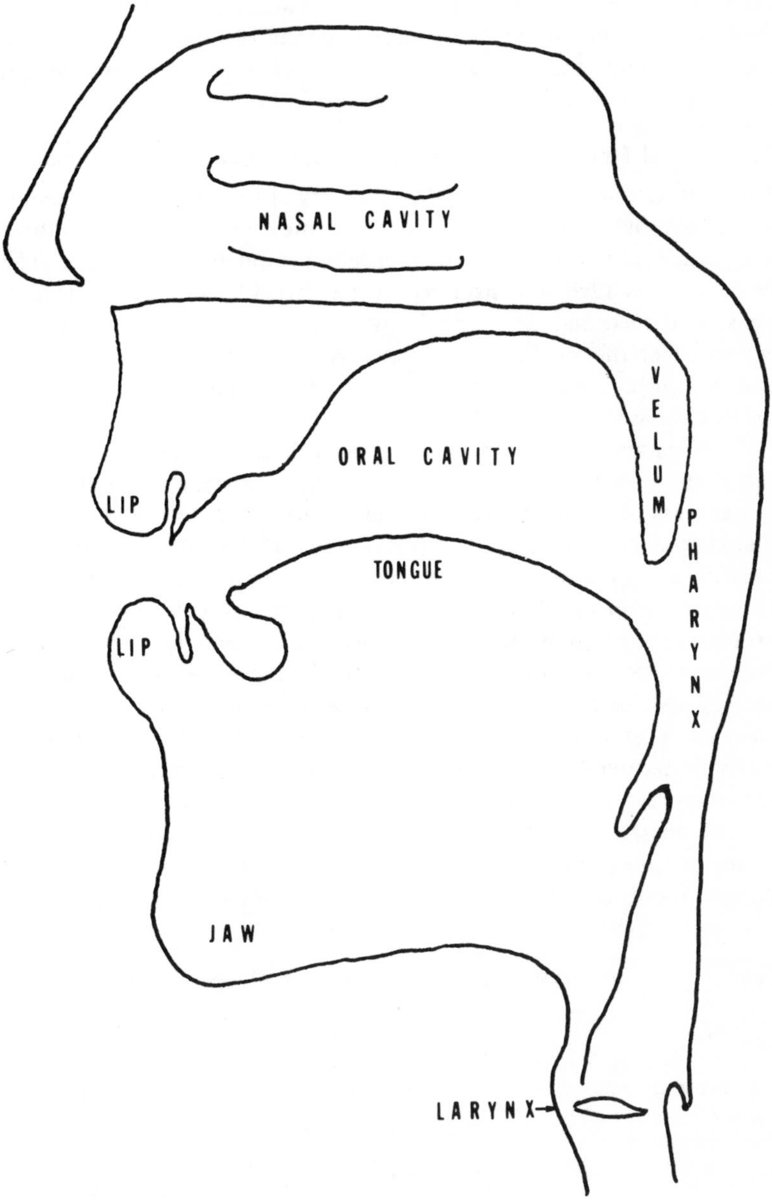

Figure 2-14. Articulatory structures of speech.

dealing with this part of the central nervous system. Table 2-1 summarizes the activities of these various cranial nerves relative to articulation. From this table we may see that the highly coordinated activity we refer to as articulation is effected through several neural pathways.

The Central Nervous System and Speech/Language Formulation

The central nervous system (CNS) consists of the brain and its major extension, the spinal cord. The brain may be divided into three major parts, the cerebrum, the cerebellum, and the brain stem. The brain stem is further considered to be divisible into the midbrain, pons, and medulla. The spinal cord is a long, slender, rod-shaped extension of the medulla and contains descending motor pathways and ascending sensory tracts with paired spinal nerves exiting at various levels.

Information in the form of electrochemical impulses reaches the CNS by way of the peripheral nervous system. Incoming impulses passing through the peripheral nervous system are modality bound to a specific sensory pathway and can be inhibited or facilitated to a limited degree. Once these neural impulses reach the CNS they fan out in all directions and go through a much more complex process of inhibition, facilitation, processing, and interaction with previously stored information. Eventually these incoming impulses are encoded or translated into response behaviors. Thus, in a complex series of interconnections every part of the CNS connects directly or indirectly with a final motor neuron and forms the basis, for instance, for such complex behaviors as speech and language.

Meninges The brain and spinal cord are covered by three layers of tissue: the dura matter, the arachnoid layer, and the pia mater. The dura matter is outermost and lines the inner surface of

Table 2-1. Cranial nerves serving articulatory structures

Structure	Motor nerve	Sensory nerve
Face and lips	VII	V
Jaw	V	V
Tongue	XII	V
Soft palate	VII, IX	V, IX
Pharynx	IX, X	IX, X

Sources: Chusid (1970) and Nishio et al. (1976).

the skull and spinal column as a tough fiberous sheet. In the skull the dura matter folds between the cerebral hemispheres at the longitudinal fissure and forms a pocket around the cerebellum. The arachnoid layer is a delicate, web-like structure through which, in the subarachnoid space, cerebrospinal fluid circulates. The innermost layer, the pia mater, invests every convolution and groove in the CNS and is richly endowed with blood vessels.

Brain

Cerebrum This structure consists of right and left hemispheres which are joined at the midline by a broad band of neural fiber tracts known as the corpus callosum. The surface of each hemisphere is folded into ridges (gyri) and grooves (sulci and fissures) which may be used as landmarks. The fissures of the cerebrum are deeper and fewer in number than the sulci. Other than the longitudinal fissure which incompletely divided the two hemispheres, each half of the brain has a lateral fissure (of Sylvius), a central fissure (of Rolando), and a parieto-occipital fissure. These fissures serve as boundaries between more general hemispheric regions known as lobes (Figure 2-15).

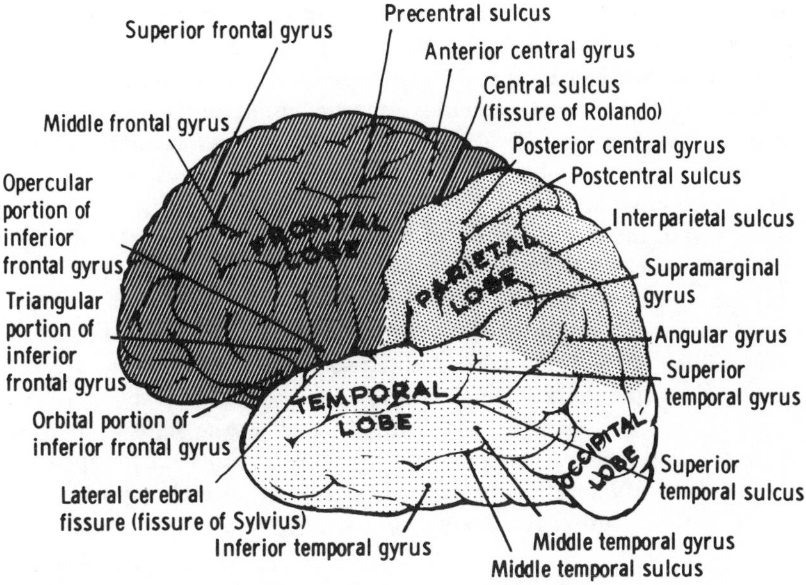

Figure 2-15. Lobes of the brain. (Source: Chusid, 1970.)

The four lobes of each hemisphere are named after the bones of the cranium which cover them. The frontal lobe is the largest and comprises all of the cortex anterior to the fissure of Rolando and above the fissure of Sylvius. The parietal lobe extends from the fissure of Rolando posteriorly to the parieto-occipital fissure and above the Sylvian fissure. The temporal lobe lies below the fissure of Sylvius and continues back to an imaginary line extending downward from the parieto-occipital fissure. The occipital lobe consists of the remaining portion of the cerebrum posterior to the parieto-occipital demarcation.

Certain gyri deserve mention because of their known association with the processes of speech, hearing, and language. The percentral gyrus contains large neurons (Betz cells) from which the pyramidal tracts arise (the primary motor pathway). The various parts of the body are topographically represented as shown in Figure 2-16, with centers for the larynx, face, and tongue being nearer to the fissure of Sylvius. The postcentral gyrus in each hemisphere serves as the primary sensory cortex for the parts of the body and is topographically arranged in parrallel with the precentral gyrus. The inferior frontal convolution, immediately in front of the lower precentral gyrus area, is known as Broca's area and functions as a neural-motor encoding center for speech. The auditory cortex in each hemisphere is located on the superior temporal gyrus (Heschl's). The auditory cortex has a general tonotopic organization; that is, certain areas tend to receive specific acoustic information. Two other gyri, the supramarginal and angular, together with portions of the superior temporal lobe, function as association areas which contribute to language use.

Within the brain a series of cavities form the lateral, third, and fourth ventricles. The largest ventricles, the lateral, extend into each hemisphere of the brain and resemble the letter "C" when viewed from the side. The third ventricle is a rectangular cavity located at the midline of the brain between the two thalami. The fourth ventricle is triangular shaped, lying between the pons and cerebellum, extending into the medulla, and continuing as a long narrow column in the spinal cord. An opening in the fourth ventricle (foramen of Magendi) at the level of the medulla permits the cerebrospinal fluid manufactured within the brain's ventricles to escape into the subarachnoid space.

The major blood supply of the brain enters at the base of the skull by way of the vertebral and internal carotid arteries. Anatom-

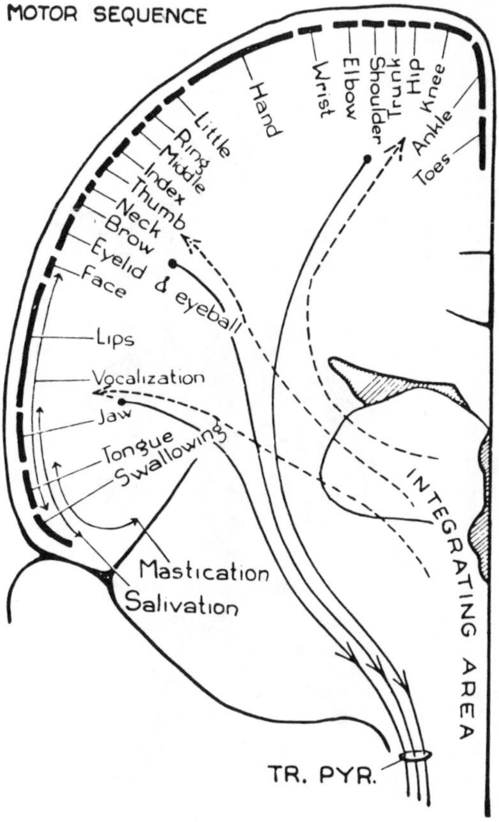

Figure 2-16. Voluntary motor tracts. Cross-section through right hemisphere along the plane of the precentral gyrus. The pathway of control of voluntary movement is suggested from gray matter, somewhere in the higher brain stem, by the broken lines to the motor transmitting strip of the precentral gyrus. From there it runs down the corticospinal tract, as shown by the unbroken lines toward the muscles. The sequence of responses to electrical stimulation on the surface of the cortex (from above down, along the motor strip from toes through arm and face to swallowing) is unvaried from one individual to another. (Source: Penfield and Jasper, 1954.)

ically these arteries are two separate systems connected by an anterior and two posterior communicating arteries. These branches along with the major vessels entering at the base of the brain form an arterial structure known as the circle of Willis (Figure 2-17). Three major pairs of arteries along with lesser branches exit from the circle of Willis to nourish the brain. The major pairs of arteries are the anterior cerebral, the posterior cerebral, and middle cer-

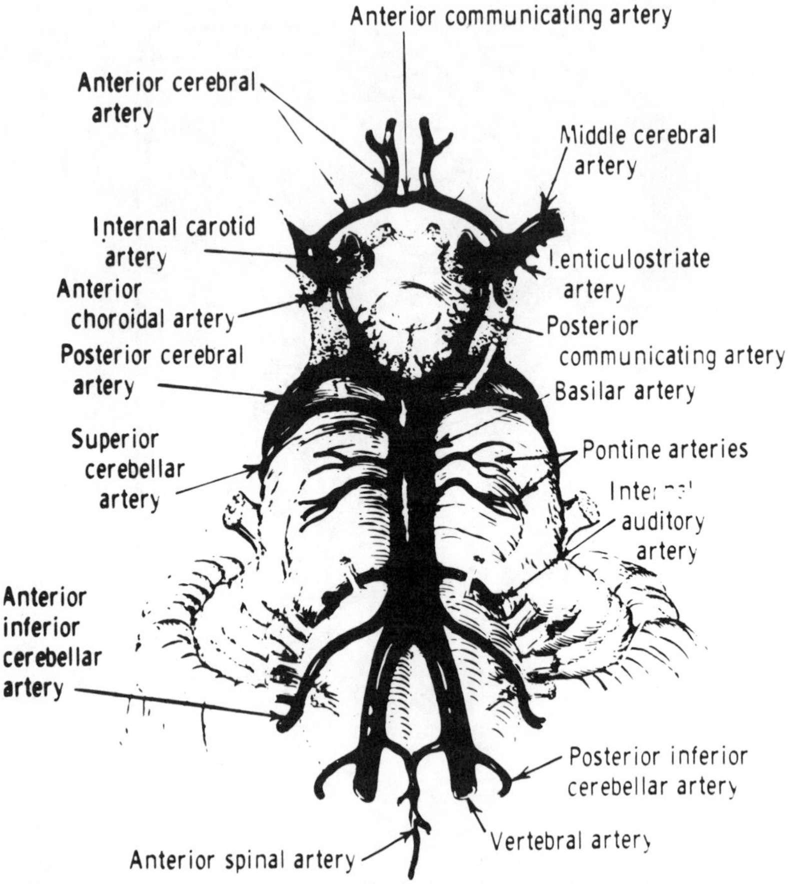

Figure 2-17. The circle of Willis. (Source: Chusid, 1970.)

ebral. Of these three pairs the middle cerebral arteries are probably the most vital for speech and hearing functions. As the middle cerebral arteries leave the circle of Willis a number of small, but important, branches are given off which enter the brain tissues and supply the internal capsule, thalamus, and basal ganglia with blood. Once the middle cerebral arteries reach the cerebral cortex they traverse the fissure of Sylvius on either hemisphere and branch to those areas of the cortex known to be involved with speech, hearing, and language functions (Figure 2-18). It has been estimated that a young healthy adult brain consumes about 8% of the total oxygen

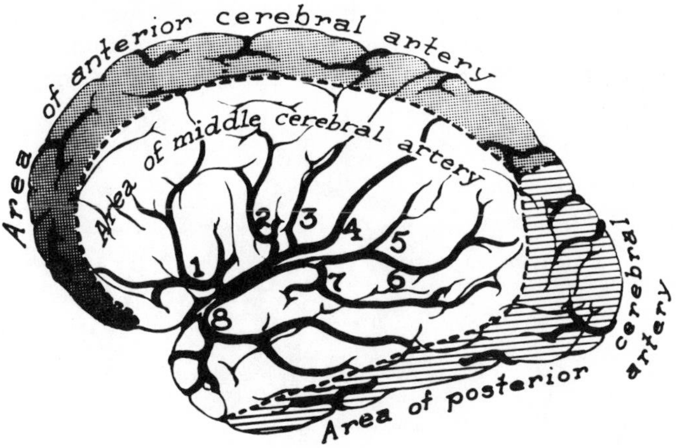

Figure 2-18. Cortical branches of the middle cerebral artery. (Source: Chusid, 1970; Bailey, 1948. Courtesy of Charles C Thomas, Springfield, Ill.)

available in the body at any given moment, or about 46 ml of oxygen per minute (Chusid, 1970). Without a constant blood supply neural cells with cease to survive and be irreplaceably lost within a matter of a few minutes. Chusid (1970) points out that in advanced age, circulation and oxygen consumption are reduced to as much as 30% below average young adult levels. Factors which may contribute to this reduced circulation in the aged brain are: lowered blood pressure, cerebrovascular resistance, blood viscosity, and cerebral vessel status – especially of the arterioles (see Chapter 3).

Beneath the cerebral hemispheres, two centrally located and elongated masses of ganglionic nuclei make up the organs of the brain known as the thalami. These two ovoid structures are situated on either side of the third ventricle and are connected by a neural bridge, the massa intermedia. Each thalamus is composed of a number of discrete nuclei. Some of these nuclei receive direct sensory input, others project to lower brain centers such as the basal ganglia, and still others have direct radiations to the cortex. Hence, the thalami function as shunting points for neural impulses of all types. In this role the thalami integrate and coordinate all sensory information that reaches the cortex except for the sense of smell. It is also important to note that all thalamic projections are ipsilateral; that is, each thalamus only radiates fibers to structures located on the same side of the brain.

The major components of the basal ganglia are the lenticular nuclei (the putamen and globus pallidus) and the caudate nucleus (Figure 2-19). These nuclei interact with portions of the cerebral

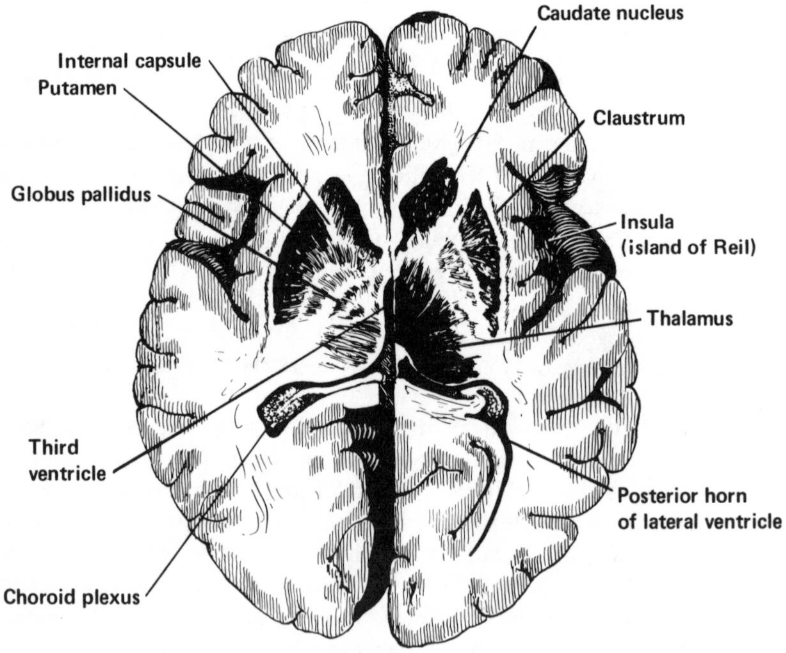

Figure 2-19. Basal ganglia of the brain. (Source: Chusid, 1970.)

cortex and the cerebellum to regulate motor activity in the body. The interneuronal connections of the basal ganglia are complex, with many interconnections, and comprise part of the extrapyramidal motor pathways. For example, it is known that the basal ganglia receive projections from the cortex, thalamus, substantia nigra, and to and from each other. The basal ganglia also radiate fibers to the subthalamic nuclei, hypothalamus, substantia nigra, red nucleus, and cerebellum. Depending on the site, lesions occurring in the basal ganglia can produce Parkinson's disease, chorea, and a form of cerebral palsy (athetosis).

Cerebellum Like the cerebrum, the cerebellum consists of two hemispheres, one on either side of the brain stem. The surface of the cerebellum is marked by narrow horizontal ridges known as folia. Three peduncles or stalks attach the cerebellum to the brain stem through which efferent and afferent neural pathways pass to higher and lower centers of the central nervous system. About three times as many fibers enter the cerebellum as leave it. This three to one reduction is indicative of the integrative function of this part of the brain.

The work of Snider and Stowell (1944) has substantially clarified the role of the cerebellum. These authors point out that information from our senses of sight, hearing, touch, and muscle and joint states are monitored and integrated by the cerebellum with motor commands into a coordinated or synergistic output. Since the function of the cerebellum is synergistic, deficits produced by cerebellar disease or damage are related to asynergy or a lack of coordination. Asynergy is manifested in speech by abrupt movements, "speech problems," and in some instances loss of muscle tonus (hypotonia). Typically, all signs and symptoms are produced on the same side of the body as the lesion.

Brain Stem As mentioned earlier, the brain stem consists of the midbrain, pons, and medulla (medulla oblongata). This portion of the brain also contains all of the cranial nerve nuclei and a complicated network of nerve cells known as the reticular formation. The brain stem is functionally important because all the sensory and motor pathways of the body pass through this structure. In addition, supraspinal reflexes and subconscious or vegetative activities such as respiration, blood pressure regulation, and heart rate are monitored here.

Midbrain The midbrain, a short segment located between the thalamus and pons, forms the uppermost post of the brain stem.

This structure contains the red (ruber) nucleus and substantia nigra which are important for locomotion and muscle tonus in the body. The descending motor pathways traverse this portion of the brain stem in addition to all of the neural fibers ascending to the thalamus. The mesencephalic portion of the Vth (trigeminal) nucleus, which is important for proprioception in the mandibular joint and muscles of mastication, is also located here along with the IIIrd and IVth (cranial) nerve nuclei, which serve to innervate muscles of the eye. Only the IIIrd (occulomotor) and IVth (trochlear) cranial nerves exit from the midbrain, however.

Pons The pons or bridge is a prominent bulge which covers both halves of the brain stem. The pons is made up of descending motor fibers which carry impulses to the spinal cord (corticospinal) and cerebellum (corticopontine). The latter tracts enter the cerebellum via the middle cerebellar peduncle for coordination of voluntary and involuntary postural movements. In this regard the function of the pons is intimately associated with that of the cerebellum. The pons also contains the nuclei of the Vth (trigeminal), VIth (abducens), VIIth (facial), and VIIIth (auditory) cranial nerves. The Vth (trigeminal) has both motor and sensory nuclei which serve the muscles of the jaw and facial sensation. Motor activity of the face is regulated by the VIIth (facial) nerve nuclei. Both the VIIth (facial) and VIIIth (auditory) cranial nerves exit from the pons at the cerebellar-pontine angle.

Medulla The medulla (medulla oblongata) begins at the caudal border of the pons and extends downward to the foramen magnum of the skull where it is continuous with the spinal cord. On the ventral side of the medulla two longitudinal ridges comprising the pyramidal (corticospinal) tracts descussate or cross over at the extreme caudal end. Just below the pons four pairs of cranial nerves leave the medulla, all of which are important for speech. These are the IXth (glossopharyngeal), Xth (vagus), XIth (accessory), and XIIth (hypoglossal) cranial nerves. Hence, all of the cranial nerves exit from the central nervous system above the level of pyramidal decussation. The nuclei associated with the Xth (vagus) are also associated with visceral input and output, vegetative functions, and respiration.

Language Processes

Grammar system Language is usually regarded as consisting of both grammar and lexical systems. The lexicon represents an internalized dictionary of words used by the grammar system. The grammar system is conventionally regarded as being composed of four components (Critchley, 1970), namely:

Syntax: the strategies used to determine word order

Semantics: the meaning of a set of symbols; meaning may be derived from word order (surface structure) and from nonverbal cues and vocal intonations which may modify the meaning of an utterance (deep structure)

Morphemics: morphemes are the minimal units of meaning within a word; the strategies for their use include tense, pluralization, and possession

Phonology: phonemes are the distinctive sound elements of a word; the strategies for the use of these elements determine which sound combinations are permissible in a particular language

In addition to the grammatical strategies of a language system, there are at least two identifiable levels of language use: propositional and nonpropositional (Jackson, 1874/1913). Propositional language is used to communicate specific meanings or elicit a particular response. Nonpropositional language uses the linguistic system in an uncreative fashion; that is, this type of speech tends to be automatic and organized from habit. Hence, propositional utterances are superior speech formulations and usually require more extensive cognitive operations. Nonpropositional utterances tend to be inferior, emotion charged, involve the use of cliches, and are usually triggered by external stimuli.

A neurolinguistic model Through the use of a model some relationships may be illustrated between language and its neurologic correlation. The model shown in Figure 2-20 is similar to Hughlings Jackson's (1878) theory of central nervous system function. Jackson postulated that the central nervous system was organized as a series of hierarchically controlled levels with lower levels subserviant to higher levels. This particular model (Figure 2-20), suggested by Hutchinson and Beasley (1976), postulates that the highest level, ideation, is the most complex and probably utilizes all areas of the cortex to generate thoughts, ideas, desires, etc., which the person wishes to express. In this sense the first level of activity is a process of conceptualization or intellectualization. The second level of central neuronal activity, symbolization, uses the grammar system to codify these conceptualizations by arranging the phonemes, syllables, or words in a proper and meaningful order. As part of this

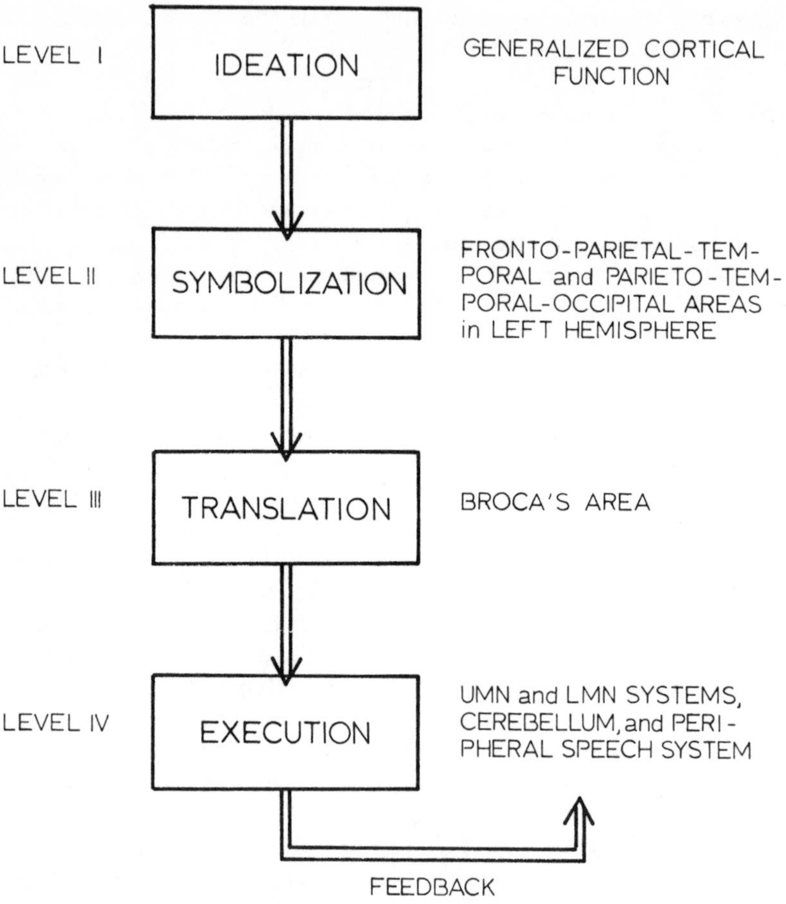

Figure 2-20. A neurolinguistic model of speech production. (Source: Hutchinson and Beasley, 1976.)

process the desired words are retrieved from the lexicon. This activity is probably accomplished in that part of the cortex referred to as Wernicke's area (Figure 2-21). At some stages in the neurologic process, conceptual units which have been linguistically encoded must be converted into neuromuscular command patterns and sent to the structures which produce speech (respiratory system, larynx, vocal tract). This translation activity, level III, is essentially a programming operation and occurs in that part of the cortex known as Broca's area (Figure 2-21). Once the linguistic message has been

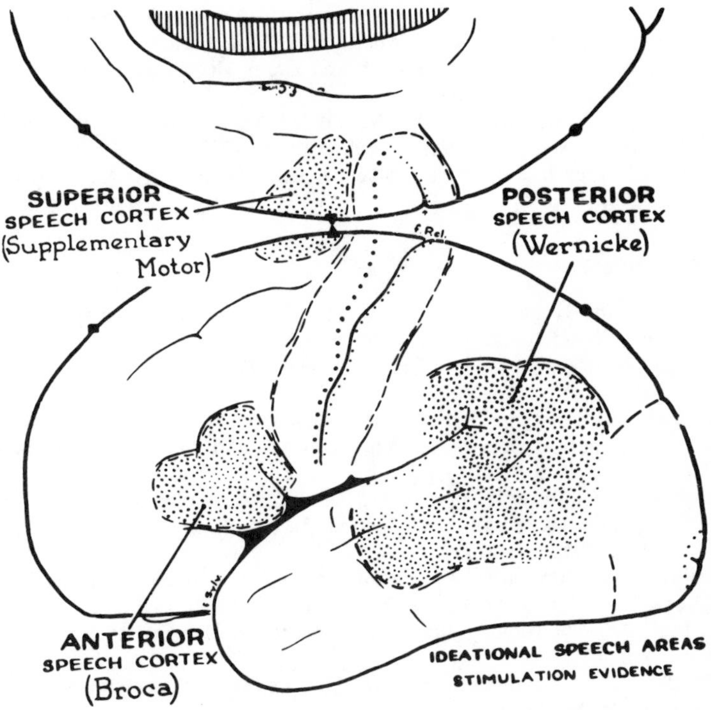

Figure 2-21. Ideational speech areas of the cortex. (Source: Penfield and Roberts, 1959.)

translated into the proper neural code, it is sent out to the peripheral speech mechanism for execution (level IV). This pathway utilizes the upper and lower motor neuron systems, the cerebellum, cranial nerves, some spinal nerves, and the final neurons which innervate the muscle systems for speech. Execution of the speech motor program at the periphery consists of an interactive and highly coordinated participation of the respiratory system, phonatory mechanism, and the articulating structures of the vocal tract.

SUGGESTED READINGS

Durrant, J., and Lovrinic, J. Bases of Hearing Science. Baltimore: Williams & Wilkins, 1977.

Hutchinson, J. M., and Beasley, D. S. Speech and language functioning among the aging. In H. J. Oyer and E. J. Oyer (eds.), Aging and Communication. Baltimore: University Park Press, 1976.

Minifie, F. D., Hixon, T. J., and Williams, F. Normal Aspects of Speech, Hearing, and Language. Englewood Cliffs, N.J.: Prentice-Hall, 1973.

Penfield, W., and Roberts, L. Speech and Brain Mechanisms. London: Oxford University Press, 1959.

Rasmussen, G., and Wendle, W. Neural Mechanisms of the Auditory and Vestibulary Systems. Springfield, Ill.: Charles C Thomas, 1960.

Zemlin, W. Speech and Hearing Science. Englewood Cliffs, N.J.: Prentice-Hall, 1968.

REFERENCES

Anson, B., and Donaldson, J. A. Surgical Anatomy of the Temporal Bone and Ear. Philadelphia: W. B. Saunders, 1973.

Bailey, P., Intracranial Tumors (2nd Ed.). Springfield, Ill.: Charles C Thomas, 1948.

Broad, D. J. Phonation. In F. D. Minifie, Hixon, T. J., and Williams, F. (eds.), Normal Aspects of Speech, Hearing, and Language. Englewood Cliffs, N.J.: Prentice-Hall, 1973.

Campbell, E. Motor pathways. In W. Fenn and H. Rahm (eds.), Handbook of Physiology (Respiration 1, Section 3). Washington D.C.: American Psychological Society, 1964.

Chusid, J. G. Correlative Neuroanatomy and Functional Neurology. Los Altos, Calif.: Lange Medical Publications, 1970.

Critchley, M. Aphasiology and Other Aspects of Language. London: Edward Arnold, 1970.

DeWeese, D. D., and Saunders, W. H. Textbook of Otolaryngology. St. Louis: C. V. Mosby, 1968.

Draper, M. H., Ladefoged, P., and Whitteridge, D. Respiratory muscles of speech. Journal of Speech and Hearing Research, 2, 16–27 (1959).

Durrant, J., and Lovrinic, J. Basis of Hearing Science. Baltimore: Williams & Wilkins, 1977.

Hixon, T. J., Goldman, M. D., and Mead, J. Kinematics of the chest wall during speech production. Journal of Speech and Hearing Research, 16, 78–115 (1973).

Hutchinson, J. M., and Beasley, D. S. Speech and language functioning among the aging. In J. H. Oyer and E. J. Oyer (eds.), Aging and Communication. Baltimore: University Park Press, 1976.

Jackson, J. H. On the nature of the duality of the brain. Medical Press Circular, Vol. 1 (1874). Reprinted in Brain, 38, 80–95 (1913).

Jackson, J. H. On affections of speech from disease of the brain. Brain, 1, 304–330 (1878).

Minifie, F. D., Hixon, T. J., and Williams, F. Normal Aspects of Speech, Hearing, and Language. Englewood Cliffs, N.J.: Prentice-Hall, 1973.

Myers, D., Schlosser, W. D., and Winchester, R. A. Otologic diagnosis and the treatment of deafness. Clinical Symposia, 14, 1962. Published by CIBA Pharmaceutical Co., Summit, N.H.

Nishio, J., Matsuya, T., Machida, J., and Miyazaki, T. The motor nerve supply of the velopharyngeal muscles. Cleft Palate Journal, 13, 20–30 (1976).

Palmer, J. Anatomy for Speech and Hearing. New York: Harper and Row, 1972.

Penfield, W., and Jasper, H. H. Epilepsy and the Functional Anatomy of the Human Brain. Boston: Little, Brown, 1954.

Penfield, W., and Roberts, L. Speech and Brain Mechanisms. Princeton, N.J.: Princeton University Press, 1959.

Schuknecht, H.F. Pathology of the Ear. Cambridge, Mass.: Harvard University Press, 1974.

Snider, R. S., and Stowell, A. Receiving areas of tactile, auditory, and visual systems in the cerebellum. Journal of Neurophysiology, 95, 331–357 (1944).

Sobatta, J. Atlas of Descriptive Human Anatomy (Vol. 3, Ed. 5; trans. by E. Uhlenhuth). New York: Hafner, 1954).

Sobotta, J., and McMurrich, J. P. Atlas and Textbook of Human Anatomy (Vol. 2). Philadelphia: W. B. Saunders, 1906.

Stevens, S. S. (ed.) Handbook of Experimental Psychology. New York: John Wiley & Sons, 1951.

Stone, R. E., Jr., and Nuttal, A. L. Relative movements of the thyroid and cricoid cartilages assessed by neural stimulation in dogs. Acta Otolaryngologica, 78, 135–140 (1974).

van den Berg, J. Myoelastic-aerodynamic theory of voice production. Journal of Speech and Hearing Research, 1, 227–243 (1958).

Wyke, D. Deus ex machina vocis: An analysis of the laryngeal reflex mechanisms of speech. British Journal of Disorders of Communication, 4, 3-25 (1969).

Zemlin, W. Speech and Hearing Science: Anatomy and Physiology. Englewood Cliffs, N.J.: Prentice Hall, 1968.

Chapter 3
The Normal Aging Process

The purpose of this chapter is to provide a limited review of some of the issues central to gerontology. This review should provide a reasonable background concerning the process of aging against which disorders of communicative function can be properly discussed. Specifically, five topic areas are reviewed: 1) biologic changes, 2) sensoriperceptual changes, 3) psychomotor changes, 4) intelligence and memory changes, and 5) psychological changes.

Any complete discussion of speech, language, and hearing impairments characteristic of aging individuals must be considered within the general framework of the aging process itself. The impact of communicative impairments is more easily appreciated when viewed within the context of biologic, psychoemotional, and sociologic alterations which typify the aged person. It is safe to state that nearly all people, as they grow older, experience physical, psychological, and interpersonal difficulty of one sort or another. Sometimes communicative handicaps cause such problems and sometimes they are the result of these impairments. For example, an older man may experience a progressive decrement in hearing acuity that causes fear and embarrassment, thereby precipitating a withdrawal from social situations. In this case, one common communicative handicap associated with aging results in a psychosocial problem. Alternatively, another older person might evidence the diffuse central nervous system atrophy frequently seen among the aged and that often impairs intelligence and memory. As a result, word recall may be impaired, thereby influencing the fluency of most spoken messages. In this instance, one common physiologic change associated with aging results in a communicative handicap. These considerations motivated the present chapter. Obviously, it is beyond the scope of this discussion to present a detailed literature review. Rather, the central purpose is to provide an overview of several aspects of aging which, we hope, will serve as a meaningful background for the chapters to follow.

BIOLOGIC CHANGES ASSOCIATED WITH ADVANCING AGE

It is well understood that with advancing age all organisms seem more susceptible to disease and deterioration and less able to initiate and sustain the process of self-repair. It is also well understood that some of the physical deterioration associated with an aging organism is genetically predetermined and some of the deterioration is a function of environmental influences. Birren (1964) has argued that, in the case of man, hereditary factors may be of lesser importance to longevity than environmental influences. Some support for such a position was provided by Jones (1959), who compared the life-span adjustments which would result from various hereditary and environmental factors (see Table 3-1). Inspection of this table reveals that many "reversible" conditions can dramatically reduce life expectancy (e.g., smoking, obesity, elevated lipoproteins, etc.).

Aging of Cells

At the most fundamental level, hereditary and environmental factors influence cellular function in body tissues. Two general problems associated with aging may be observed at a cellular level. First, it is well documented that many cells die within several of the critical organs of the body (Wolff, 1959), and replacement of these cells is either reduced or absent among the elderly. Second, remaining cells may not operate at peak efficiency in older organisms. Collectively, these two conditions result in reduced functional capacity in many organs of the body. Birren (1964) has suggested that aging may selectively influence highly differentiated cells that cannot undergo further mitosis. If this were true, such cellular organizations as the nervous, vascular, and muscular systems should be particularly susceptible to the effects of senescence; this is indeed the case.

One commonly accepted explanation for cell deterioration is that over time there is damage to the DNA (deoxyribonucleic acid) component of chromosomes. With damage to DNA, defective messenger molecules (RNA or ribonucleic acid) may be generated which are unable to synthesize the necessary enzymes for maintaining cell operation. As a result, cells die or cannot undertake proper division (Birren, 1964).

Aging of General Body Systems

At a more general level, experimentalists have marshalled a substantive body of knowledge regarding the effects of cellular aging in several of the body systems. For purposes of the present review, only four systems are considered as examples: cardiovascular, muscular, endocrine, and neurologic.

Certainly, the cardiovascular system has been one of the most widely investigated because of the often lethal problems that result from diseases of the heart and circulatory system. In this regard, perhaps the most common problem characteristic of aging persons is circulatory impairment caused by cardiac insufficiency attributable to valvular heart disease; hypertension; pulmonary, metabolic, or infectious diseases; and localized ischemia resulting from arteriosclerosis (Simonson, 1965). Of course, cardiovascular disturbances have a profound impact on other bodily systems, particularly the nervous system. As we will see later, many of the deficits in sensorimotor performance associated with aging may be attributed to cardiovascular disease.

Another rather obvious change associated with advancing age is atrophy of skeletal muscles. According to Wolff (1959), it is not entirely clear whether the decrease in muscle mass is attributable to a loss of fibers, a decrease in muscle fiber diameter, or both. Of course, the reduction in skeletal muscle mass characteristic of advanced age explains much of the decreased muscle strength observed among older persons. Birren (1959) has noted that some muscles do not evidence a dramatic decline in strength (e.g., the hand), probably because of continued high levels of use.

It is interesting to note that the endocrine system is relatively less susceptible to the aging process (Birren, 1964). For example, Freeman (1959) observed that the pituitary-adrenal mechanism functioned at normal or near normal expectancy even in the very old. However, it is accepted that certain hormone productions such as insulin may decrease with advanced age. In addition, gonadal failure is common among older persons. Wolff (1959) has summarized the influence of aging on endocrine activity by stating:

> ... it is generally believed that, in the aging body, there is persistence of the integrity of the pituitary-adrenal mechanism; there is maintenance of the functional capacity of the catabolism-mediating glands in contrast to a progressive loss of capacity in the glands with anabolic activities ... (p. 16).

Table 3-1. Physiologic age and life-span differences considered permanent and reversible

Reversible: Comparison	Reversible: Years	Permanent: Comparison	Permanent: Years
Country versus city dwelling †	+5	Female versus male sex †	+3
Married status versus single, widowed, divorced	+5	Familial constitutions: ‡	
Overweight §		2 grandparents lived to 80 yr	+2
25 per cent overweight group	−3.6	4 grandparents lived to 80 yr.	+4
35 per cent overweight group	−4.3	Mother lived to age 90 yr.	+3
45 per cent overweight group	−6.6	Father lived to age 90 yr.	+4.4
55 per cent overweight group	−11.4	Both mother and father lived to age 90 yr.	+7.4
67 per cent overweight group	−15.1	Mother lived to age 80 yr.	+1.5
Or: an average effect of 1 percent overweight	−0.17	Father lived to age 80 yr.	+2.2
Smoking ‖		Both mother and father lived to age 80 yr.	+3.7
1 package cigarettes per day	−7	Mother died at 60 yr.	−0.7
2 packages cigarettes per day	−12	Father died at 60 yr.	−1.1
Atherosclerosis #		Both mother and father died at age 60 yr.	−1.8
Fat metabolism		Recession of childhood and infectious disease over past century in Western countries	+15
In 25th percentile of population having "ideal" lipoprotein concentrations	+10	Life Insurance *Impairment Study* **	
Having average lipoprotein concentrations	0	Rheumatic heart disease, evidenced by:	
In 25th percentile of population having elevated lipoproteins	−7		

In 5th percentile of population having highest elevation of lipoproteins	−15 ††	Heart murmur	−11
Diabetes ‡‡		Heart murmur + tonsillitis	−18
Uncontrolled, before insulin, 1900	−35	Heart murmur + streptococcal infection	−13
Controlled with insulin		Rapid pulse	−3.5
1920 Joslin Clinic record	−20	Phlebitis	−3.5
1940 Joslin Clinic record	−15	Varicose veins	−0.2
1950 Joslin Clinic record	−10	Epilepsy	−20.0
		Skull fracture	−2.9
		Tuberculosis	−1.8
		Nephrectomy	−2.0
		Trace of albumin in urine	−5.0
		Moderate albumin in urine	−13.5

Source: Jones (1959).

† Central Bureau of Statistics (Statistiska Centralbyran) (1917, 1953); National Health Service of Denmark (1914, 1921; 1937, 1949); Federal Security Agency (1940–1955).

§ Dublin, et al. (1951).

|| Hammond and Horn (1954).

Gofman (1956).

** Society of Actuaries (1951).

†† This 70 percent difference in distribution of lipoproteins, between 25 percent versus 5 percent highest, is equivalent to a total of 25 years in relative displacement of physiologic age.

‡ As measured in 1900. These effects may be measurably less now, as environment is changing to produce greater differences between parents and progeny.

‡‡ Joslin, et al. (1952).

Aging of the Nervous System

Particular attention to the impact of aging on the nervous system is warranted because of its critical importance to all aspects of communicative function. It is well understood that the nervous system is highly susceptible to aging, and at least three reasons may be offered to account for this. First, as suggested earlier, neurons in the central nervous system are not replaced by division of the remaining cells. Accordingly, any loss of cells in the central nervous system (CNS) is cumulative with age (Wright and Spink, 1974). Second, the brain is highly sensitive to a lack of oxygen, and, therefore, temporary interruptions in the blood supply will likely result in the death of neurons. It has already been established the the process of aging is accompanied by cardiac-circulatory insufficiency. In addition, there are common changes in the blood vessels of the brain that collectively may be termed cerebral arteriosclerosis (Busse, 1959). These changes can reduce blood supply to certain areas of the brain or even result in occlusion of a cerebral artery. Third, there is a proclivity for pigment deposits (lipofuscin) in cells of the aging brain (Bondareff, 1959; Brizzee and Johnson, 1974). It has been commonly thought that the accumulation of lipofuscin may have an effect on the physiologic capabilities of neurons and may even result in the death of such cells (Brizzee and Johnson, 1974).

Perhaps one of the most obvious changes in the gross anatomy of the nervous system associated with aging is a decrease in brain weight (Bondareff, 1959). For example, Appel and Appel (1942) documented an 11% decrease in brain weight between ages 25 and 96 years. Bondareff (1959) has described a decrease in brain volume relative to skull capacity as a function of advancing age. This gives the brain a shrunken appearance with an exaggerated pattern of cortical convolutions characterized by narrowed gyri and widened sulci. For purposes of illustration an advanced case of frontal lobe atrophy is presented in Figure 3-1. The brain shown here is associated with a case of Pick's disease (see Chapter 15), and it must be understood that most aging brains will not manifest such a circumscribed and exaggerated pattern of cortical atrophy. In addition to these changes in cortical surface structure, there may be thickening of the meninges, atrophy of the corpus callosum, shrinking of the basal ganglia, distended ventricles, and an increase in cerebrospinal fluid (Bondareff, 1959).

Microscopically, a number of studies have documented a decrease in CNS neurons with advancing age. Several of these were

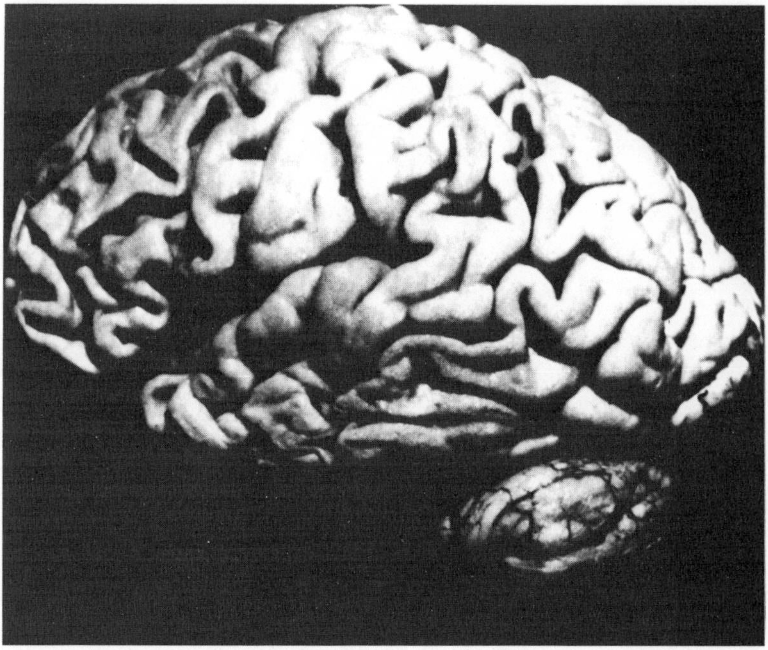

Figure 3-1. Lateral view of the cerebrum in a patient with Pick's disease. Note circumscribed atrophy of parts of frontal, temporal, and parietal lobes. (Source: Malamud, 1972.)

summarized by Wright and Spink (1974) and are presented in Figure 3-2. Of particular interest is Brody's (1955) observation of a marked decline in neuronal cell density in the cerebral cortex as a function of age for 20 brains. He noted the greatest cell loss in the superior temporal gyrus with lesser reductions in the precentral gyrus, area striata, inferior temporal gyrus, and postcentral gyrus. Neuron cell loss has also been recorded in the peripheral nervous systems of older subjects. Specifically, there appears to be a reduction in the number of larger fibers (Corbin and Gardner, 1937; Magladery, 1959). It is interesting to note the reduction in neurons within the auditory and speech production mechanisms (see Chapters 4 and 5). Birren (1964) has argued that aging will have a progressively more serious influence on the less primitive aspects of the nervous system. That is, later evolved structures such as the cortex will be more susceptible to the effects of senescence than will more primitive structures such as the vegetative centers of the brain stem.

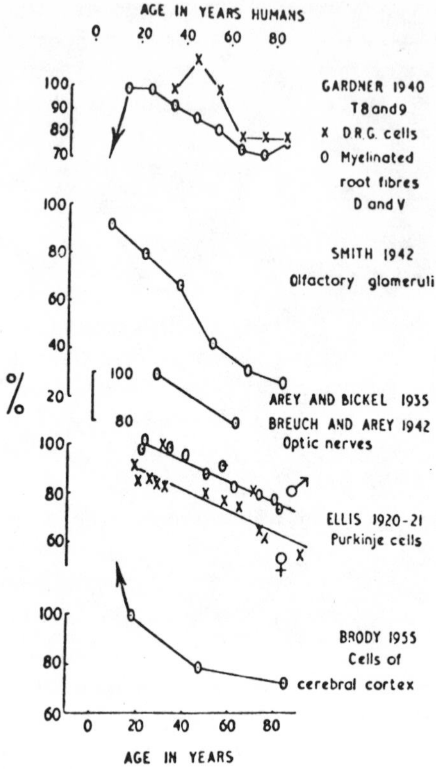

Figure 3-2. Data relating total nerve cell count to age in humans. All counts have been standardized as percentages of the highest count between the ages of 15 and 34 years, except in the data of Smith, where the counts in the newborn were taken as 100%. The arrows are directed toward the counts found at birth. (Source: Wright and Spink, 1974.)

SENSORIPERCEPTUAL CHANGES ASSOCIATED WITH ADVANCING AGE

Undoubtedly, studies of sensory and perceptual changes in the elderly are among the most voluminous in the scientific literature on gerontology. Therefore, since only an overview is provided in this section, the reader is referred to Braun (1959), Weiss (1959), Birren (1964), Corso (1971), and Botwinick (1973) for more detailed information. In this chapter, initial attention concerning this topic focuses on the special senses of vision, taste, smell, touch, and pain. Because of its importance to the central theme of this book, the topic of hearing is covered in substantive detail in Chapter 4. Following this review, a discussion of perceptual performance in elderly subjects is provided. For purposes of this chapter, sensation is considered to be awareness of stimuli through the exteroceptive systems (eyes, ears, taste buds, etc.) and perception is relegated to the interpretation and integration of sensations and patterns of sensation.

The Special Senses

Vision Perhaps one of the principle tests of visual adequacy is acuity, which is measured with respect to the smallest object that can be perceived at a given distance. Birren (1964), Weale (1965), and Botwinick (1973) have all noted that there is generally little change in acuity from roughly age 15–50. However, precipitous declines in acuity are typically observed beyong age 50 and "... by age 70, without correction, poor vision is a rule rather than the exception" (Botwinick, 1973, p. 121). In part, this visual deterioration can be attributed to pupil size which diminishes with age, thereby reducing the amount of light reaching the retina. This is illustrated in Figure 3-3, which is a reproduction of the data reported by Birren, Casperson, and Botwinick (1950).

Another indication of visual sensory integrity has been termed "accommodation," which refers to the ability of the eye to focus on objects at different distances. Several classic studies have documented that maximum accommodation is observed in childhood and decreases with advancing age. For example, Weiss (1959) suggested that maximum accommodation is roughly 20 diopters at age 5 and decreases at the rate of 0.3 diaopter/year until minimum accommodation of 0.5 diopter is reached at age 60.

Still another indicator of visual efficiency is dark adaptation which, according to Botwinick (1973), has two dimensions: 1) the time it takes to reach maximum acuity in the dark, and 2) the acuity level finally reached. There is consistency among investigations that the acuity level ultimately achieved deteriorates with age. However, there is some controversy with respect to the first dimension. For example, Domey, McFarland, and Chadwick (1960) reported a slower rate of dark adaptation with advancing age while Birren and Shock (1950) and Weale (1962) did not.

Other aspects of vision such as required illumination level, contrast discrimination, color vision, and critical flicker fusion have also been shown to deteriorate with advancing age (Weiss, 1959; Birren, 1964; Botwinick, 1973).

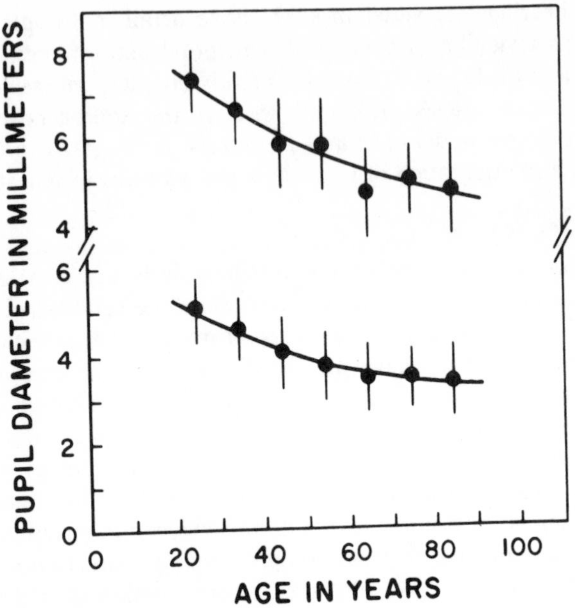

Figure 3-3. Mean pupil diameter (mm) of the eye in relation to age. The upper curve was derived from measurements of pupil size in the dark, the lower curve from pupil size under 1.0 millilambert brightness. Vertical lines represent ±1 standard deviation. (Source: Birren, Casperson, and Botwinick, 1950.)

The reasons for deterioration in visual performance among the elderly are many and include retinal decay, reduction in pupil diameter, opacities and bubbles in the lens and vitreous humour, and loss of lens elasticity. Some of these eye problems result from degenerative diseases such as senile macular degeneration (Ruiz, 1975), and others may be of vascular, metabolic, or endocrine origin (Knox, 1975).

Taste The study of taste changes with advancing age has been minimal, and interpretation of results has been difficult for several reasons. In general, most research suggests that sensitivity for the major taste qualities of salty, sour, bitter, and sweet decreases in older subjects (Cooper, Bilash, and Zubek, 1959). Schiffman (1977) observed that elderly subjects were significantly less able to identify unseasoned blended foods than younger subjects. However, it should be noted that Cohen and Gitman (1958) did not observe such a decline and Balogh and Lelkes (1961) concluded that sensitivity for bitterness actually increases with age. Reasons for equivocal research outcomes might include history of smoking, olfactory sensitivity, and attitudes toward food and eating (Botwinick, 1973). Moreover, aging appears to have a differential impact on taste buds in certain areas of the tongue (Schiffman, 1977).

Olfaction As with taste, few experimental data on olfactory sensitivity and aging are available. Birren (1964) reported a decrease in the number of olfactory nerve fibers with advancing age, implying a reduction in the sense of smell. Indeed, nearly all of the experimental evidence would support that conclusion (Chalke and Dewhurst, 1957; Kimbrell and Furchtgott, 1963; Schiffman, 1977). However, factors such as history of smoking, presence of nasal obstructions, and occupational conditions may contaminate many efforts to assess the effects of senescence on olfaction.

Touch and Pain As might be expected, the experimental literature rather uniformly establishes that touch and pain sensitivity decreases in older subjects. Specifically, stereognosis (Thompson, Axelrod, and Cohen, 1965), sensitivity to von Frey hairs (Birren, 1964), vibratory sensitivity (Cosh, 1953), and radiant heat pain sensitivity (Sherman and Robillard, 1960) have all been shown to decrease with advancing age. However, as Botwinick (1973) has pointed out, some of the diminished sensitivity reported in the literature may be a function of caution. That is, older subjects tend to exhibit more conservative thresholds for many sensory tests because of the need for certainty regarding the presence of the stimulus. It should be noted that diminished touch sensitivity may have some impact on speech; this is explored in Chapter 5.

Perception

It must be appreciated that sensation and perception cannot be easily separated in most experimental tasks because an impairment of one usually influences the adequacy of the other. However, in this section, a review of events assumed to involve processing, decoding, or interpretation at levels other than that of the peripheral input is discussed. For this review, selected examples are offered to illustrate the general conclusion that perceptual performance diminishes with advancing age.

Some Experimental Examples Several experiments have documented decrements in visual processing among the elderly. For example, tachistoscopic experiments such as those of Wallace (1956),

Riegel (1956), Rajalashmi and Jeeves (1963), and Malepeai and Hutchinson (1977) have established that older subjects require much greater exposure times to identify designs, words, and pictures. In addition, the age effects are usually more profound when interfering visual stimuli and reduced contrasts are introduced.

Basowitz and Korchin (1957) conducted an investigation regarding age differences in the perception of complex visual stimuli. Subjects were required to isolate smaller figures concealed within larger visual patterns. It was determined that older subjects performed much poorer than younger subjects. Using a somewhat different experimental strategy, Botwinick, Robbin, and Brinley (1959) presented young and old subjects with ambiguous, reversible pictures (e.g., the common "young or old woman" picture). Both studies illustrated that younger subjects were much better able to reorganize an original precept and see the alternate figure.

Another example of perceptual deterioration common among older persons was offered by Botwinick (1973) in his description of age performance on the Hooper Visual Organization Test. This test requires subjects to name drawings of objects which have been "cut apart" in jigsaw fashion. Correct naming can result only if the subject is successful in a spatial reorganization and integration of the parts. With increased age, there is a decreased ability to integrate spatially these line drawings.

In an interesting study by Landahl and Birren (1959) subjects ranging in age from 18 to 85 were presented a standard weight of 100 g in one hand and a variable weight (100–115 g) in the other and asked to decide which was heavier. Discrimination performance was clearly inferior among older participants.

Some Conclusions Although this review of perceptual experiments is quite impoverished when considering the vast research literature available, some concluding observations are possible. First, because of anatomic changes in the sensory systems, the CNS receives less information upon which processing decisions may be made. Second, threshold responses to tasks such as tachistoscopic recognition may be elevated in part because of caution in responding. Third, as a result of CNS alterations during aging, the ability to integrate information from several senses or within one sense may deteriorate. Fourth, for the same reason, the elderly may display a rigidity in responding and a reduced ability to alter original percepts (e.g., the ambiguous picture experiment).

PSYCHOMOTOR CHANGES ASSOCIATED WITH ADVANCING AGE

Partially as a result of deteriorations in sensory and perceptual function, the elderly exhibit slower responses to environmental stimuli. Many experts consider reductions in psychomotor speed to be a principal indicator of nervous system senescence (Birren, 1964). In view of the theoretical importance of response slowing to the entire issue of aging, a selected review of reaction time and movement time data is warranted.

Reaction Time/Movement Time Experiments

One of the earliest research efforts was that of Koga and Morant (1923), and their data are still of considerable value today. As a part of a larger study Koga and Morant measured reaction time to both auditory and visual stimuli. An example of the results for the auditory cue is found in Figure 3-4. As can be seen, reaction time decreases with increasing age to about 20 years and steadily decreases beyond that time. Similar results were observed for reactions to a sudden light stimulus. Since this early research, a plethora of studies has confirmed increased reaction time with advancing age (see Welford (1959) and Botwinick (1973) for complete reviews of this experimental effort).

Despite these rather consistent research findings, it has been documented that an increase in age may not always result in increased reaction times. For example, Botwinick and Thompson (1968) discovered that young, athletic subjects had faster reaction times than did young, nonathletic subjects. Spirduso (1975) investigated this issue further and concluded that life style appeared to play a greater role in determining reaction time than did the process of aging.

It should also be noted that Smith and Green (1962) demonstrated that tasks frequently performed were less affected by aging than those performed less frequently. This type of reasoning led Botwinick and Thompson (1967) to test the hypothesis that slower reaction times among the aged may decrease with repeated trials. Their results for 52 elderly subjects confirmed this probability. Later, Murrel (1970), who measured the response initiation times to a light signal in three subjects, showed that decrements in reaction time ascribed to the elderly can largely be eliminated with practice.

Of course, one might argue that reaction time deficits in older

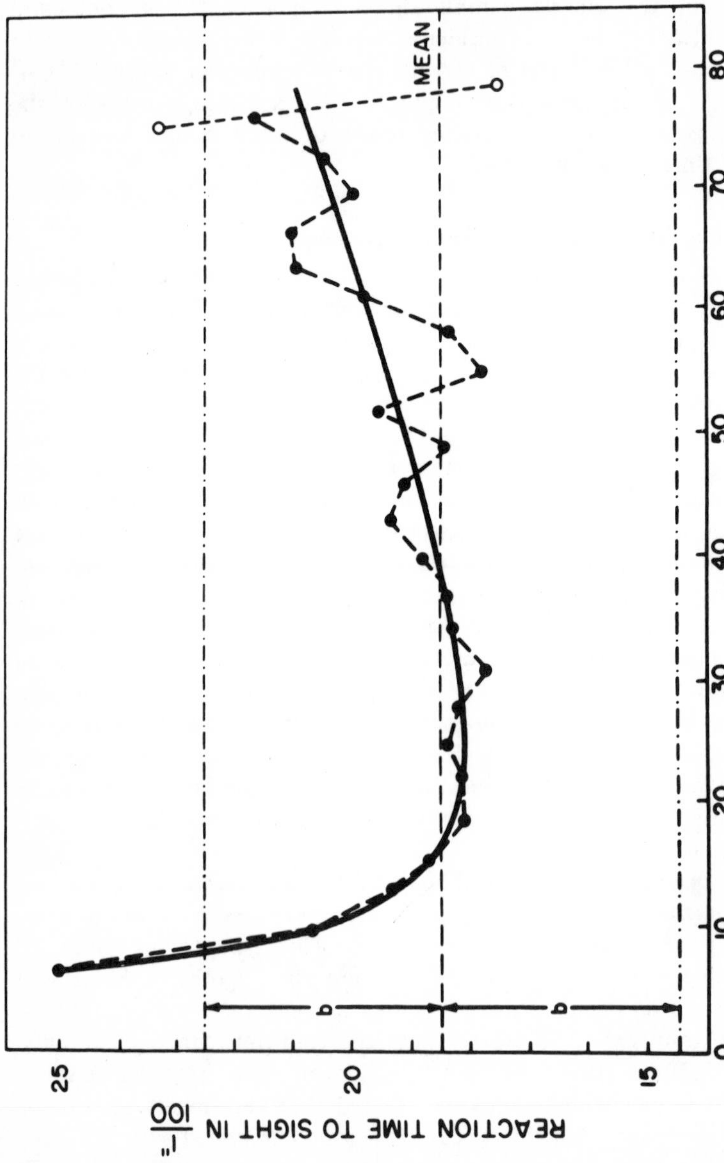

Figure 3-4. Reaction time to auditory signals in relation to age. (Source: Koga and Morant, 1923.)

subjects could be attributable to considerable slowness in muscular movement rather than decreased reaction per se. Whereas movement times are slower in the elderly (Pierson and Montoye, 1958), Birren (1964) has argued that:

> . . . a number of experiments suggest that by far the largest portion of the increased time with age is in the reaction time—i.e., the time from the appearance of a signal to the beginning of the movement—rather than in the movement time. (p. 118)

Several years ago, one of the central questions posed by experimenters concerned the principal locus of reaction time increments in the elderly. Could these elevations be attributed primarily to peripheral function or primarily to central delays in integrating and processing? Today, there are some reasonable answers to this question, and a summary of current reasoning follows.

Peripheral Mechanisms

Whereas it is well documented that perceptual speed is slower among older subjects, it is interesting to note that increasing stimulus intensity for the elderly in a reaction time experiment can minimize age-related differences (Botwinick, 1972). This suggests that factors other than those associated with input must be primary contributors to decreased reaction time. A second avenue of investigation concerned peripheral nerve conduction rates in the old versus the young. By way of summary, at least three major studies (Birren and Wall, 1956; Hügen, Norris, and Shock, 1960; Lafratta and Canestrari, 1966) have documented that while a small decrease in nerve conduction velocity may be seen in the elderly, it must be considered a trivial component of the elevated reaction time typically seen in these subjects.

Central Mechanisms

In view of the relatively insignificant role of peripheral factors in accounting for the direct relationship between reaction time and age, it would appear likely that central deficits must therefore account for the greatest portion of psychomotor slowness in the elderly. Welford (1965) presented four changes in the CNS which can be expected to influence psychomotor performance during senescence. First, the known reduction in the number of functional neuron cells will reduce signal strength and processing capacity. Second, there may be an increase in random neural activity in the older brain that acts as noise during the processing of certain stimulus-response events. Third, the aged may evidence longer "aftereffects" of neural activity which interfere or blur new signals coming to the brain, thereby reducing the ability of the brain to process these more recent activities. Fourth, arousal levels may be diminished in the central nervous systems of older persons and optimum activity levels in central neurons or neuron sets are diminished. This would have the overall effect of reducing signal strength and functional capacity.

INTELLIGENCE AND MEMORY CHANGES ASSOCIATED WITH ADVANCING AGE

As Miller (1977) noted, much of the research on intellectual and memory performance among the elderly was completed some time ago, and productivity in this experimental area has diminished in recent years. For excellent reviews of the literature regarding intellectual and memory functioning in older persons, the reader is referred to Jones (1959), Birren (1964), Botwinick (1967), Botwinick (1973), and Miller (1977).

Intelligence Test Data

There is tremendous uniformity among investigations that the elderly do not perform as well on traditional intelligence tests when compared with younger subjects. For example, Figure 3-5 illustrates a typical inverse relationship between age and test scores for the WAIS (Wechsler Adult Intelligence Scale). This particular intelligence test consists of 11 subtests, which may be grouped into two larger units: the verbal subtests (Information, Comprehension, Arithmetic, Similarities, Digit Span, Vocabulary) and the performance subtests (Digit Symbol, Picture Completion, Block Design, Picture Arrangement, Object Assembly). When analyzing the scores for older people on these two groupings, there emerges what Botwinick (1967, 1973) has called a "classic pattern." Without exception, the experiments reveal a much greater age-dependent decrement in the performance subtests. An illustration of this typical profile is seen in Figure 3-6.

Problems with Traditional Intelligence Test Data

It would be very hazardous to view these experimental data as true of all individual cases of aging. It must be remembered that the results portrayed in Figures 3-5 and 3-6 constitute a statistical repre-

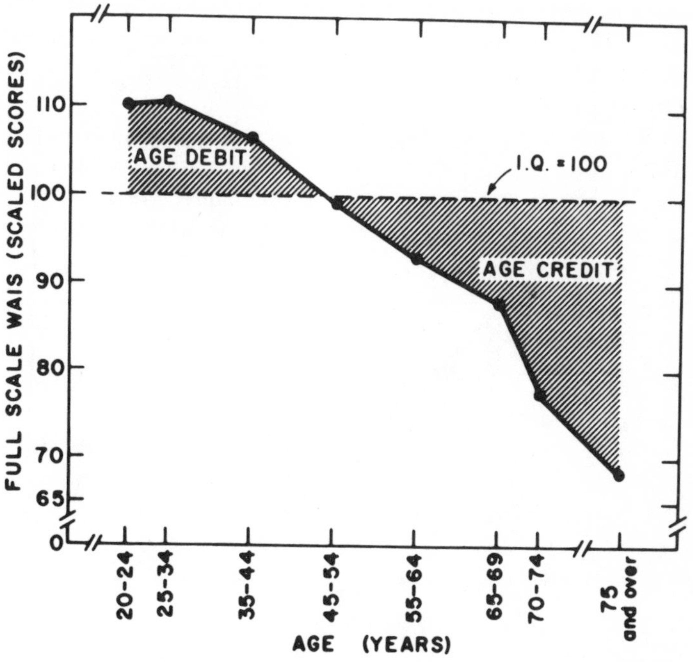

Figure 3-5. Full scaled scores as a function of age. Data were obtained from Table 18 of the WAIS Manual (1955, pp. 82–97) by culling scaled scores of IQs of 100. The broken line represents the conversion of the scaled scores to IQs. (Source: Botwinick, 1967.)

sentation of the gerontologic population. A number of important variables should be considered when interpreting these findings.

First, education has proved to be an important factor in the aforementioned intelligence test experiments. Birren and Morrison (1961) re-evaluated WAIS scores along two dimensions, age and educational level. They discovered that education level is more important than age in determining mental capacity and that failure to account for this factor greatly inflates the age-related decrement in intelligence test scores. Second, the health of subjects appears to have a significant impact on test scores. As evidence of this, Botwinick and Birren (1963) tested two groups of elderly using the WAIS. One group exhibited excellent health and the other was a typical representation of older subjects without incapacitating health problems. Though their results were not statistically impressive, Botwinick and Birren confirmed that healthier subjects perform

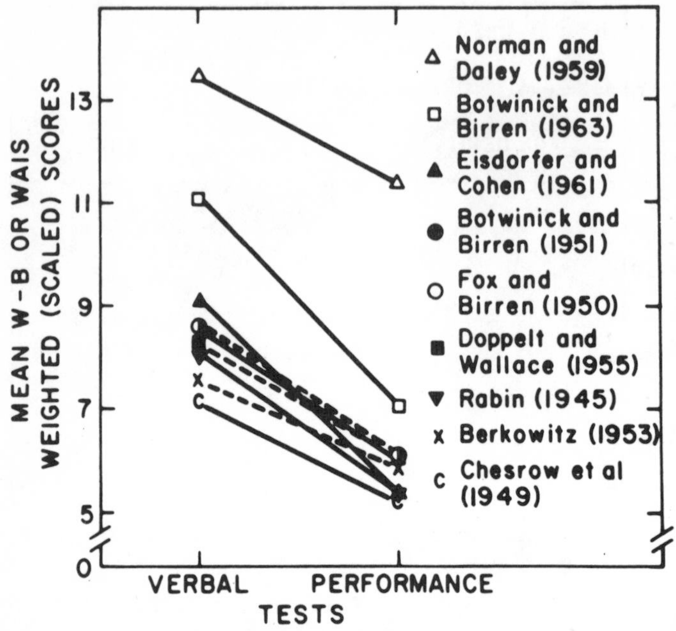

Figure 3-6. Mean verbal and mean performance WAIS subtest scores obtained from nine studies which reported results with elderly subjects. Note that greater decline is indicated in each study with the performance subtests than with the verbal ones. The expected verbal and performance scores of young adults of average intelligence are both 10. (Source: Botwinick, 1967.)

better on such tests. Third, it should be noted that, for obvious reasons, most intelligence test experiments involve cross-sectional designs with respect to the age factor. Miller (1977) argued that longitudinal studies should provide a better index of intellectual decline. After reviewing the limited number of published longitudinal experiments, Miller concluded that cross-sectional experiments overestimate the rate of intellectual decline as a function of age.

The apparent differential abilities for verbal and performance subtests in the elderly may be explained in part by the speed factor required in the performance skills. As already noted, response speed declines with advancing age and this is reflected in intelligence testing. Miller (1977) has also reasoned that "... subtests showing most change seem to involve memory or the ability to adduce new relationships, whilst those at the other end of the scale are more concerned with acquired knowledge" (p. 16).

An Interpretation of Intelligence Test Data

In amplifying upon the differential subtest scores seen among elderly subjects, Miller (1977) reintroduced the concepts of "fluid" and "crystallized" abilities originally proposed by Cattell (1943). Fluid intelligence refers to the ability of the individual to adapt to new situations, adduce new relationships, or acquire new ideas. On the other hand, crystallized intelligence is understood to mean learned intellectual skills. It is Miller's contention that fluid intelligence is more susceptible to aging than crystallized abilities. He used the results of Cunningham, Clayton, and Overton (1975) as support for this view. Briefly, Cunningham et al. showed that older subjects performed relatively poorer on the Raven's Progressive Matrices (fluid intelligence) when compared with scores for the Wechsler Vocabularly Scale (crystallized intelligence).

If this hypothesis is accurate, several other indices of intellectual functioning such as problem-solving skill, creative thinking, and development of new ideas might be expected to decline in older subjects when such tasks require considerable fluid skills. Indeed, most of the experimental data marshalled so far would confirm this expectation (Botwinick, 1967, 1973).

Memory

For purposes of this discussion, it is assumed that memory involves at least two fundamental levels: 1) a temporary short-term storage of limited capacity and rapid decay, 2) a long-term storage with considerable capacity and relatively more permanent fixation of traces. In general, experimental results (e.g., Gilbert, 1941; Davis and Obrist, 1966; Gilbert and Levee, 1971; etc.) have confirmed that older people do not perform as well as younger people on various tests of memory.

However, as with intelligence testing, several factors must be considered when interpreting such data. For example, memory test scores may be influenced by factors such as stimulus intensity, speed of stimulus presentation, attention, and sensory modality used. That is, there may be many variables which retard or prevent information from reaching the initial short-term memory storage. Furthermore, as Botwinick (1973) has pointed out, learning and memory cannot be differentiated in most memory tests. It is interesting to note that when extent of learning is controlled such that both young and old subjects reach a criterion level of learning, memory deficits between ages are largely eliminated up to at least 1 week post-training. After 1 week, it would appear that the elderly begin to exhibit more serious decaying in the long-term storage (Botwinick, 1973).

PSYCHOLOGICAL CHANGES ASSOCIATED WITH ADVANCING AGE

When discussing issues such as psychological factors characteristic of advancing age, it must be recognized that general statements become very difficult to offer. A variety of influences including family size, family attitude, health, site of residence, ethnic and religious background, socioeconomic status are all critically important in determining the psychological profile of an older individual. Despite the importance of these variables, it is possible to present some general concluding statements regarding this topic. For purposes of initiating this discussion, some attention to personality changes is warranted.

Personality Changes

One rather important issue which spans both psychological and sociological considerations has been termed "disengagement." This theoretical position is important because it has prompted a number of important research efforts. The crux of disengagement theory is the observation that older people tend to withdraw or become relatively more introverted (Botwinick, 1973). Initially, Cumming and Henry (1961) argued that disengagement was a natural, almost preprogrammed phenomenon wherein an individual becomes much more preoccupied with himself and less concerned with interpersonal contact. Inherent within such a speculation was the notion that societal forces play a relatively trivial role in forcing withdrawal upon aging people. Cumming and Henry reasoned further, that since disengagement is a natural event, the disengaged elderly will usually be satisfied, happy, and well adjusted.

However, subsequent research efforts rather seriously tortured the disengagement theory as formulated by Cumming and Henry. As a result, there has developed a more mature understanding of disengagement and its influence on happiness. In summarizing the rather extensive literature spawned by early formulations, Botwinick (1973) stated:

> . . . the disengagement-happiness relationship is dependent upon the age of the person, the health status (both physical and mental), the personality, the social role, the type of activity in which the person engages, and whether or not there is a confidant. (p. 55)

It is rather important that health professionals and particularly specialists in communicative disorders be cognizant of the disengagement phenomenon and the factors determining its influence on the adjustment of elderly people.

Two other dimensions of personality which have been considered characteristic of senescence are cautiousness and rigidity. Evidence of cautiousness is perhaps more abundant. The reader is again referred to Botwinick (1973) for an excellent treatment of this topic. Briefly, however, it has been documented that older subjects are much more cautious in "life decisions." For example, Wallach and Kogan (1961) discovered that the elderly would be more cautious in decisions involving financial risk even when the potential for marked financial gain was present. Further evidence of cautiousness in decision making has been reported by many investigators in a variety of experimental tasks (Miller, 1977). As a point of interest, the factor of caution can influence clinical assessments of the elderly. As is explored in more detail later, cautious responses are probably responsible for part of the elevated hearing thresholds commonly reported for older people.

The issue of rigidity is somewhat more equivocal. By definition, rigid behavior implies stereotyped response patterns and resistance to change. To a first approximation, it is accurate to say that older people tend to exhibit such inflexibility. However, so many factors influence rigidity, such as life-long personality characteristics, educational history, intellectual skills, cultural factors, etc., that rigidity among the elderly must be considered an oversimplification (Botwinick, 1973).

Yet another personality characteristic commonly attributed to the aged is depression. Several obvious reasons for depressive episodes may be offered, including loss of peers and spouse through death, declining health, economic restrictions, reduced feeling of self-worth, and social isolation. Certainly, health professionals can do much to combat feelings of depression by helping to restore feelings of self-worth, encouraging social contact, and restructuring life goals (Botwinick, 1973).

Beyond these general dimensions of personality, it is very difficult to isolate any other definite age-related personality factors. It has beeen stated with some regularity that a variety of issues will influence personality structure in older subjects and perhaps some attention should be directed to them.

Factors Influencing Personality Characteristics of the Elderly

Fozard and Thomas (1975) have claimed that "personality is remarkably stable over the adult years in most respects" (p. 139). Such a statement implies that life-long patterns of behavior and attitude will remain relatively well preserved in advancing age. Certainly one of the most critical determinants of personality change will be continued health and vitality. Long, debilitating diseases present little promise for happy life in the remaining years. Two other related factors are family relationship and family attitudes. Strong ties to living spouses, brothers, sisters, and/or children will provide an opportunity for emotional support and interpersonal contact. Of course, financial security also predisposes the elderly to happier retirement years. Finally, the issue of relocation, particularly to institutions, bears importantly on emotional well-being and warrants special consideration.

The Issue of Relocation

Often, because of poor health, elderly people are relocated from their home environments. Very frequently the new residence is an institution such as a nursing home. If the relocated person is mentally alert and properly oriented, the relocation may be perceived quite negatively. Miller and Lieberman (1965) reported that relocation may result in severe depression characterized by feelings of having been cheated, of having a meaningless life, and of having a dim future with no possibility of happiness.

Reactions to the End of Life

The final topic to be considered briefly in this section is how psychological changes and aging affect reactions to the end of life. There is little in the way of systematic research on the psychology of the last stages of life. However, it is well known that many elderly people who are emotionally healthy and mentally alert will engage in a life review. This review has been characterized by Birren (1964) as "an active, or purposeful, examination of the events of one's life accompanying an impression of impending death. The intent of the life review is to reconcile one's values with the behavior of one's life and to leave behind an acceptable image" (p. 287). Of course, not all people react to an impression of impending death by undertaking a life review. Some deny the impression, some react passively to it, and some become rather seriously depressed.

In recent years, there has been a growing interest in the topic of death and dying. For more complete reviews of this issue, the reader is referred to Kübler-Ross (1969, 1974, 1975), Glaser and Strauss (1968), and Hinton (1967). In summarizing her rather extensive research with terminally ill patients, Kübler-Ross (1975) discovered that some were in relatively good spirits and able to talk about the issue of death. She further noted that one of the critical variables in this "well adjusted" attitude was the way in which the physician responded to the terminally ill patient. Since most health professionals, including speech pathologists and audiologists, often interact with dying patients, Kübler-Ross' observations regarding an ideal physician's approach warrant review. Essentially, seven common denominators were recorded (1975, p. 533):

1. Personal experience in their own families with terminal illness, suffering, and death. They had learned through these personal experiences to become more comfortable in dealing with death.
2. As soon as the diagnosis was confirmed, they sat with their patients and their families and informed them about the seriousness of the illness.
3. They were then able to wait until the patient was emotionally ready to "hear more," i.e., when patients asked more details or more specific questions pertaining to their illness or prognosis. All questions were answered in a language which the patient was able to understand.
4. Combined with the bad news, these physicians gave hope and conveyed to the patient that they did not plan to desert them later on (this refers implicitly to the time when the patient is beyond medical help).
5. They continued to visit them in the same manner and with the same care from the beginning of the hospitalization to the time of their death. When a patient was transferred to a nursing home or to his own home, they continued the contact by personal visits or by phone.
6. They did not avoid questions from patient or family members.
7. Finally, and significantly, they saw to it that adequate pain

relief minimized the suffering and they did not hesitate to ask social services, ministers, or others for help when indicated.

With respect to the patients themselves, Kübler-Ross observed five common stages in the reaction of dying: 1) denial, 2) anger, 3) depression, 4) bartering, and 5) acceptance. It must be realized that not all people with terminal illness go through these stages and not all achieve a state of acceptance. Some evidence bitter or angry resignation and a sense of utter despair. All health professionals should cooperate and respond to dying patients so that they might achieve a positive attitude toward death and feel a sense "of being wanted, needed, and loved" (Kübler-Ross, 1975, p. 537).

SUGGESTED READINGS

Birren, J. E. (ed.). Handbook of Aging and the Individual. Chicago: University of Chicago Press, 1959.
Birren, J. E. The Psychology of Aging. Englewood Cliffs, N.J.: Prentice-Hall, 1964.
Botwinick, J. Cognitive Processes in Maturity and Old Age. New York: Springer, 1967.
Botwinick, J. Aging and Behavior. New York: Springer, 1973.
Miller, E. Abnormal Ageing. London: John Wiley & Sons, 1977.
Welford, A. T., and Birren, J. E. (eds.). Behavior, Aging, and the Nervous System. Springfield, Ill.: Charles C Thomas, 1965.

REFERENCES

Appel, F. W., and Appel, E. M. Intracranial variation in the weight of the human brain. Human Biology, 14, 48–68 (1942).
Balogh, K., and Lelkes, K. The tongue in old age. Gerontologica Clinica, 3, Supplement, 38–54 (1961).
Basowitz, H., and Korchin, S. J. Age differences in the perception of closure. Journal of Abnormal and Social Psychology, 54, 93–97 (1957).
Birren, J. E. Principles of research on aging. In J. E. Birren (ed.), Handbook of Aging and the Individual: Psychological and Biological Aspects. Chicago: University of Chicago Press, 1959.
Birren, J. E. The Psychology of Aging. Englewood Cliffs, N. J.: Prentice-Hall, 1964.
Birren, J. E., Casperson, R. C., and Botwinick, J. Age changes in pupil size. Journal of Gerontology, 5, 216–221 (1950).
Birren, J. E., and Morrison, D. F. Analysis of the WAIS subtests in relation to age and education. Journal of Gerontology, 16, 363–369 (1961).
Birren, J. E., and Shock, N. W. Age changes in rate and level of visual dark adaptation. Journal of Applied Physiology, 2, 407–411 (1950).
Birren, J. E., and Wall, P. D. Age changes in conduction velocity, refractory period, number of fibers, connective tissue space, and blood

vessels in sciatic nerve of rats. Journal of Comparative Neurology, 104, 1–16 (1956).

Bondareff, W. Morphology of the aging nervous system. In J. E. Birren (ed.), Handbook of Aging and the Individual: Psychological and Biological Aspects. Chicago: University of Chicago Press, 1959.

Botwinick, J. Cognitive Processes in Maturity and Old Age. New York: Springer, 1967.

Botwinick, J. Sensory-perceptual factors in reaction time in relation to age. Journal of Genetic Psychology, 121, 173–177 (1972).

Botwinick, J. Aging and Behavior. New York: Springer, 1973.

Botwinick, J., and Birren, J. E. Cognitive processes: Mental abilities and psychomotor responses in healthy aged men. In J. E. Birren et al. (eds.), Human Aging: A Biological and Behavioral Study. Washington, D.C.: U.S. Government Printing Office, 1963.

Botwinick, J., Robbin, J. S., and Brinley, J. F. Reorganization of perceptions with age. Journal of Gerontology, 14, 85–88 (1959).

Botwinick, J., and Thompson, L. Practice of speeded response in relation to age, sex, and set. Journal of Gerontology, 22, 72–76 (1967).

Botwinick, J., and Thompson, L. Age differences in reaction time: An artifact? Gerontologist, 8, 25–28 (1968).

Braun, H. W. Perceptual processes. In J. E. Birren (ed.), Handbook of Aging and the Individual: Psychological and Biological Aspects. Chicago: University of Chicago Press, 1959.

Brizzee, K. R., and Johnson, F. A. Depth distribution of lipofuscin in cerebral cortex of albino rat. In E. A. Wright et al. (eds.), Brain Structure and Aging. New York: MSS Information Corp., 1974.

Brody, H. Organization of the cerebral cortex. III. A study of aging in the human cerebral cortex. Journal of Comparative Neurology, 102, 511–556 (1955).

Busse, E. W. Psychopathology. In J. E. Birren (ed.), Handbook of Aging and the Individual: Psychological and Biological Aspects. Chicago: University of Chicago Press, 1959.

Cattell, R. B. The measurement of adult intelligence. Psychological Bulletin, 3, 153–193 (1943).

Chalke, H. D., and Dewhurst, J. R. Coal gas poisoning: Loss of sense of smell as a possible contributory factor with old people. British Medical Journal, 2, 1915–1917 (1957).

Cohen, T., and Gitman, L. Studies in the gastrointestinal tract of the aged. Journal of Gerontology, 13, Abstract, 441 (1958).

Cooper, R. M., Bilash, I., and Zubek, J. P. The effect of age on taste sensitivity. Journal of Gerontology, 14, 56–58 (1959).

Corbin, K. B., and Gardner, E. D. Decrease in number of myelinated fibers in human spinal roots with age. Anatomical Record, 68, 63–74 (1937).

Corso, J. F. Sensory processes and age effects in normal adults. Journal of Gerontology, 26, 90–105 (1971).

Cosh, J. A. Studies on the nature of vibration sense. Clinical Science, 12, 131–151 (1953).

Cumming, E., and Henry, W. Growing Old: The Process of Disengagement. New York: Basic Books, 1961.

Cunningham, W. R., Clayton, V., and Overton, W. Fluid and crystallized intelligence in young adulthood and old age. Journal of Gerontology, 30, 53–55 (1975).

Davis, S. H., and Obrist, W. D. Age differences in learning and retention of verbal material. Cornell Journal of Social Relations, 1, 95–103 (1966).

Domey, R. G., McFarland, R. A., and Chadwick, E. Dark adaptation as a function of age and time: II. A derivation. Journal of Gerontology, 15, 267–279 (1960).

Fozard, J. L., and Thomas, J. C. Psychology of aging. In J. G. Howels (ed.), Modern Perspectives on the Psychiatry of Old Age. New York: Brunner/Mazel, 1975.

Freeman, J. T. The mechanisms of stress and the forces of senescence. Journal of the American Geriatrics Society, 7, 71–78 (1959).

Glaser, B. G., and Strauss, A. L. Time for Dying. Chicago: Aldine, 1968.

Gilbert, J. G. Memory loss in senescence. Journal of Abnormal and Social Psychology, 36, 73–86 (1941).

Gilbert, J. G., and Levee, R. F. Patterns of declining memory. Journal of Gerontology, 26, 70–75 (1971).

Hinton, J. M. Dying. Baltimore: Penguin, 1967.

Hügen, F., Norris, A. H., and Shock, N. W. Skin reflex and voluntary reaction times in young and old males. Journal of Gerontology, 15, 388–391 (1960).

Jones, H. E. Intelligence and problem-solving. In J. E. Birren (ed.), Handbook of Aging and the Individual: Psychological and Biological Aspects. Chicago: University of Chicago Press, 1959.

Kimbrell, G. M., and Furchtgott, E. The effect of aging on olfactory threshold. Journal of Gerontology, 18, 364–365 (1963).

Knox, D. L. Disorders of vision: Vascular, metabolic, and endocrine. In W. S. Fields (ed.), Neurological and Sensory Disorders in the Elderly. New York: Stratton Intercontinental Medical Book Corp., 1975.

Koga, Y., and Morant, G. M. On the degree of association between reaction times in the case of different senses. Biometrika, 15, 355–359 (1923).

Kübler-Ross, E. On Death and Dying. New York: Maxmillan, 1969.

Kübler-Ross, E. Questions and Answers on Death and Dying. New York: Macmillan, 1974.

Kübler-Ross, E. Facing death. In J. G. Howells (ed.), Modern Perspectives in the Psychiatry of Old Age. New York: Brunner/Mazel, 1975.

LaFratta, C. W., and Canestrari, R. E. A comparison of sensory and motor nerve conduction velocities as related to age. Archives of Physical Medicine and Rehabilitation, 47, 286–290 (1966).

Landahl, H. D., and Birren, J. E. Effects of age on the discrimination of lifted weights. Journal of Gerontology, 14, 48–55 (1959).

Magladary, J. W. Neurophysiology and aging. In J. E. Birren (ed.), Handbook of Aging and the Individual: Psychological and Biological Aspects. Chicago: University of Chicago Press, 1959.

Malamud, N. Neuropathology of organic brain syndromes associated with aging. In C. M. Gaitz (ed.), Aging and the Brain. New York: Plenum Press, 1972.

Malepeai, B. B., and Hutchinson, J. M. Word retrieval and visual processing skills among the elderly. Paper presented at the Annual Convention of the American Speech and Hearing Association, Chicago, 1977.

Miller, D., and Lieberman, M. A. The relationship of affect state and adaptive capacity to reactions to stress. Journal of Gerontology, 20, 492–497 (1965).

Miller, E. Abnormal Ageing. London: John Wiley & Sons, 1977.

Murrel, F. The effect of extensive practice on age differences in reaction time. Journal of Gerontology, 25, 268–274 (1970).

Pierson, W., and Montoye, H. Movement time, reaction time, and age. Journal of Gerontology, 13, 418–421 (1958).

Rajalashmi, R., and Jeeves, M. Changes in tachistoscopic form perception as a function of age and intellectual status. Journal of Gerontology, 18, 275–278 (1963).

Riegel, K. A study of verbal achievement of older persons. Journal of Gerontology, 14, 453–456 (1956).

Ruiz, R. S. Disorders of vision: Degenerative diseases. In W. S. Fields (ed.), Neurological and Sensory Disorders in the Elderly. New York: Stratton Intercontinental Medical Book Corp., 1975.

Schiffman, S. Food recognition by the elderly. Journal of Gerontology, 32, 586–592 (1977).

Sherman, E. D., and Robillard, E. Sensitivity to pain in the aged. Canadian Medical Association Journal, 83, 944–947 (1960).

Simonson, E. Performance as a function of age and cardiovascular disease. In A. T. Welford and J. E. Birren (eds.), Behavior, Aging, and the Nervous System. Springfield, Ill.: Charles C Thomas, 1965.

Smith, K., and Green, D. Scientific motion study and aging process in performance. Ergonomics, 5, 155–164 (1962).

Spirduso, W. Reaction and movement time as a function of age and physical activity level. Journal of Gerontology, 30, 435–440 (1975).

Thompson, L. W., Axelrod, S., and Cohen, L. D. Senescence and visual identification of tactual-kinesthetic forms. Journal of Gerontology, 20, 244–249 (1965).

Wallace, J. Some studies of perception in relation to age. British Journal of Psychology, 47, 283–297 (1956).

Wallach, M. A., and Kogan, N. Aspects of judgment and decision making: Interrelationships and changes with age. Behavioral Science, 6, 23–36 (1961).

Weale, R. A. Photo-chemical changes in the dark-adapting human retina. Vision Research, 2, 25–33 (1962).

Weale, R. A. On the eye. In A. T. Welford and J. E. Birren (eds.), Behavior, Aging, and the Nervous System. Springfield, Ill.: Charles C Thomas, 1965.

Weiss, A. D. Sensory functions. In J. E. Birren (ed.), Handbook of Aging and the Individual: Psychological and Biological Aspects. Chicago: University of Chicago Press, 1959.

Welford, A. T. Psychomotor performance. In J. E. Birren (ed.), Handbook of Aging and the Individual: Psychological and Biological Aspects. Chicago: University of Chicago Press, 1959.

Welford, A. T. Performance, biological mechanisms, and age. In A. T.

Welford and J. E. Birren (eds.), Behavior, Aging, and the Nervous System. Springfield, Ill.: Charles C Thomas, 1965.

Wolff, K. The Biological, Sociological, and Psychological Aspects of Aging. Springfield, Ill.: Charles C Thomas, 1959.

Wright, E. A., and Spink, J. M. A study of the loss of nerve cells in the central nervous system in relation to age. In E. A. Wright et al. (eds.), Brain Structure and Aging. New York: MSS Information Service, 1974.

Chapter 4
Presbycusis

The structural alterations commonly observed within the auditory system as a result of the process of aging are identified and reviewed. Also included is an overview of the auditory dysfunctions which are associated with presbycusis.

The effects of aging on man's auditory system have been noted in the literature since the late 1800s (Zwaardemaker, 1894). Early investigations of this process focused on the structural changes found to occur within the cochlea, and for an extended period of time it was generally believed that the effects of aging on audition were confined to this particular portion of the hearing mechanism (Davis, 1970). Presbycusis, the term most often utilized when referring to the deterioration in auditory functioning associated with aging, was therefore thought for some time to involve only the peripheral auditory mechanism, specifically the structures of the inner ear.

More recent investigations by numerous researchers, including Hinchcliffe (1962), Crabbe (1963), Schuknecht (1964), and Hansen and Reske-Nielsen (1965), have disclosed that no one portion of the auditory system of man is immune to senescent alterations. The pathology of presbycusis has been shown to involve all of the major divisions of both the peripheral and central auditory mechanisms.

Schuknecht, in particular, has contributed the most toward what is currently known concerning presbycusis. This is especially true of the structural changes that can be associated with aging within the inner ear and the neural structures of the auditory system. After extensive investigation, Schuknecht (1955) published a description of two distinct types of presbycusis. The first he termed "epithelial atrophy," which involves the degeneration of essentially all of the structures contained within the cochlea from its basal end through to the apex. It was Schuknecht's opinion that these changes were similar to those observed in all tissues of the body during aging. The second type of presbycusis Schuknecht described was "neural atrophy." This form is associated with the degeneration of spiral ganglion cells and the neurons of the higher auditory pathway. In 1964 Schuknecht again presented further information concerning presbycusis, this time identifying and describing four types of presbycusis. "Sensory presbycusis" (formerly termed "epithelial atrophy") is characterized by atrophy of the organ of Corti and the auditory nerve in the basal portion of the cochlea. "Neural presbycusis" (formerly "neutral atrophy") is associated with a loss of nerve fibers or cells in the auditory pathway of the central nervous system. "Metabolic presbycusis" refers to those defects in biochemical or biophysical processes involved in the transducer mechanism of the cochlea and is directly linked with atrophy within the stria vascularis. Schuknecht's last type was called "mechanical presbycusis" and was linked with the motion properties of the cochlear duct.

The influence of genetic and environmental factors on presbycusis has been studied at some length. The work of Rosen, Bergman, Plester, El-Mofty, and Satti (1962) and Rosen, Plester, El-Mofty, and Rosen (1964) suggested that environmental factors, such as exposure to noise during one's lifetime, may contribute to the general loss of hearing commonly observed in presbycusis. To more accurately express this, the term "sociocusis" has been proposed by Glorig and Nixon (1962) to indicate a loss of hearing resulting from a lifetime of exposure to noise in today's modern society.

Whatever the etiology might be, the fact remains that substantial alterations do occur in the entire auditory system of the elderly. The next portion of this chapter identifies and discusses those changes thought to take place in the major divisions of the hearing mechanism.

STRUCTURAL ALTERATIONS

Outer Ear

Although structural changes which occur here do not have any substantial effect on the hearing of the aging, the alterations which do occur are still worthy of note. As discussed later in Chapter 6, anatomic alterations in the outer ear can influence the administration of specific audiometric tests and also can be of some importance when consideration is given to the fitting of a hearing aid.

Pinna Any individual having occasion to examine the outer ear structures of the elderly will soon note that there are many abnormally large auricles in this age group. Research by Tsai, Chou, and Cheng (1958), as discussed by Willeford (1971), tends to support this observation. In their investigation the authors investigated the length of the pinna as a function of both age and sex. They found that the average length of the pinna in the male group increased more than 5 mm and in width by 2 mm as the age of the subjects was varied from the 20s to the 50s. Similar changes were also observed in the females.

As noted by Guild (1942) and Willeford (1971), the pinna of the aged is also often characterized by the presence of a considerable amount of stiff, wiry hair on or near a number of landmarks of the auricle. Senescence may also lead to excessive freckling of the pinna (Senturia, 1957). Close inspection of the pinna also reveals that it is decidedly more stiff and rigid than what is normally observed in younger individuals.

External Auditory Meatus In separate studies Babbitt (1947) and Rosenwasser (1964) reported that the tissues lining the external auditory meatus undergo some degree of atrophic alterations during the process of senescence. This may, as suggested by Babbitt (1947) and Magladery (1959), lead to a narrowing of the width of the ear canal. However, the experience of the present authors, as well as Fowler (1944), would indicate that changes associated with aging may result in actually widening the external meatus in many of the elderly.

Rosenwasser (1964) also noted a general thinning of the skin lining the ear canal and, along with Senturia (1957), pointed out the tendency for diminished elasticity in these tissues as well. A pronounced dryness of the epidermis of the canal may also be observed in some aged individuals (Senturia, 1957). These factors may serve to explain the cracking of the skin, the crusting, and the tendency for bleeding referred to by Rosenwasser (1964).

Middle Ear

Senescent changes of a significant magnitude also occur in this division of the auditory system, with certain of these alterations resulting in some degree of auditory dysfunction.

Tympanic Membrane Although the eardrum is felt by some investigators to be altered in the presbycusic, the exact nature of this alteration appears to be somewhat uncertain at this time. Covell (1952), in discussing changes which occur in the conductive apparatus of the middle ear, pointed out that among the alterations which occur are the thinning and loss of rigidity of the tympanic membrane. Likewise, Rosenwasser (1964) noted that the drum membrane of the elderly is often thin and translucent. In older patients having chronic rheumatism and arthritis, Klotz (1963) reported that a sclerotic thickening or a nonreflective eardrum may be present.

Ossicles Substantial evidence exists regarding the development of increased rigidity of the three bones of the ossicular chain. Rosenwasser (1964) discussed the ossification of the malleoincudal joint with calcification in the articular cartilage. He also noted the presence of ossicular atrophy, particularly in the crura of the stapes. Klotz (1963) and Crabbe (1963) have also concluded that sclerosis of the joints of the ossicles occurs, resulting in increased rigidity of these bones. Although stating that arthritic changes in the ossicular joints increase with age, Etholm and Belel (1974) concluded that these modifications do not appear to affect hearing.

In addition to the development of abnormal rigidity of the ossicular chain, mention is made by Covell (1952) of the possibility of excessive wearing of the joints of the ossicles. However, no substantial evidence to support this contention has been presented.

Muscles and Ligaments As observed with many of the other muscles of the body, a general degeneration and atrophy take place in the tensor tympani and stapedius muscles of the middle ear and in the numerous ligaments present. Covell (1952) and Rosenwasser (1964) are among those who have described these alterations. Deterioration of the two middle ear muscles may lessen the amount of protection provided the structure of the ear during the contraction of these muscles in the presence of intense noise. This is supported by the evidence presented by Thompson, Sills, and Bui (1976) concerning the acoustic reflex in young and old ears.

Davis (1970) has pointed out the potential effect of the atrophy of the ligaments attached to the ossicles on hearing in the elderly. He reported that degenerative changes in these structures may result in the ossicles not operating as efficiently, conceivably causing minor decreases in hearing acuity and producing some degree of distortion within the conductive mechanism. Davis also noted the potential for the atrophy of the ligaments and muscles of the ossicles to result in the production of less tension on the tympanic membrane, making the membrane somewhat flabby and less able to respond to incoming sound waves.

Eustachian Tube The breakdown of tissue shown to occur in older persons makes it plausible to suspect that the normal operation of the Eustachian tube may be altered to some extent. Although no specific investigation of this notion has been carried out, it would appear that if the muscles specifically responsible for the opening of the tube (levator and tensor palatini) undergo atrophy, as occurs with most muscle tissue in older individuals, and do not function efficiently, then the ability of the Eustachian tube to open properly may be impaired. An inability for the tube to open effectively may lead to some undesirable consequences within the middle ear, such as the creation of negative pressure in the middle ear cavity.

Although no direct research on the status of the Eustachian tube in the elderly has been conducted, a study recently done in a nursing home setting by Nerbonne, Schow, Goset, and Bliss (1976) has revealed some evidence to suggest the possibility of some malfunction of this important structure. A total of 16.5% of the elderly ears evaluated by means of tympanometry in their study yielded results indicative of the presence of an abnormal negative pressure in the middle ear cavity, which is suggestive of some degree of Eustachian tube inadequacy. Further exploration of this issue appears warranted.

Inner Ear

Although not all investigators believe that the primary location for presbycusic alterations is the inner ear (Hinchcliffe, 1962), it is generally agreed that the degeneration of certain structures within the inner ear during the process of senescence has a substantial effect on the process of hearing in elderly people. The deterioration appears to affect most of the critical components of the cochlea, and a review of these modifications follows.

General Atropy of the Organ of Corti A number of investigators have reported on the senescent alterations of the organ of Corti as a whole. Saxen and von Fiendt (1937) were among the earliest to document the degeneration of this structure within the inner ear. In their research Saxen and von Fiendt found that the organ of Corti was severely atrophied in more than one-half of the temporal bones of the 33 patients they examined. Jorgensen (1961) also noted that the organ of Corti is often found in a collapsed state, and is reduced to a small bulge on the basilar membrane.

It is, at this stage of degeneration, virtually impossible to discern any anatomic details. Jorgensen found that this process, although associated with the inner ear of the elderly, can be seen in certain cases at a relatively young age. This overall atrophy of the organ of Corti is generally observed in a very specific area of the basal end of the cochlea (Schuknecht, 1955).

Hair Cells The early works of Crowe, Guild, and Polvogt (1934), and later of Schuknecht (1955), were instrumental in establishing the strong association which exists between aging and a loss of hair cells. Their research pointed out, however, that the correlation between visible hair cell degeneration and hearing loss is less than perfect, suggesting that hair cell deterioration does not, by itself, serve to explain totally the presence of hearing loss in the elderly. Further evidence regarding hair cell alterations in the aging ear has been supplied by Pestalozza and Shore (1955) and Gacek (1975). it was Gacek who stated that while the etiology of hair cell degeneration was not clear, evidence suggests that changes in the metabolic activity of the lysosomes in the hair cells coincide with a decrease in enzymatic activity, which leads eventually to the death of the hair cell.

Basilar Membrane Alteration in the stiffness of the basilar membrane which accompanies aging has been suggested by a number of individuals, including Mayer (1919–1920) and Crowe et al. (1934), as an important factor in the creation of hearing loss in the elderly. Further support for this contention has been offered by Schuknecht (1964), with his labeling of "mechanical presbycusis." Schuknecht (1967) has also discussed the atrophy of the basilar membrane and the rupture of this structure, with thinning of the membrane occurring at the location of the rupture.

Stria Vascularis Structural atrophy of the stria vascularis has been shown by Crowe et al. (1934), Saxen and von Fiendt (1937), and Schuknecht (1964) to occur frequently in older persons, resulting in substantial interruption of the transducer activity within the cochlea. Because the stria vascularis is felt to be the source for the production of endolymph (Zemlin, 1968), and because it is also felt to be the source of the DC potential so important in the processing which occurs in the inner ear, its degeneration is thought to be a major factor in explaining the depression in acuity observed in the presbycusic. Goodhill and Guggenheim (1971) have stated that alterations in the chemical composition of endolymph can appear concurrently with presbycusis.

Auditory Nerve

The loss of ganglion cells in the spiral ganglion is consistently cited as one of the most significant alterations that occurs within the entire auditory system during the presbycusis process. Crowe et al. (1934) and Saxen and von Friendt (1937) were among the first investigators to identify and describe this modification and to point out that its primary location was within the basal portion of the cochlea. Schuknecht (1955) further described the degeneration of ganglion cells of the auditory nerve pathway, initially terming this "neural atrophy." This term was changed to "neural presbycusis" in subsequent writing by Schuknecht (1964).

The loss of neurons throughout the entire central nervous system has been shown to begin early and to continue throughout life (Brody, 1955). It apparently has no significant effect on hearing until much later in life when the neuron loss is massive. Schuknecht and Woellner (1955) found that spiral ganglion losses must approach 75% before any significant changes in threshold occur.

Also of relevance to the degeneration of the auditory nerve structures is the narrowing of the internal auditory meatus in the elderly, attributable to progressive deposition of connective tissue, osteoid, and bone at the base of the internal auditory meatus (Krmpotic-Nemanic, 1971). It is suggested that this may serve to compress fibers of the auditory nerve, leading to atrophy of the affected fibers. In connection with this, Rasmussen (1940) counted the nerve fibers in cross-sections of the auditory nerve and found 2200 fewer fibers in the cochlear division of persons from 44 to 60 years of age than for younger age groups.

The net result of nerve degeneration appears to be a substantial decrease in speech discrimination abilities, with less effect on auditory acuity (Pestalozza and Shore, 1955; Hinchcliffe, 1962). More discussion regarding this form of degeneration is presented later.

Brain Stem and Cortical Structures

The loss of neurons as the result of aging extends into all portions of the central nervous system. As suggested by Schuknecht (1955, 1964), deficits in the number of functional neural units exist in second-, third-, and fourth-order neurons in addition to the atrophy of first-order neurons described earlier.

Specific alterations occurring in the auditory pathways of the central nervous system have been discussed by numerous investigators. Kirkae, Sato, and Shitara (1964) found atrophy of neural structures in the ventral cochlear nuclei, the superior olivary complex, the lateral lemniscus, the inferior collicular and medical geniculate nuclei, and in the auditory cortex itself. Similar types of histologic changes were also observed by Hansen and Reske-Nielsen (1965). Structures within this portion of the auditory system clearly experience severe atrophy, with an accompanying reduction in neural cells within the auditory cortex of the brain.

AUDITORY MANIFESTATIONS OF PRESBYCUSIS

By virtue of the diffuse distribution of the atrophic effects which aging has within the auditory system, a considerable degree of diversity is seen in the alterations which occur in the auditory functioning of the elderly. Some amount of deterioration is usually seen in the most basic auditory functions, such as acuity, and is also generally observed in the complex aspects of auditory perception. The rest of this chapter briefly identifies and discusses the auditory manifestations of presbycusis currently known to occur. Further discussion associated with this material can also be found in subsequent chapters dealing with auditory assessment and disorders.

Incidence of Hearing Loss Associated with the Aged

Attempts have been made in the past to establish the incidence of hearing loss as a function of age. The Metropolitan Life Insurance Company has periodically published data (from the U.S. Health Interview Survey) regarding hearing loss in the general population. Its most recent report (1976, p. 7) states: "From 13 per 1000 at ages under 17, the prevalence rate generally doubled or tripled from one age group to the next, reaching a peak of 399 per 1000 at ages 75 and over." Table 4-1 contains specific information on prevalence of hearing loss as a function of age.

Although the above prevalence figures from the Metropolitan Life Insurance Company accurately reflect the percentage of elderly in the general population with hearing loss, they cannot be used to represent the incidence rates of hearing loss in the elderly residing within residential institutionalized settings. Research by Wunderlich (1965), Bloomer (1960), Alpiner (1963), Chafee (1967), and others has shown that the percentage of institutionalized elderly with hear-

Table 4-1. Prevalence of hearing loss as a function of age

Age period (years)	Rate per 1000 persons
All ages	71.6
Under 17	13.0
17–44	42.4
45–64	114.1
65–74	231.1
75 and over	398.6

Source: Based upon data from the Metropolitan Life Insurance Company (1976).

ing loss is generally higher than that observed in similar age groups in the general population. Estimates of the incidence of hearing loss in nursing home residents have varied considerably, however, ranging from 20 (Wunderlich, 1965) to 97% (Miller and Ort, 1965).

Schow and Nerbonne (1976) pointed out that this variability in the estimates of the incidence of hearing loss in nursing home residents may stem from one or more of three variables: 1) the type of nursing home from which subjects are drawn, 2) the definition of hearing loss, and 3) the methods used to assess hearing. In an investigation involving 163 residents from five different nursing homes, Schow and Nerbonne found that if a strict definition of normal hearing was employed (best pure tone average of 25 dB hearing threshold level (HTL) or better), 80% of the residents were categorized as having a hearing loss. When a different definition was used for normal hearing (best pure tone average of 40 dB HTL), which more accurately reflects the point of communication difficulty for the institutionalized, the percentage of individuals with hearing losses dropped to 54%.

These data on incidence should be interpreted carefully for, as Botwinick (1973) pointed out, some of the diminished sensitivity reported may result from a conservative response strategy. It should also be noted, however, that the attempts thus far to estimate the incidence of hearing loss in the aged have been based primarily on the measurement of auditory acuity for pure tones. Little attention has been placed on other important aspects of hearing, such as speech perception, in determining incidence figures. Because presbycusis manifests itself in many ways other than loss of acuity, the incidence figures given above may not, therefore, be an accurate indicator of the prevalence of hearing loss in the elderly. These estimates, in fact, may underestimate the extent of the problem.

Auditory Acuity

Far more is known about the effects of aging on auditory sensitivity than about any other type of hearing dysfunction observed in older persons. The method of measurement utilized in assessing auditory sensitivity has been the audiogram, where absolute thresholds are obtained for pure tone signals presented at a variety of frequencies. The first investigators to employ this procedure in the evaluation of hearing acuity as a function of age include Zwaardemaker (1894), Bezold (1894), and Bunch (1929, 1931). These investigations were instrumental in establishing the close association which exists between age and auditory acuity.

Later research (Beasley, 1938; Glorig, Wheeler, Quiggle, Grings, and Summerfield, 1957; Corso, 1959; Hinchcliffe, 1959a, b) served to provide further support concerning the influence of age and also provided documentation regarding the effect of sex on the progressive loss of acuity seen in the elderly. The pure tone threshold results obtained in the National Health Survey of 1962 as a function of age and sex are shown in Figure 4-1. These data demonstrate a number of characteristics concerning the diminution of acuity. The initial deterioration in sensitivity occurs relatively early in life, with measurable changes observed in early adulthood. Males experience sensitivity decrements at an earlier age than females, with relatively large differences in thresholds occurring between the sexes by the third decade of life. The hearing loss is more pronounced in the higher frequencies, particularly in men.

Much of the emphasis in early investigations involving age and hearing acuity was on persons 65 years of age or younger, and this resulted in a lack of information specific to the over 65 age group. Information that was available (Sataloff and Menduke, 1965; Hinchcliffe, 1959a, b) tended to suggest little additional decrease in sensitivity beyond 65–70 years. A subsequent investigation by Goetzinger, Proud, Dirks, and Embrey (1961) served to demonstrate further sensitivity decrements of a substantial nature well into the 80s (see Figure 4-2). This progression was also evident in the institutionalized elderly, as shown by the work of Schow and Nerbonne (1976) (see Figure 4-3). As previously indicated, poorer thresholds are found in the nursing home residents as compared to the general

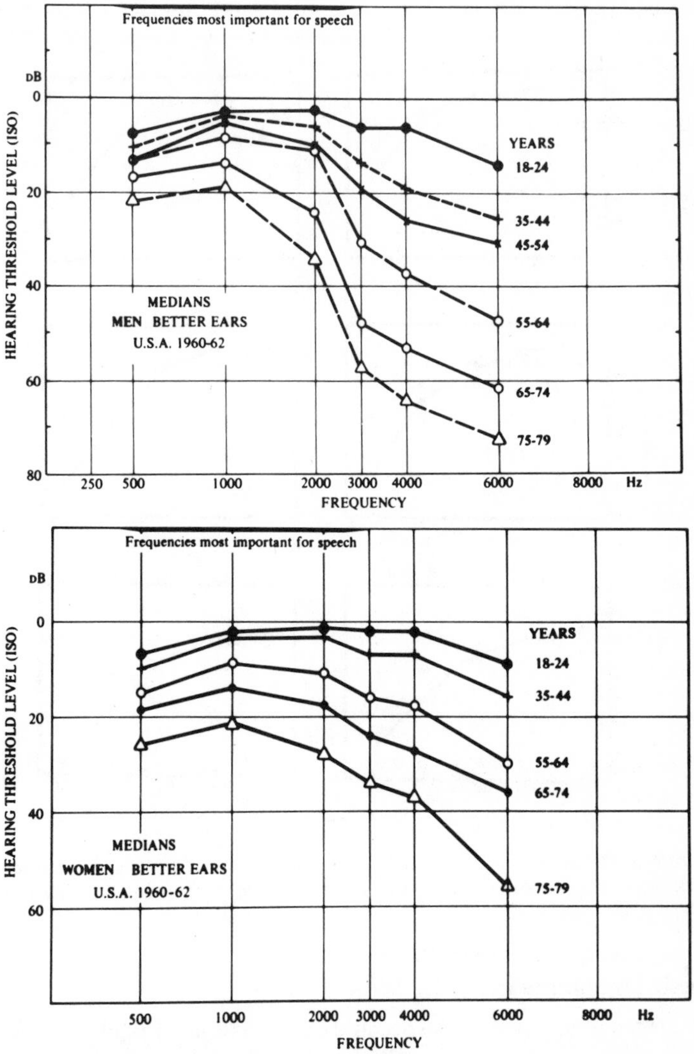

Figure 4-1. Composite audiograms for the better ear in men (A) and women (B), by age groups. The values plotted are the medians or 50-percentile values (re ISO, 1964). (Source: Hearing Levels of Adults by Age and Sex in the United States 1960–1962. Public Health Service, Washington, D.C., Publication 1000, Series 11, No. 11.)

population, and an examination of Figure 4-4 substantiates this fact.

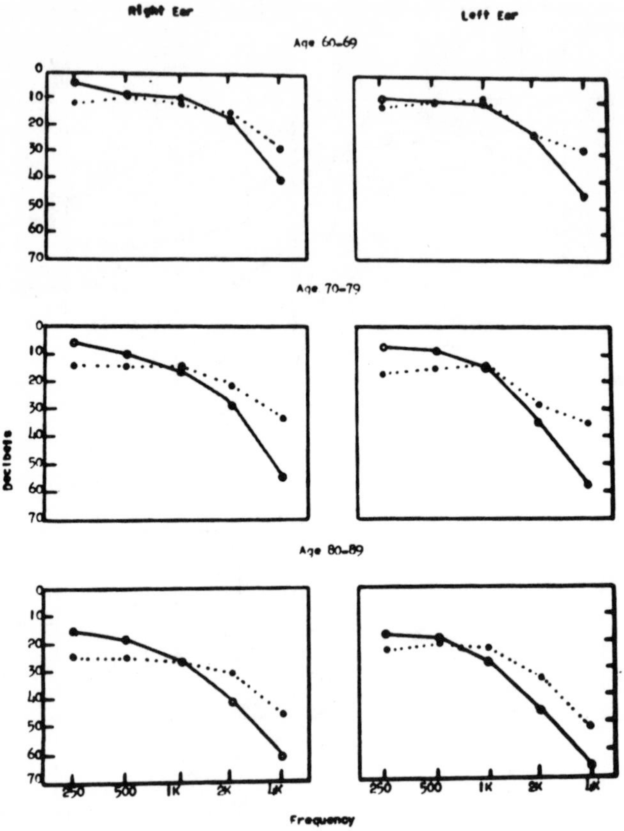

Figure 4-2. Mean air conduction thresholds for right and left ears of subjects (re ASA). Open circles represent men; closed circles, women. (Source: Goetzinger et al., 1961.)

Speech Discrimination

The presence of significant speech discrimination difficulty in people with presbycusis has been well documented in the literature, particularly in the case of neural degeneration (Schuknecht and Igaraski, 1964). As indicated by Gaeth (1948), severe discrimination abilities may be present without any corresponding decrement in auditory acuity. This condition has been described by Gaeth as "phonemic regression." Further substantiation for the presence of speech discrimination abnormalities has been provided by Pestalozza and Shore (1955), Harbert, Young, and Menduke (1966), and

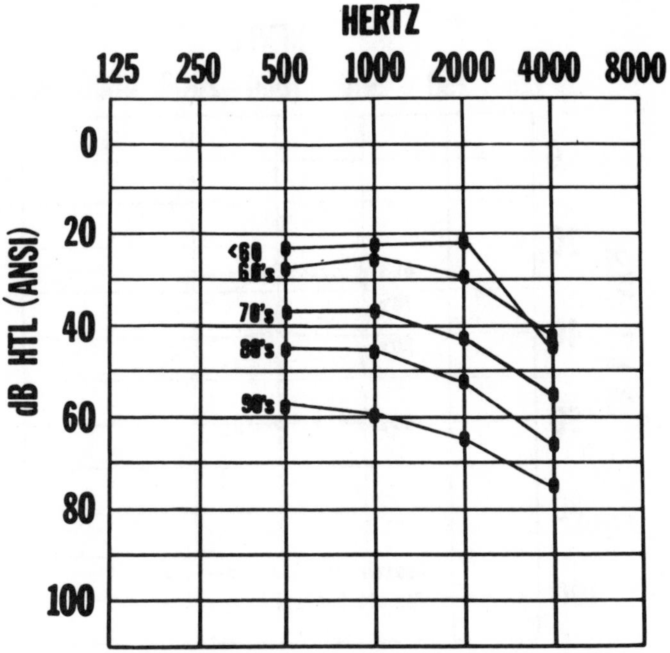

Figure 4-3. Mean air conduction pure tone thresholds for 163 nursing home residents as a function of age. (Source: Schow and Nerbonne, 1976.)

Punch and McConnell (1969). Goetzinger and Rousey (1959) demonstrated the decrement in discrimination observed as a function of age, and their results are shown in Table 4-2. The W-22 and Rush-Hughes discrimination tests were used to assess speech discrimination in their subjects, with the percentage correctly perceived being computed for each 50-word list presented. The change in discrimination ability with age may be more dramatic when the material is more difficult, as shown in the scores on the Rush-Hughes test.

Other Areas of Audition

Numerous other auditory manifestations of presbycusis have been noted in the literature, though some may have not received an adequate amount of attention to allow for a complete description at this time.

Studies by Calearo and Lazzaroni (1957), de Quiras (1964), Sticht and Gray (1969), Schon (1970), and Jerger (1973b) have

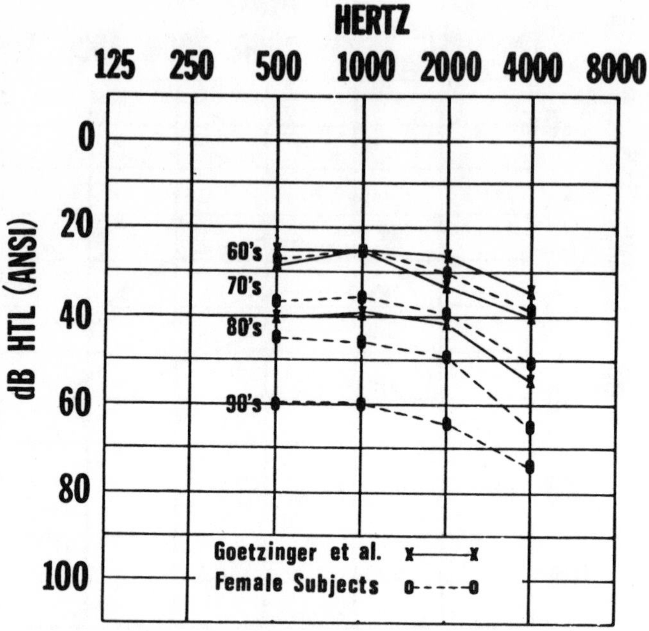

Figure 4-4. Mean pure tone thresholds for female nursing home subjects from Schow and Nerbonne (1976) as compared to data for females from Goetzinger et al. (1961) as a function of age.

demonstrated that the aged encounter difficulty in the discrimination of time-distorted speech. These investigations have found that time-compressed speech will create more errors in elderly listeners when compared with the performance of young listeners with similar hearing acuity. A recent investigation by Konkle, Beasley, and Bess

Table 4-2. Means and standard deviations for the recorded W-22 and Rush-Hughes tests for normal hearing subjects with reference to age

Number of ears	Mean chonologic age (years)	Mean speech reception threshold	W-22		Rush-Hughes	
			Mean	SD	Mean	SD
30	11.5	Normal	94.3	1.8	75.1	5.2
40	27	5.0	97.0	2.1	81.0	4.6
10	46	1.2	97.8	1.7	81.6	4.4
64	66	12.8	88.0	10.2	67.8	12.0
64	74	15.9	81.2	12.7	58.0	14.9
64	84	26.5	78.1	8.5	43.8	14.5

Source: Adapted from Goetzinger and Rousey (1959).

(1977) has provided further description of the effects of the aging process on the perception of temporally altered speech stimuli, with specific reference to the influence which the variables of presentation level and rate of time compression have on the resulting intelligibility of the material with the elderly.

Speech signals which have been altered in other ways also have been shown to result in substantial perceptual difficulties for the elderly. These modifications include a reduction in the frequency and intensity parameters of the material (Berlin, 1972; Jerger, 1973a).

Studies by Warren (1961), Warren and Warren (1966), and Obusek and Warren (1973) have all shown a gradual decline in the number of verbal transformations which occur in older subjects. Warren (1976) has suggested that the reduction may be attributable to a reduced capacity for short-term storage of verbal information.

The aging process also appears to result in somewhat variable alterations in loudness and pitch perception. In an evaluation of the loudness function in presbycusic subjects, Jerger, Shedd, and Harford (1959) and Goetzinger et al. (1961) found that while not all of their elderly listeners demonstrated abnormal loudness discrimination, a large percentage did. Konig (1957), among others, has shown that pitch discrimination abilities also deteriorate in the aged person.

As described by Willeford (1971), the possibility of excessive auditory adaptation exists in older listeners, though the pattern is highly inconsistent.

SUMMARY

It is evident that the presbycusic alterations which occur within the auditory system reveal themselves auditorially in many different ways. It is important, therefore, to emphasize that the precise auditory manifestations of presbycusis will depend largely upon the particular type(s) of presbycusis involved in a given case and that these manifestations will be highly variable in severity. Merely to state that an individual has presbycusis is not sufficient to convey the true nature of the person's auditory disorder.

SUGGESTED READINGS

Naunton, R. Presbycusis. In M. Paparella and D. Shumrick (eds.), Otolaryngology (Volume 2: Ear). Philadelphia: W. B. Saunders, 1973.

Willeford, J. The Geriatric Patient. In D. Rose (ed.), Audiological Assessment. Englewood Cliffs, N.J.: Prentice-Hall, 1971.
Yarington, C., Jr. Presbycusis. In J. Northern (ed.), Hearing Disorders. Boston: Little, Brown, 1976.

REFERENCES

Alpiner, J. Audiological problems of the aged. Geriatrics, 18, 19-26 (1963).

Babbitt, J. The endaural surgery of chronic suppurations. In S. Kapetzky (ed.), Looseleaf Surgery of the Ear. New York: Nelson and Sons, 1947.

Beasley, W. Generalized age and sex trend in hearing loss. Hearing Study Series Bulletin No. 7. National Health Survey. Washington, D.C.: U.S. Public Health Service, 1938.

Berlin, C., and Lowe, S. Temporal and dichotic factors in central auditory testing. In J. Katz (ed.), Handbook of Clinical Audiology. Baltimore: Williams & Wilkins, 1972.

Bezold, F. Investigations concerning the average hearing power of the aged. Archives of Otolaryngology, 23, 214-227 (1894).

Bloomer, H. Communication problems among aged county hospital patients. Geriatrics, 15, 291-295 (1960).

Botwinick, J. Aging and Behavior. New York: Springer, 1973.

Brody, H. Organization of the central cortex: III. Study of aging in human cerebral cortex. Journal of Comparative Neurology, 102, 511-556 (1955).

Bunch, C. Age variations in auditory acuity. Archives of Otolaryngology, 9, 625-636 (1929).

Bunch, C. Further observations on age variations in auditory acuity. Archives of Otolaryngology, 12, 178-180 (1931).

Calearo, C., and Lazzaroni, A. Speech intelligibility in relation to the speed of the message. Laryngoscope, 67, 410-419 (1957).

Chafee, C. Rehabilitation needs of nursing home patients: A report of a survey. Rehabilitation Literature, 28, 377-382 (1967).

Corso, J. Age and sex differences in pure-tone thresholds. Journal of the Acoustical Society of America, 31, 498-507 (1959).

Covell, W. Histological changes in the aging cochlea. Journal of Gerontology, 7, 173-177 (1952).

Crabbe, F. Presbycusis. Acta Otolaryngologica, Supplement 183, 24-26 (1963).

Crowe, S., Guild, S., and Polvogt, L. Observations on the pathology of high tone deafness. Bulletin of Johns Hopkins Hospital, 54, 315-379 (1934).

Davis, H. Abnormal hearing and deafness. In H. Davis and R. Silverman (eds.), Hearing and Deafness. New York: Holt, Rinehart and Winston, 1970.

de Quiras, J. Accelerated speech audiometry, an examination of test results (Trans. by J. Tanndorf). Transactions of the Beltone Institute of Hearing Research, No. 17. Chicago: Beltone Institute of Hearing Research, 1964.

Etholm, B., and Belel, A. Senile changes in the middle ear joints. Annals of Otolaryngology, 23, 49-54 (1974).

Gacek, R. Degenerative hearing loss in aging. In W. Fields (ed.), Neurological and Sensory Disorders in the Elderly. New York: Stratton International Medical Book Corp., 1975.

Gaeth, J. A study of phonemic regression associated with hearing loss. Unpublished doctoral dissertation, Northwestern University, Evanston, Ill. 1948.

Glorig, A., and Nixon, J. Hearing loss as a function of age. Laryngoscope, 72, 1562–1610 (1962).

Glorig, A., Wheeler, D., Quiggle, R., Grings, W., and Summerfield, A. 1954 Wisconsin State Fair Hearing Survey. Monograph, American Academy of Opthalmology and Otolaryngology (1957).

Goetzinger, C., Proud, G., Dirks, D., and Embrey, J. A study of hearing in advanced age. Archives of Otolaryngology, 73, 662-674 (1961).

Goetzinger, C., and Rousey, C. Hearing problems in later life. Medical Times, 87, 771-780 (1959).

Goodhill, V., and Guggenheim, P. Pathology, diagnosis and therapy of deafness. In L. Travis (ed.), Handbook of Speech Pathology and Audiology. New York: Appleton-Century-Crofts, 1971.

Guild, S. The ear. In E. Cowdry (ed.), Problems of Ageing. Baltimore: Williams & Wilkins, 1942.

Hansen, C., and Reske-Nielsen, E. Pathological studies in presbycusis. Archives of Otolaryngology, 82, 115–132 (1965).

Harbert, F., Young, I., and Menduke, H. Audiologic findings in presbycusis. Journal of Auditory Research, 6, 297–312 (1966).

Hinchcliffe, R. The threshold of hearing as a function of age. Acustica, 9, 303-308 (1959a).

Hinchcliffe, R. Correction of pure tone audiograms for advancing ages. Journal of Laryngology, 73, 830–832 (1959b).

Hinchcliffe, R. The anatomical locus of presbycusis. Journal of Speech and Hearing Disorders, 27, 301-310 (1962).

Jerger, J. Diagnostic audiometry. In J. Jerger (ed.), Modern Developments in Audiology (2nd. Ed.). New York: Academic Press, 1973a.

Jerger, J. Audiological findings in aging. Advances in Oto-Rhino-Laryngology, 20, 115-124 (1973b).

Jerger, J., Shedd, J., and Harford, E. On the detection of extremely small changes in sound intensity. Archives of Otolaryngology, 69, 200–211 (1959).

Jorgensen, M. Changes of aging in the inner ear. Archives of Otolaryngology, 74, 56-62 (1961).

Kirikae, I. Sato, R., and Shitara, T. A study of hearing in advanced age. Laryngoscope, 74, 205–220 (1964).

Klotz, P. La surdite du troisieme age. Readoption, 102, 27–31 (1963).

Konig, E. Pitch discrimination and age. Acta Otolaryngologica, 48, 475–489 (1957).

Konkle, D., Beasley, D., and Bess, F. Intelligibility of time-altered speech in relation to chronological aging. Journal of Speech and Hearing Research, 20, 108-115 (1977).

Krmpotic-Nemanic, J. A new concept of the pathogenesis of presbycusis. Archives of Otolaryngology, 93, 161–166 (1971).

Magladery, J. Neurophysiology of aging. In J. Birren (ed.), Handbook of Aging and the Individual: Psychological and Biological Aspects. Chicago: University of Chicago Press (1959).

Mayer, O. Das anatomische Substrat der Alterschwerhorigkeit. Arch. Ohr. Nas. Kehlkopfheilk, 105, 1-13 (1919-1920).

Metropolitan Life Insurance Company. Hearing impairments in the United States. Metropolitan Life Insurance Statistics, 57, 7-9 (1976).

Miller, M., and Ort, R. Hearing problems in a home for the aged. Acta Otolaryngologica, 59, 33-44 (1965).

Nerbonne, M., Schow, R., Goset, F., and Bliss, A. Prevalence of conductive pathology in a nursing home population. Unpublished study, Idaho State University, Pocatello, 1976.

Obusek, C., and Warren, R. A comparison of speech perception in senile and well preserved aged by means of the verbal transformation effect. Journal of Gerontology, 28, 184–188 (1973).

Pestalozza, G., and Shore, I. Clinical evaluation of presbycusis on the basis of different tests of auditory function. Laryngoscope, 65, 1136-1163 (1955).

Punch, J., and McConnell, F. The speech discrimination function of elderly adults. Journal of Auditory Research, 9, 159-166 (1969).

Rasmussen, A. Studies of the VIIIth cranial nerve of man. Laryngoscope, 50, 67-83 (1940).

Rosen, S., Bergman, M., Plester, D., El-Mofty, A., and Satti, M. Presbycusis study of a relatively noise-free population in the Sudan. Annals of Otology, Rhinology and Laryngology, 71, 727–743 (1962).

Rosen, S., Plester, D., El-Mofty, A., and Rosen, H. High frequency audiometry in presbycusis. A comparative study of the Mabaan tribe in the Sudan with urban populations. Archives of Otolaryngology, 79, 18-32 (1964).

Rosenwasser, H. Otitic problems in the aged. Geriatrics, 19, 11-17 (1964).

Sataloff, J., and Menduke, H. Presbycusis: Air and bone conduction thresholds. Laryngoscope, 75, 889-901 (1965).

Saxen, A., and von Fiendt, H. Pathologic und klinik der Altersschwerhorigkeit. Acta Otolaryngologica, Supplement 23, 1–85 (1937).

Schon, T. The effects of speech intelligibility of time-compression and expansion on normal hearing, hard of hearing, and aged males. Journal of Auditory Research, 10, 263-268 (1970).

Schow, R., and Nerbonne, M. Hearing levels in nursing home residents. Research Laboratory Reports 1, pp. 1-10. Department of Speech and Audiology, Idaho State University, Pocatello, 1976.

Schuknecht, H. Presbycusis. Laryngoscope, 65, 402-419 (1955).

Schuknecht, H. Further observations on the pathology of presbycusis. Archives of Otolaryngology, 80, 369-382 (1964).

Schuknecht, H. The effect of aging on the cochlea. In B. Graham (ed.), Sensorineural Hearing Processes and Disorders. Boston: Little, Brown, 1967.

Schuknecht, H., and Igaraski, M. Pathology of slowly progressive sensorineural deafness. Transactions of the American Academy of Ophthalmology and Otolaryngology, 68, 222-242 (1964).

Schuknecsht, H., and Woellner, R. Experimental and clinical study of deafness from lesions of the cochlear nerve. Journal of Laryngology, 69, 75-97 (1955).

Senturia, B. Diseases of the External Ear. Springfield, Ill.: Charles C Thomas, 1957.

Sticht, T., and Gray, B. The intelligibility of time-compressed words as a function of age and hearing loss. Journal of Speech and Hearing Research, 12, 443–448 (1969).

Thompson, D., Sills, J., and Bui, D. Acoustic reflex growth in aging ears. Paper presented at the Annual Convention of the American Speech and Hearing Association, Houston, 1976.

Tsai, H., Chou, F., and Cheng, T. On changes in ear size with age, as found among Taiwanese-Formosans of Kukienese extraction. Journal of the Formosan Medical Association, 57, 105–111 (1958).

Warren, R. Illusory changes of distinct speech upon repetition—the verbal transformation effect. British Journal of Psychology, 52, 249–258 (1961).

Warren, R. Auditory illusions and perceptual processes. In N. Lass (ed.), Contemporary Issues in Experimental Phonetics. New York: Academic Press, 1976.

Warren, R., and Warren, R. A comparison of speech perception in childhood, maturity, and old age by means of the verbal transformation effect. Journal of Verbal Learning and Verbal Behavior, 5, 142–146 (1966).

Willeford, J. The geriatric patient. In D. Rose (ed.), Audiological Assessment. Englewood Cliffs, N.J.: Prentice-Hall, 1971.

Wunderlich, G. Characteristics of residents in institutions for the aged and chronically ill. National Health Survey, Series 12:2, Washington, D.C.: Department of Health, Education, and Welfare, 1965.

Zemlin, W. Speech and Hearing Science. Englewood Cliffs, N. J.: Prentice-Hall, 1968.

Zwaardemaker, H. The range of hearing at various ages. Journal of Psychology, 7, 10–28 (1894).

Chapter 5
Speech and Language Changes Among the Aging

This chapter explores the literature regarding normal changes in speech and language function of advancing age. Specifically, attention is directed to disturbances in message generation, symbolic function, motor programming, and peripheral execution of the speech process. The last topic is discussed with reference to known structural and physiologic alterations in the peripheral speech mechanisms of gerontologic subjects.

It is quite reasonable to assume that the physiologic and structural changes associated with senescence will influence the speech and language characteristics of the elderly. Indeed, perceptual experiments have documented that listeners can rather easily discern recorded samples of older talkers from those of younger subjects. This chapter examines some of the experiments relating to speech and language processing of older subjects who do not have any history of neurologic disease or any disorders in the speech production system.

As mentioned in Chapter 2, it is both conventional and convenient to characterize language according to three components: 1) syntax (structure), 2) semantics (meaning), and 3) phonology (nature of sound system). Furthermore, the utterance of any message involves some form of central generation of an idea through cortical activity. Once the generative process has been undertaken, the idea must undergo a transformation such that it is cast into the symbolic code of the speaker's native language. Again, this processing appears to be largely a function of cortical operations in the dominant (usually left) hemisphere. Luria (1966) described the next level of language encoding as the "kinetic organization of the motor act" (p. 196). That is, the symbolic representation is further transformed into a motor program for proper execution by the peripheral speech mechanism. This function has been relegated to Broca's area of the brain, which is the base of the third frontal convolution of the dominant hemisphere. The final stage in the encoding process is the execution of the central motor program by the peripheral speech mechanism.

It is within this general framework that typical disturbances in the encoding process associated with normal aging are discussed. It must be recognized that experimental evidence regarding language functioning among the elderly is scarce, though more information exists concerning the actual speech production process.

TYPICAL DISTURBANCES

Message Generation

Most of the experimental evidence regarding central language formulation among the elderly has focused on vocabulary performance. After a rather lengthy review of studies involving standardized vocabulary tests, Jones (1959) suggested that the normal aged maintain relatively high levels of performance on tasks which reflect accumulated experience, particularly vocabulary. For example, Shakow and Goldman (1938) investigated 348 subjects between the ages 18 and 89 years. The subjects were divided into three groups according to educational achievement. It was determined that there was no effect of age on vocabulary score until the sixth decade, with a small subsequent decline until age 90. Fox (1947) evaluated the vocabulary abilities of individuals within the 70–79 year age range. The results of this investigation indicated that the average vocabularly size was essentially the same for the two groups. In addition, Lewinsky (1948) investigated the relationship between vocabulary, advancing age, education, and intelligence in 1000 males between the ages of 17 and 62 years. It was determined through this investigation that vocabulary use was a relatively stable function in adulthood with no well defined changes in vocabulary scores as a function of advancing age.

Using a somewhat different experimental strategy, Elias and Kinsbourne (1974) instructed elderly subjects between the ages of 63 and 77 years and young subjects between the ages of 23 and 33 years to match two successive visual stimuli on the basis of "sameness." In one condition, the messages were nonverbal (arrows) and in the other condition the messages were verbal (letters). The results indicated that the mean of the reaction time for verbal skills was significantly shorter than for nonverbal skills in the elderly.

It should be noted that other vocabulary-related aspects of verbal achievements among the elderly reveal inferior performances as compared to those of younger subjects. For example, Birren, Riegel, and Robbin (1962) instructed 30 young subjects (18–33 years) and 21 elderly subjects (60–80 years) to give continuous word associations as rapidly as possible. The results demonstrated that the elderly subjects exhibited poorer performance on the continuous word associations. The findings did not indicate that speech rate was a factor. Rather, central processing problems were implicated.

Malepeai and Hutchinson (1977) evaluated the speed of picture naming among the elderly through an examination of visual processing performance. The variables of naming latency, visual detection threshold, visual processing time, and word retrieval time were investigated for 30 elderly (70–79 years) and 30 young (20–29 years) adults. Durations recorded for the elderly were increased with respect to all variables. However, the elderly subjects were not observed to be disproportionally slower on any component of naming latency (visual detection threshold, visual processing time, or word retrieval).

The impact of these findings on the spontaneous oral language performance of the elderly is unknown. If word association and word retrieval times are slower, one possible effect would be an overall slowing in speech rate as well as the appearance of more dysfluency, particularly meditative hesitations and interjections, revisions, and repetitions. Some initial support for these speculations was provided by Mysak and Hanley (1958), who discovered an overall reduction in speaking rate for elderly subjects. In addition, Yairi and Clifton (1972) reported a significantly greater number of dysfluencies in the speech of elderly subjects (69–87 years) when compared with high-school seniors. In particular, interjections, word repetitions, and dysrhythmic phonations were more frequent in the older subjects.

Symbolic Function

One of the few investigations of symbolic functioning among the elderly was provided by Gordon, Hutchinson, and Allen (1976). They evaluated discourse samples from ten young adult (mean age, 23 years) and ten elderly adult (mean age, 80 years) subjects for frequency of "uncertainty behaviors" (revisions, hesitant interjections and fillers, unfinished utterances not revised, and number of prompts by the examiner), frequency and location of pauses, and various utterance length characteristics. The results showed that gerontologic subjects differed from young adults only with regard to uncertainty behavior. Specifically, older subjects exhibited significantly more hesitant interjections and fillers. The two subject groups did not differ in terms of pause location or utterance length characteristics. These results were interpreted as evidence that semantic-syntactic complexity and the organization of verbal behavior are well preserved with advancing age. The increased number of hesitant interjections and fillers observed for the gerontologic group was thought to reflect word retrieval problems.

Motor Programming

As pointed out by Hutchinson and Beasley (1976), it would appear that no experimental effort has been undertaken with respect to problems of motor programming for speech among the elderly. Such problems, collectively termed apraxia, are apparently spared by typical central nervous system deteriorations associated with aging. It is possible that some of the hesitation, interjection, and repetition behavior observed in discourse samples of older subjects is indicative of the search for appropriate motor programming. However, such a speculation must await further research for confirmation.

Peripheral Execution of Speech

Experimental Evidence A great deal more experimental evidence has been generated with respect to speech production in gerontologic subjects. It should be noted that most of the investigations have focused on the acoustic and perceptual correlates of speech with relatively less attention to peripheral physiologic alterations. The initial portion of this review examines the experimental evidence and the second portion offers some anatomic and physiologic data concerning speech mechanism changes known to occur in aging.

One of the earliest studies of aging was completed by Mysak (1959), who required male subjects ranging in age to read a short prose passage. Measures of phonation/time ratio (percentage of total utterance involved in voicing), words/minute, fundamental frequency, and range of fundamental frequency were obtained. The results demonstrated a progressive increase in average fundamental frequency from about age 50 to 85. There was a trend toward greater pitch variability as a function of advancing age. Mysak also reported reduced speaking rate and reduced phonation/time ratios among the elderly. (MS)

Using a similar experimental strategy, McGlone and Hollien (1963) obtained oral reading samples from elderly women. In contrast to the findings of Mysak (1959), McGlone and Hollien reported no significant effects of age on fundamental frequencies of women. Furthermore, there was a slight decrease in pitch variability for elderly women when compared with younger subjects. Similar findings were reported by Charlip (1968). McGlone and Hollien argued that the differences in fundamental frequency observed for men by Mysak may relate to the relatively more profound anatomic changes in the laryngeal structures of men during puberty.

In an effort to evaluate changes in fundamental frequency across a broad range of adult ages, Hollien and Shipp (1972) sampled the speech of 25 subjects in the seven decade spans from age 20 to 89. They noted that fundamental frequency decreased slightly from age 20 to 50 and, in accordance with Mysak's observation, increased progressively from 50 to 89. From the results of several studies, Hollien (1977) has noted no evidence of a change in phonational frequency range of adult subjects as a function of age. This latter finding disagrees with that of Ptacek, Sander, Maloney, and Jackson (1966), who did find decrements in range of fundamental frequency among gerontologic subjects.

Beyond the issue of fundamental frequency and range of fundamental frequency, there has been little effort to ascertain the effects of aging on other acoustic aspects of speech. Ryan (1972) completed a rather extensive evaluation of 20 subjects in each of four decade spans from 40 to 70. These subjects, who had normal hearing, evidenced an increase in vocal intensity with advancing age, but statistical significance for the vocal intensity data was not obtained until the 70-year-old group was compared with the younger subject samples. In accordance with findings of Mysak reviewed earlier, Ryan documented a reduction in speaking rate for old subjects.

A final acoustic evaluation of the speech of gerontologic subjects was reported by Hutchinson, Robinson, and Nerbonne (in press). They examined velopharyngeal function by recording ratios of nasal sound pressure to total (nasal plus oral) sound pressure. The results clearly established that aging was associated with elevated nasal/total scores which was interpreted as evidence of a mild velopharyngeal incompetence.

Speculations on Anatomic and Physiologic Substrates Given these experimental findings, the question arises as to what anatomic and physiologic changes occur in the peripheral speech mechanism that might cause such age effects in speech production. To date, few experimental data are available to provide a direct assessment of the impact of structural changes on the speech production of the elderly. Consequently, much of the present review is speculative in nature. The present writers are indebted to Meyerson (1976) for his careful treatment of this subject.

Respiration It is well understood that the respiratory system provides the driving air source for speech production and there are some known changes in respiratory function with advancing age. Several investigators have reported decrements in various spirometric functions among the elderly (Berglund, Birath, Bjure, Grimby, Kjellmer, Sandquist, and Soderholm, 1963; Ericsson and Irnell, 1969; Weg, 1973). One of the best evaluations of spirometric function was provided by Morris, Koski, and Johnson (1971), who studied 988 healthy nonsmoking men and women who had insignificant exposure to any form of air pollution. They observed a progressive decline in ventilatory function with age characterized by reductions in forced vital capacity, forced expiratory flow, forced midexpiratory flow, and forced expiratory volume. Several explanations may be offered to account for these respiratory effects, including air flow caused by airway narrowing or airway collaspe (Morris et al., 1971), tissue atrophy, rib cage stiffening, and reduced respiratory muscle force (Agostini and Margania, 1962).

In addition to these normal aging phenomena, elderly people are much more susceptible to respiratory disease, particularly if they have been life-long smokers or worked in environments with significant air pollution. For example, the general incidence of chronic obstructive pulmonary disease (emphysema, chronic bronchitis, asthma, etc.) increases dramatically in the fifth decade of life (Addington and Agarwal, 1974).

As mentioned earlier, the influence these respiratory changes will have on the aging voice is unknown. Ptacek et al. (1966) argued that their observed reductions in intraoral air pressure and maximum vowel durations for older subjects could be attributed in part to the concomitant reduction in vital capacity. This is undoubtedly true, but three clarifying comments are warranted. First, maximum values for intraoral air pressure and vowel duration greatly exceed the requirements for speech production. Consequently, these reduced performances among the elderly observed by Ptacek et al. may have no significant effect on the speech of older subjects. Second, in the case of maximum vowel duration, it must be recognized that the laryngeal system serves as a valving device for respiratory flow. If this valving is inefficient among the elderly, there will be laryngeal air wastage and a commensurate reduction in sustained vowel duration. Finally, speech is generally accomplished within midrange lung volumes (35–60% of the vital capacity) according to Hixon (1973). Therefore, the aging person can sustain a fair reduction in vital capacity before speech will be observed to suffer. Perhaps the best concluding statement, given the contemporary evidence, was provided by Meyerson (1976):

> In summary, those tissue changes that appear to occur in the normal aging process of the respiratory mechanism have no serious demonstrable effects on voice or any other aspect of communication. (p. 30)

Phonation In considering laryngeal function, the rather well documented changes in voice characteristics for aging males may be attributed to several factors. Mysak (1959) and Hollien and Shipp (1972) argued that atrophy of the vocal fold muscles resulting in reduced vibrating mass was the probable cause for elevated fundamental frequencies among gerontologic males. Indeed, some histologic support for atrophic muscular changes within aging larynges was provided by Bach, Lederer, and Dinolt (1941). Zemlin (1968) has also noted that the aging laryngeal cartilages undergo notable ossification and calcification. The factor accompanied by the stiffening of laryngeal cartilage joints (resulting from a loss of elasticity in the ligaments and possible arthritic changes) and reduction of adductor-tensor muscle strength (Luchsinger and Arnold, 1965) probably accounts for any potential deteriorations in pitch range and voicing control. With respect to voicing control, it must be recognized that much more research is necessary to determine potential age-related changes in voice onset time, voice adjustment time, etc. It is quite conceivable that deteriorations in these aspects of vocal control will be observed among the elderly partially as a result of reductions in sensory receptors responsible for providing afferent data for laryngeal motor control. In this context, Mallard (1974) reported that topical anesthesia of the vocal folds will result in slight deteriorations in voice adjustment time.

Two other conditions associated with senescence may result in voice problems for the elderly. First, for several reasons (allergic conditions, chronic bronchitis, etc.), the tissues in the larynx and trachea oversecrete mucus, which may form on the vocal folds and affect vibration (Luchsinger and Arnold, 1965). Second, endocrine changes associated with advancing age may have some influence on voice production, but the dynamics are not well established (Luchsinger and Arnold, 1965).

Articulation Very little research has been completed concerning structural changes in the articulatory system as a function of advancing age. There is some evidence that speed and accuracy of oral gesturing does deteriorate among older subjects. In addition to the reduced rate of speech and mild loss of velar control discussed earlier, Ptacek et al. (1966) reported reduced diadochokinetic rates for lip and tongue movements among subjects over age 65. Frequently, these changes in articulatory function have been attributed to deteriorations in peripheral neuromuscular control (Mysak and Hanley, 1958; Mysak, 1959; Ryan, 1972; Hutchinson et al., in press), reduced sensory feedback (Mysak, 1959; Ryan and Burk, 1974; Hutchinson et al., in press), and central processing deficits (Mysak and Hanley, 1958; Ryan and Burk, 1974; Hutchinson et al., in press).

It should be noted that at least one paper has suggested essentially normal neuromuscular speech control among gerontologic subjects. Blonsky, Logemann, Boshes, and Fisher (1975) evaluated cineradiographic films of swallowing and acoustic records of vocal function for 100 patients with Parkinson's disease, 10 patients with benign essential tremor, and 10 normal gerontologic subjects. Their conclusion was that the gerontologic subjects "maintained normal neuromuscular control for speech" (p. 302). In addition, they observed no motility disorders and only slightly elevated transit times for swallowing among the normal older subjects. These conclusions are perhaps a bit strong considering the data reported. Certainly, in comparison to patients with diagnosed neurologic problems, the normal subjects would be judged much superior. However, proper experimental control would have included normal young adults as well. Furthermore, in view of the limited sample size and minimal research effort concerning speech production and aging, it is somewhat premature to conclude that older subjects exhibit "normal neuromuscular control for speech."

PERCEPTUAL STUDIES OF SPEECH PRODUCTION AMONG THE AGING

As mentioned earlier in this chapter, it is rather easy even for naive listeners to discern utterances made by elderly subjects from those made by younger speakers. This observation has prompted several published experiments which warrant review because of the insights offered concerning the normal aging process.

The first studies were designed to document the accuracy of listeners in identifying older speakers. One of these initial investigations was completed by Ptacek and Sander (1966), who asked 10 listeners to discriminate "old" speakers (greater than age 65) from "young" speakers (less than age 35). After judging recordings of sustained vowels and readings of a prose passage, the listeners exhibited 99% accuracy in identifying the ages when forward playing of the samples was used. The listeners also offered some cues considered important in making accurate judgments: rate of speech, pitch, voice quality, loudness, and fluency.

A second experiment reported by Shipp and Hollien (1969) involved an elaboration of the binary decision (young versus old) required of listeners in the Ptacek and Sander paper. In this second study, recordings were obtained from 175 adult males ranging in age from 20 to 90 years. The recordings were then presented to three groups of listeners, each of whom was aked to perform a different experimental task. In the first, the listeners rendered a judgment of "young," "old," or "neither young nor old." Listeners in the second group were required to place the subject whose sample they evaluated into the proper decade of life (30s, 40s, etc). The last set of listeners assigned an actual age to the recorded subject. For all tasks, the listeners exhibited considerable accuracy, and the correlation between actual age and perceived age as judged by the third group was +0.88.

In view of the consistent reliability in age judgments reported in several experiments, Ryan and Burk (1974) reasoned that a hierarchy of acoustic cues must exist in the samples of older speakers that permits such accurate age estimates. Accordingly, they embarked upon a two-stage experiment designed to test this hypothesis. In the first stage, recordings of 40 elderly subjects, who were reliably and accurately judged with respect to perceived age, were presented to 18 trained speech pathologists. These professionals were asked to judge the presence or absence of ten speech and voice disorder characteristics. In addition, Ryan and Burk calculated mean intensity level, mean fundamental frequency, standard deviation of fundamental frequency, and words per minute for each subject. In the second stage of the experiment, the perceptual and acoustic data were combined to form predictor variables in a multiple regression analysis wherein chronologic age served as the criterion. The results revealed six predictor variables which accounted for most of the variance (.92): 1) laryngeal air loss, 2) laryngeal tension, 3) voice tremor, 4) mean fundamental frequency, 5) slow articulation rate, and 6) imprecise consonants. It may be observed that the first four variables were indicative of problems in laryngeal function, and this point was amplified considerably by Ryan and Burk. Such a finding lends credence to the need for further study of laryngeal adjustment and laryngeal control suggested earlier in this chapter.

A FINAL COMMENT

It is clear from the foregoing review that the contribution of speech pathology, linguistics, and speech science to gerontology is at best embryonic. It is imperative that a much more expansive research effort be undertaken to assess the impact of aging on language and speech functioning. Very much related to this issue is the potential role of speech and language pathologists in treating normal elderly subjects. This latter issue has sparked controversy in the communicative disorders profession—a controversy reviewed in some detail in Chapter 20.

SUGGESTED READINGS

Hutchinson, J. M., and Beasley, D. S. Speech and language functioning among the aging. In H. J. Oyer and E. J. Oyer (eds.), Aging and Communication. Baltimore: University Park Press, 1976.

Meyerson, M. The effect of aging on communication. Journal of Gerontology, 31, 29–38 (1976).

REFERENCES

Addington, W. W., and Agarwal, M. K. Managing reversible complications of chronic obstructive pulmonary disease in ambulatory patients. Geriatrics, 29, 76–83 (1974).

Agostini, E., and Margaria, R. Aspects and problems of respiratory physiology in the aged. In H. T. Blumenthal (ed.), Medical and Clinical Aspects of Aging. New York: Columbia University Press, 1962.

Bach, A. C., Lederer, F. L., and Dinolt, R. Senile changes in the laryngeal musculature. Archives of Otolaryngology, 34, 47–56 (1941).

Berglund, E., Birath, G., Bjure, J., Grimby, G., Kjellmer, I., Sandquist, L., and Soderholm, B. Spirometric studies in normal subjects: 1. Forced expirograms in subjects between 7 and 70 years of age. Acta Medica Scandinavica, 173, 185 (1963).

Birren, J., Riegel, K., and Robbin, J. Age differences in continuous word associations measured by speech recordings. Journal of Gerontology, 17, 95–96 (1962).

Blonsky, E. R., Logemann, J. A., Boshes, B., and Fisher, H. B. Comparison of speech and swallowing function in patients with tremor disorders and in normal geriatric patients: A cinefluorographic study. Journal of Gerontology, 30, 299–303 (1975).

Charlip, W. S. The aging female voice: Selected fundamental frequency characteristics and listener judgments. Unpublished doctoral dissertation, Purdue University, Lafayette, Ind. 1968.

Elias, M., and Kinsbourne, M. Age and sex differences in processing verbal and nonverbal stimuli. Journal of Gerontology, 29, 162–171 (1974).

Ericsson, P., and Irnell, L. Spirometric studies of ventilatory capacity in elderly people. Acta Medica Scandinavica, 185, 179 (1969).

Fox, C. Vocabulary ability in later maturity. Journal of Educational Psychology, 38, 484–492 (1947).

Gordon, K., Hutchinson, J. M., and Allen, C. S. An evaluation of selected discourse characteristics among the elderly. Research Laboratory Report Department of Speech Pathology and Audiology, Idaho State University, Pocatello, 1976.

Hixon, T. J. Respiratory function in speech. In F. D. Minifie, T. J. Hixon, and F. Williams (eds.), Normal Aspects of Speech, Hearing and Language. Englewood Cliffs, N.J.: Prentice-Hall, 1973.

Hollien, H. The registers and ranges of the voice. In M. Cooper and M. H. Cooper (eds.), Approaches to Vocal Rehabilitation. Springfield, Ill.: Charles C Thomas, 1977.

Hollien, H., and Shipp, T. Speaking fundamental frequency and chronologic age in males. Journal of Speech and Hearing Research, 15, 155–159 (1972).

Hutchinson, J. M., and Beasley, D. S. Speech and language functioning among the aging. In H. J. Oyer and E. J. Oyer (eds.), Aging and Communication. Baltimore: University Park Press, 1976.

Hutchinson, J. M., Robinson, K. L., and Nerbonne, M. A. Patterns of nasalance in normal gerontologic subjects. Journal of Communication Disorders, 11, in press.

Jones, H. E. Intelligence and problem-solving. In J. E. Birren (ed.), Handbook of Aging and the Individual. Chicago: University of Chicago Press, 1959.

Lewinsky, R. Vocabulary and mental measurement: A quantitative investigation and review of research. Journal of Genetic Psychology, 72, 247–281 (1948).

Luchsinger, R., and Arnold, G. T. Voice-Speech-Language. Belmont, Cal.: Wadsworth, 1965.

Luria, A. R. Higher Cortical Functions in Man. New York: Basic Books, 1966.

Malepeai, B. B., and Hutchinson, J. M. Word retrieval and visual processing skills among the elderly. Paper presented at the Annual Convention of the American Speech and Hearing Association, Chicago, 1977.

Mallard, A. R. Sensory control of phonation. Unpublished doctoral dissertation, Purdue University, Lafayette, Ind. 1974.

McGlone, R. E., and Hollien, H. Vocal pitch characteristics of aged women. Journal of Speech and Hearing Research, 6, 164–170 (1963).

Meyerson, M. The effects of aging on communication. Journal of Gerontology, 31, 29–38 (1976).

Morris, J. F., Koski, A., and Johnson, L. C. Spirometric standards for healthy, nonsmoking adults. Respiratory Disease, 103, 57–67 (1971).

Mysak, E. D. Pitch and duration characteristics of older males. Journal of Speech and Hearing Research, 2, 46–54 (1959).

Mysak, E. D., and Hanley, T. D. Aging process in speech: Pitch and duration characteristics. Journal of Gerontology, 13, 309–313 (1958).

Ptacek, P. H., and Sander, E. K. Age recognition from voice. Journal of Speech and Hearing Research, 9, 273–277 (1966).

Ptacek, P. H., Sander, E. K., Maloney, W. H., and Jackson, C. Phonatory and related changes with advanced age. Journal of Speech and Hearing Research, 9, 353–360 (1966).

Ryan, W. J. Acoustic aspects of the aging voice. Journal of Gerontology, 27, 265–268 (1972).

Ryan, W. J., and Burk, K. W. Perceptual and acoustic correlates of aging in the speech of males. Journal of Communication Disorders, 7, 181–192 (1974).

Shakow, D., and Goldman, R. The effects of age on the Stanford-Binet vocabulary scores of adults. Journal of Educational Psychology, 2, 241–256 (1938).

Shipp, T., and Hollien, H. Perception of the aging male voice. Journal of Speech and Hearing Research, 12, 703–710 (1969).

Weg, R. B. Changing physiology of aging. In R. H. David (ed.), Aging: Prospects and Issues. Los Angeles: University of Southern California, 1973.

Yairi, E., and Clifton, N. F. Disfluent speech behavior of preschool children, high school seniors, and geriatric persons. Journal of Speech and Hearing Research, 15, 714–719 (1972).

Zemlin, W. R. Speech and Hearing Science. Englewood Cliffs, N.J.: Prentice-Hall, 1968.

Section II
DISORDERS OF HEARING

Chapter 6
Assessment of Hearing Disorders

Traditional assessment procedures are described here as used in evaluation of the hearing-impaired patient. Nonaudiometric assessment tools, namely, the case history interview and self-evaluation of handicap, are discussed. The audiometric procedures of pure tone, speech, impedance, and site of lesion testing are also described. All these methods are reviewed in terms of their use with the elderly patient.

When hearing loss is suspected in an elderly person, or any other person for that matter, it is advisable to seek the services of a physician and an audiologist. The physician is able to perform a physical examination of the ear canal and eardrum and, to some extent, observe the status of the middle ear through the translucent eardrum. However, in order to diagnose and properly treat hearing loss, the medical doctor needs much information besides that obtained from a simple physical examination. The results of basic audiologic assessment are invaluable in diagnosis. Some physicians use tuning forks and informal conversation to make a gross assessment, but turn to complete audiometry when a diagnosis is to be made. This chapter first describes methods and tests used by audiologists in assessing hearing disorders, and then focuses on how these methods apply to the elderly.

NONAUDIOMETRIC ASSESSMENT

Case History

The preliminary step in audiologic assessment is an interview with the patient to gather relevant information. In some medical settings this may not be done by the audiologist directly, but the information should be available and reviewed in connection with audiologic assessment regardless of who may interview the patient.

The following information should be obtained through the case history interview:

1. Reason for having a hearing assessment
2. Symptoms or complaints associated with hearing
3. Previous medical, rehabilitative, and family history related to hearing

Some subjects know why they are being tested; others do not. However, knowing the reason for referral can guide the audiologist in obtaining relevant information during his evaluation. The patient who reports symptoms or complaints associated with hearing loss needs to be asked if tinnitus (buzzing or ringing head noises), dizziness, or vertigo is present, and if a hearing loss is experienced. The patient who is aware of a loss should report whether it developed suddenly or gradually and whether or not it fluctuates. It is important to learn how much communication difficulty the loss causes and in what listening situations the difficulty routinely occurs. The history of previous ear infections, surgery, treatment, hearing aid use, or a family history of hearing loss will provide valuable information. Of course, other additional details of relevance may be learned during the course of this interview.

Self-Evaluation of Hearing Handicap

Another useful type of information which can be obtained prior to audiometric testing is a formal quantification of the handicap or difficulty imposed by the hearing impairment. A variety of handicap scales have been devised for this purpose (Ewertsen and Nielsen, 1973; Alpiner, Chevrette, Glascoe, Metz, and Olsen, 1974; Sanders, 1975). However, the most popular one is the Hearing Handicap Scale (HHS), which was developed by High, Fairbanks, and Glorig (1964) (see Appendix A). With this scale the patient is given a form which contains 20 items probing the extent of handicap as it occurs in various life situations. The patient may respond on each item by choosing a scaled response from 1 to 5. The higher numbers indicate greater difficulty and a percent score is computed based on all 20 items. In a study of handicap associated with various losses, Schow and Tannahill (1977) found that persons without hearing loss tended to score 0–20% on the HHS. Scores from 21 to 40 percent were classified as borderline handicap, while scores in excess of 40 percent indicated substantial handicap typical of patients who are hearing aid users (see Table 6-1).

Table 6-1. Categories and associated percentage scores for use in classifying hearing handicap performance on the HHS

Category	Scores (%)
No handicap	0-20
Mild hearing handicap	21-40
Moderate hearing handicap	41-70
Severe hearing handicap	71-100

The value of this type of scale is that with it one can quantify the way the client feels about his hearing difficulty and compare this score with scores of others who are hearing impaired. These scales also provide some measure of how the loss is affecting the person in view of his particular lifestyle and hearing demands. Guidance is often thus provided in decisions about rehabilitation.

It can be valuable to have other interested parties, such as a spouse, a son, or a daughter, fill out such a form based on their perception of the patient's difficulties. Sometimes this will help the patient to appreciate that he may be unrealistic in his estimate of handicap, and it will provide the audiologist with added useful data.

AUDIOMETRIC ASSESSMENT

When preliminary information has been gathered, the audiologist may proceed with the audiometric assessment of hearing. This generally involves at least pure tone testing and often speech testing and impedance measurement in addition. In certain cases additional specialized procedures may also be warranted.

Pure Tone Audiometry

In pure tone audiometry, a sound-generating electronic instrument called an audiometer is utilized. The auditory stimuli produced by the audiometer may be delivered to either ear from a set of earphones. This type of examination is referred to as an air conduction (AC) pure tone test, since the signal passes by air vibration through the ear canal and into the middle ear. Sounds may also be delivered from the audiometer via a bone conduction (BC) vibrator, which is generally placed on the mastoid process of the temporal bone, located behind the pinna. With this presentation method the sound passes directly by bone conduction into the inner ear.

Through these output devices, individual test tones of specific frequencies (250, 500, 1000, 2000, 4000, and 8000 Hz) are presented at various intensities (0–110 dB) to determine the softest level (lowest intensity) at which the patient is able to hear each test tone. This level is termed "threshold," and values measured at each test frequency are recorded for each ear on an audiogram similar to that shown in Figure 6-1. An audiogram has two important parameters: 1) intensity in decibels (dB) on the vertical axis of the graph; and 2) frequency of the test tones in Hertz on the horizontal scale. Recording symbols are shown in the audiogram key, and for illustrative purposes a threshold value of 20 dB is recorded in the right ear at 1000 Hz as is a threshold of 45 dB in the left ear at 2000 Hz. Thresholds found between 0 and 26 dB on the audiogram are considered to be within the normal range of hearing. Values from 27 to 40 dB indicate a slight loss of hearing, while those from 41 to 55 dB are mild, 56 to 70 dB are considered moderate, 71 to 90 are classified as severe, and thresholds over 90 dB point to a profound loss of hearing (AAOO, 1965; see Table 6-2).

The thresholds from air conduction and bone conduction pure tone testing may be compared to obtain information about the site of difficulty within the auditory system. If the problem is located within the outer or middle ear, it is termed a "conductive" hearing loss. The bone conduction thresholds will be within the normal range and the air conduction thresholds will evidence a loss. Figure

Table 6-2. Scale of hearing impairment based on levels advocated by the Committee on Conservation of Hearing of the American Academy of Ophthalmology and Otolaryngology

Degree of hearing loss	Hearing level (dB)
None	26 or less
Slight	27–40
Mild	41-55
Moderate	56–70
Severe	71-90
Profound	91 or more

Source: Adapted from AAOO (1965).

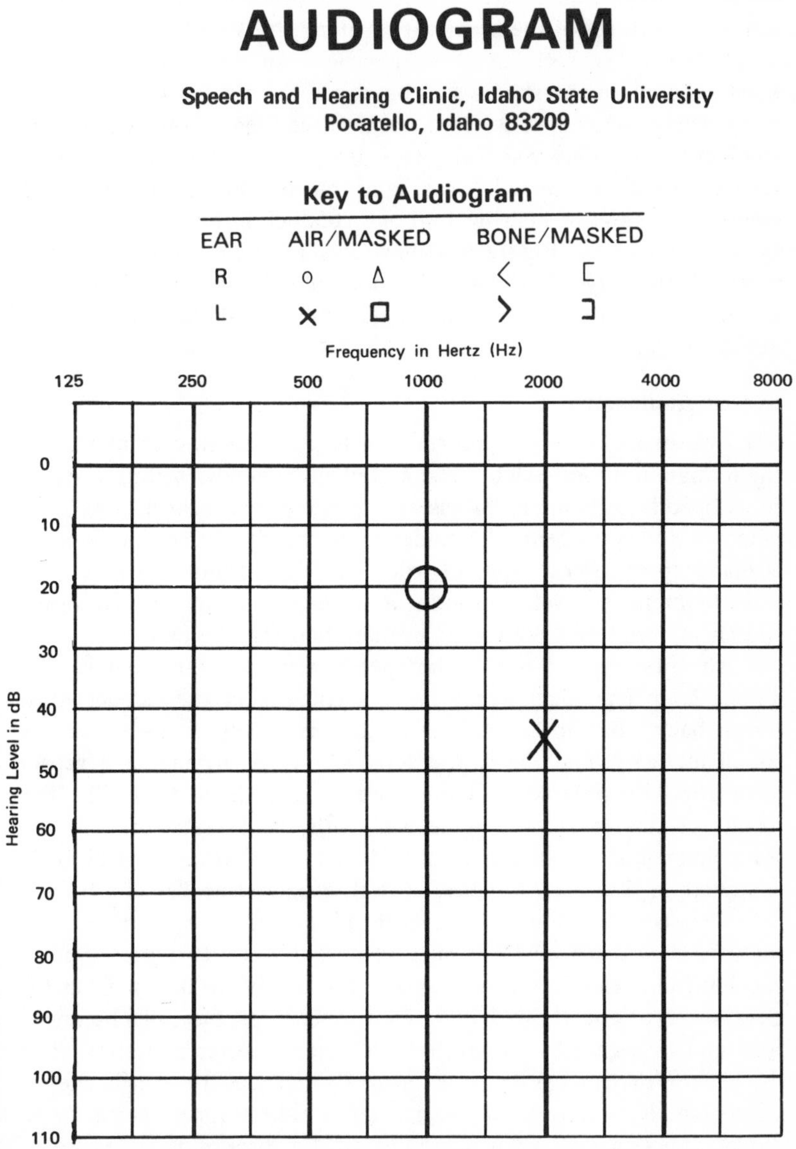

Figure 6-1. Example of an audiogram with a right ear threshold plotted at 20 dB for 1000 Hz and a left ear threshold plotted at 45 dB for 2000 Hz.

6-2 is an illustration of such a case. If the problem occurs within the sensory structures of the inner ear or along the VIIIth cranial nerve, it is called a "sensorineural" hearing loss. In this case the air and bone conduction thresholds will be about the same and will be depressed from what is considered normal (see Figure 6-3). When both conductive and sensorineural losses are present, the combination is referred to as a "mixed" loss, and on the audiogram this will emerge as a loss of hearing by bone conduction and a greater loss by air conduction. Figure 6-4 illustrates this type of loss. Central types of auditory disorders often do not show a loss of hearing, but when they do, air and bone conduction thresholds are generally about the same.

Speech Audiometry

The processing of speech information is the most important task of the human auditory system. The audiologist employs testing referred to as speech audiometry to assess the effect of a hearing loss on a person's ability to hear and understand speech. Speech audiometry is made up of several types of tests which are administered at controlled intensity levels through a speech audiometer. Recorded speech material or "live voice" presentation may be used.

The first type of test is the speech reception threshold (SRT). Two-syllable (spondee) words are presented, and the listener must repeat back what he hears. The audiologist gradually decreases the sound intensity, and the softest level where the listener can repeat back approximately 50% of the words is considered the SRT. The results of this test often agree well with the average of the pure tone thresholds obtained at 500, 1000, and 2000 Hz. The SRT scale is similar to that used for pure tone thresholds (see Table 6-2).

The second test used in speech audiometry is speech discrimination. Here a list of 25 or 50 single-syllable words is presented at a comfortable intensity level. Usually the words are drawn from the CID W-22 or the NU-6 lists, which include phonetically balanced (PB) equivalent forms for multiple list testing. After presentation of the list the percentage of words correctly repeated by the listener is calculated. For example, if the listener is able to repeat correctly 40 out of the 50 words, then he would have a discrimination score of 80%. Scores of 90% and above are generally found in cases of normal hearing or conductive losses. In sensorineural loss, discrimination scores will tend to be lower than this. Scores, of course, are influenced by the level of presentation. Most routine speech dis-

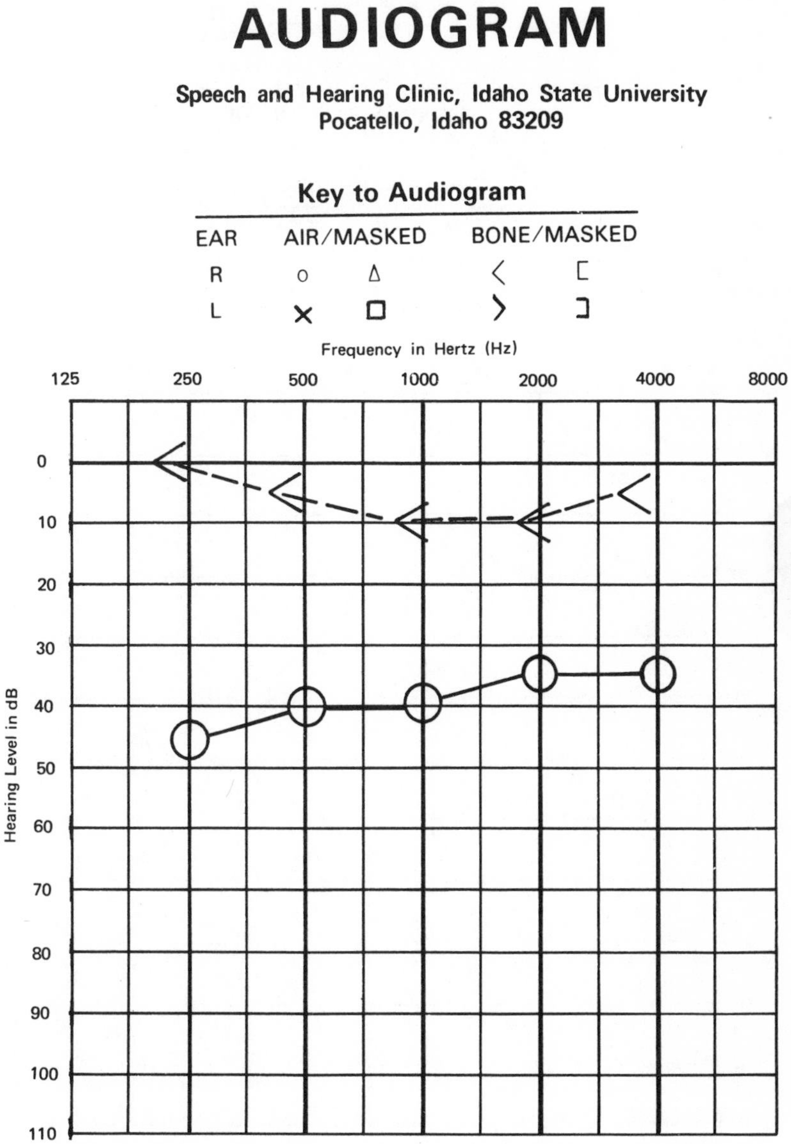

Figure 6-2. Example of an audiogram showing a conductive hearing loss.

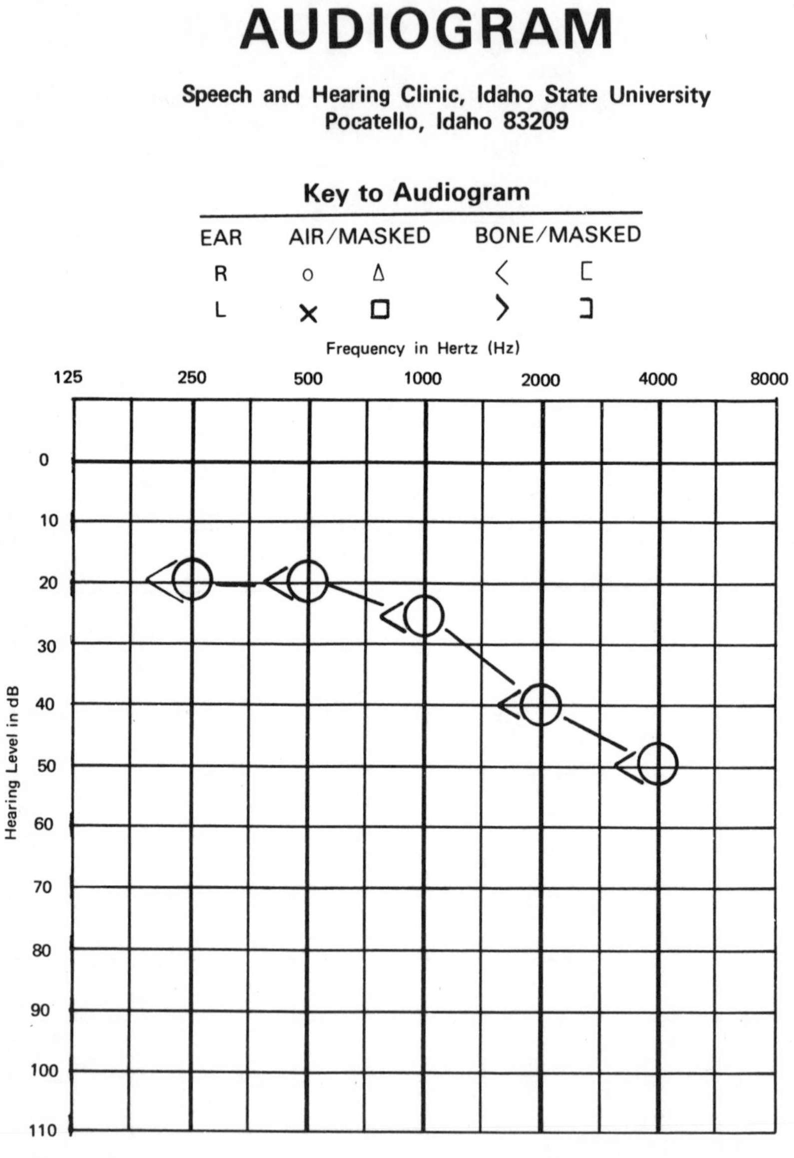

Figure 6-3. Example of an audiogram showing a sensorineural hearing loss.

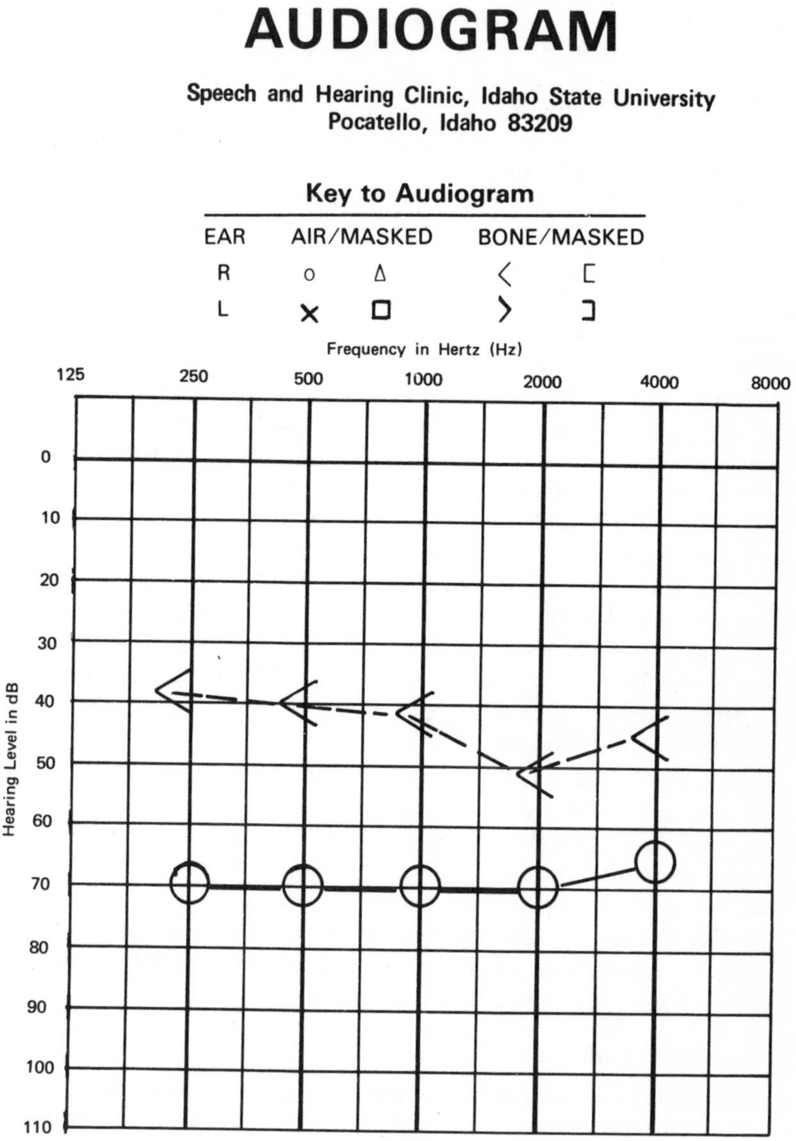

Figure 6-4. Example of an audiogram showing a mixed hearing loss.

crimination tests are given at a comfortable listening level to determine performance for each ear. However, in some cases the lists are presented at other intensities, for example, at a normal conversational loudness, or at increasing levels to determine an improvement curve. Such a graph is referred to as a PI-PB function, for performance vs. intensity of phonetically balanced words. Special synthetic "sentence-like" stimuli such as "Go change your car color is red" are also used to derive such functions (Jerger, Speaks, and Trammell, 1968).

Another procedure in speech audiometry involves the use of speech signals distorted in a variety of ways to make an unusually difficult listening task. For example, one recording of some difficult speech discrimination word lists, the Rush-Hughes version of the PAL PB 50s, is especially difficult because of the cryptic style of the speaker and the fact that the words are less familiar than the W-22s. This test is often used when a harder task is felt to be appropriate. The difference between the W-22 and the Rush-Hughes test scores can be diagnostic since it does not generally exceed 20% except in cases of advanced age or in certain other neural or central auditory disorders (Goetzinger and Rousey, 1959; Goetzinger, Proud, Dirks, and Embrey, 1961; Goetzinger and Angell, 1965). Sometimes distortion is introduced by superimposing noise on the speech signal or by removing high or low frequency parts of the signal with filters. Another variation involves the presentation of different signals to each ear as in the NU-20 Competing Message Test (Olsen and Carhart, 1967) or in the Staggered Spondaic Word (SSW) Test (Brunt, 1972). Simply deleting alternate sections of the message is another form of distortion used in speech audiometry. This will result in a shorter, time-compressed version of the stimulus items. Depending on how much of the material is deleted, the message is said to be compressed from 0% (no compression) up to 80% (listening to the message requires only 20% of the original time) and beyond (Beasley and Maki, 1976). Further explanation of special speech tests is contained in Chapter 9.

Impedance Audiometry

With impedance audiometry audiologists place a small probe tube at the entrance to the ear canal. Through it they monitor the intensity of a tone which is sent into the canal and reflected off the eardrum. When a great deal of the sound is reflected back, this indicates a high impedance of the middle ear, which is possibly associated with the presence of fluid or otosclerosis. When a great amount of sound is absorbed and little reflected, this indicates unusually low impedance as would result from an interruption of the ossicular chain.

Tympanometry is the name of one of the impedance procedures. In this case the ear canal is sealed, and pressure changes (-200 mm H_2O to $+200$ mm H_2O) are created within it to determine what effect this will have on impedance as measured at the eardrum. Usually, impedance is measured in compliance units (cc's) or susceptance units (mmho's). These refer basically to the amount of sound that is transmitted by the conductive mechanism rather than the amount impeded. Tympanometric curves (compliance versus pressure) may be classified as type A, B, or C, or they may be described in terms of pressure, compliance, and shape. This information provides valuable diagnostic data, especially in determining the status of the middle ear. For example, type A tympanograms show a high peak in compliance at or near 0 mm of pressure. Such a graph is shown in Figure 6-5. Patients with normal hearing or sensorineural loss tend to show type A tracings. Type B curves show a relatively flat pattern across the pressure range as shown in Figure 6-6. These are frequently seen in cases of otitis media, perforation, ear wax obstruction, or other conditions that render the eardrum immobile with changes in ear canal pressure. Type C patterns show a high compliance peak but at a negative pressure in excess of -50 mm H_2O (see Figure 6-7). These tracings are typically found in cases of poor Eustachian tube function and in beginning and resolving otitis media. The difference between the highest and lowest point on a tympanogram is termed the *absolute compliance* (or, in a general sense, absolute impedance). The normal range for this value is from .39 cc to 1.3 cc (Jerger, Jerger, and Mauldin, 1972).

Another impedance procedure involves the measurement of the *acoustic reflex* (the action of the middle ear muscles in response to loud acoustic stimuli). Movement of the stapedius muscle, particularly, can be monitored by the same probe tube through changes reflected in impedance. *Acoustic reflex decay* is another variation of this procedure in which the strength of the muscle response is measured over a 10-second period. Rapid decay ($\geq 50\%$) is a diagnostic sign of a tumor of the VIIIth cranial nerve. The adequacy of *Eustachian tube function* can also be monitored through impedance testing.

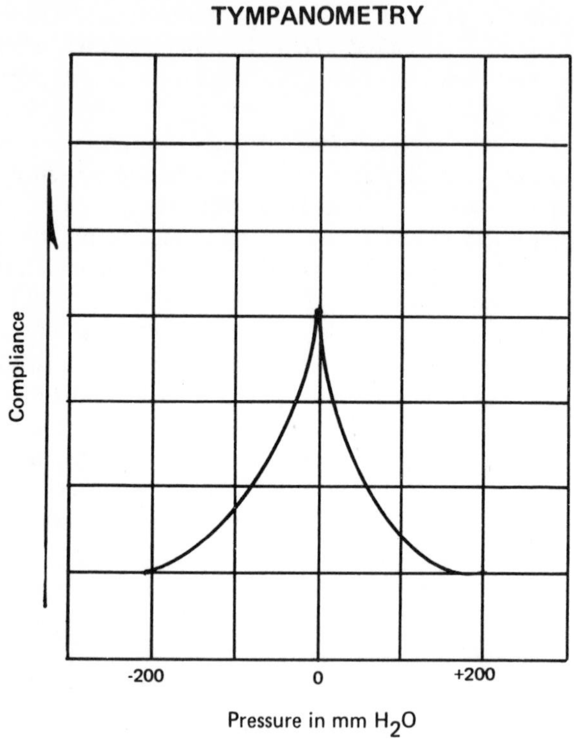

Figure 6-5. Example of a type A tympanogram.

Special Site of Lesion Test Battery

Usually it is possible to determine whether the hearing loss is conductive or sensorineural from the results of pure tone air and bone findings. Speech audiometry and tympanometry can be used to confirm this. In certain cases, however, it is desirable to know if the hearing loss is sensory (located in the cochlea), neural (in the nerve tract), central (at the cortical level), or of nonorganic (functional) origin. In these cases, audiologists may use SISI, Bekesy, loudness balance, and tone decay tests in a diagnostic test battery to isolate sensory and neural disorders or batteries of central and functional tests to determine the site of the lesion.

Conventional Four-Test Battery The SISI test requires the patient to detect a small increment in the loudness of a steady tone. An increment of 1 dB is presented 20 times, and the subject receives

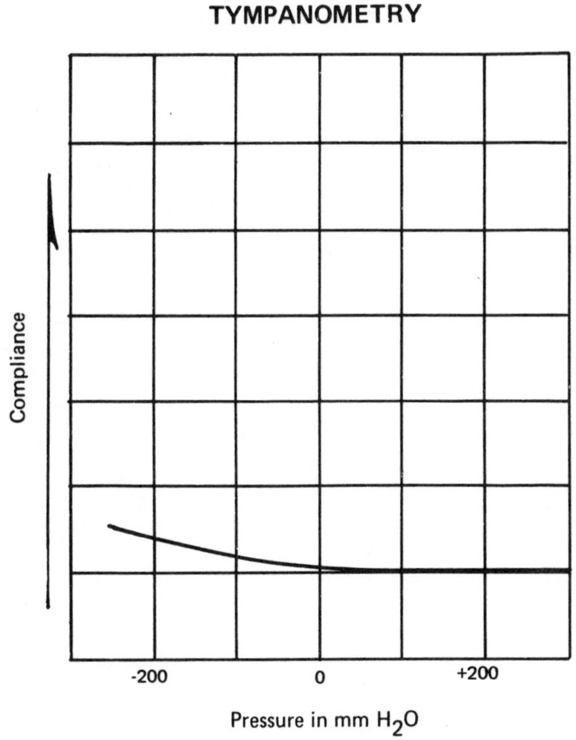

Figure 6-6. Example of a type B tympanogram.

a percentage score depending on the number of increments he detects.

In *tone decay* testing the patient is required to listen to a continuous tone at his threshold to determine if he can hear it for a total of 60 seconds. If the tone fades, the level is increased until he is able to perform the task. The decay is the amount the tone has to be increased before the patient can hear it for 60 seconds at one level.

With *Bekesy* audiometry, the patient is asked to use an automatic audiometer to trace his hearing threshold for continuous and interrupted tones. The relationship between these two tracings is used to classify the findings into one of five types. The diagnostic significance of types I–V is discussed below.

If the patient has normal hearing in one ear, *alternate binaural*

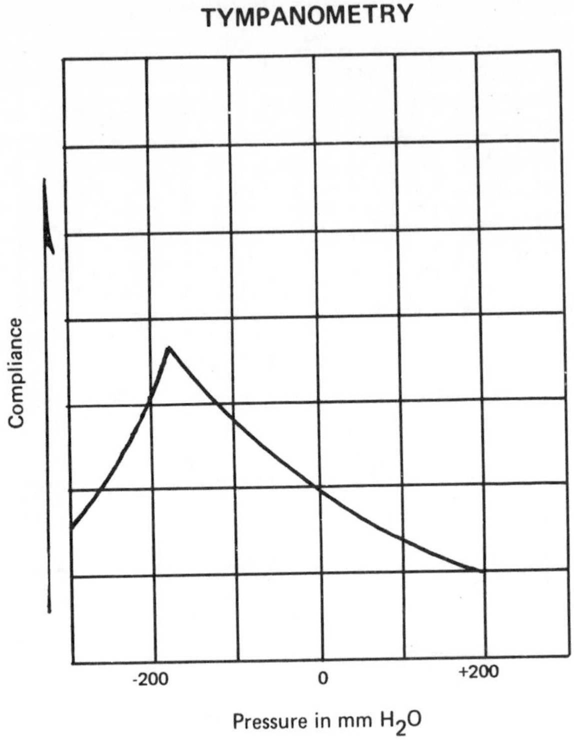

Figure 6-7. Example of a type C tympanogram.

loudness balance testing may be administered. A suprathreshold tone is presented to the good ear. Another tone is delivered to the impaired ear, and the patient is asked to adjust its intensity until the signal is equal in loudness to the tone in the good ear. The loudness perception of the tone in the nonimpaired ear is assumed to be normal. If the loudness match occurs at about the same intensity levels rather than the same level above threshold, then there is an abnormally rapid increase in loudness for the impaired ear. This indicates that *recruitment* is present. A variation of this procedure, *monaural loudness balance,* involves a loudness match between two frequencies in the same ear. Still another variation allows measurement of recruitment in connection with the acoustic reflex test.

Results from this battery of four tests are often used to pinpoint the lesion. Generally, if the loss is conductive, SISI scores will be low, there will be little (≤ 10 dB) if any tone decay, Bekesy tracings will be type I, and loudness balance will show no recruitment. If the damage is located in the cochlea, SISI scores will be high (60–100%), tone decay will be moderate (≤ 30 dB), Bekesy tracings will be type II, and loudness balance will show recruitment to be present. When the loss is located on the VIIIth cranial nerve, SISI scores will tend to be low, tone decay high (> 30 dB), Bekesy will be type III or IV, and no recruitment will be present in loudness balance testing (see summary in Table 6-3). The expected results do not always emerge on each of these tests, but a trend is usually evident among the majority of test findings. Along with pure tone, speech, and impedance tests, such a trend will contribute to differential diagnosis.

Central Test Battery Distorted or other specialized forms of speech audiometry are the most valuable assessment tools in locating and describing the effect of central auditory lesions. Included here are the previously discussed tests such as the Rush-Hughes, competing message tests, the SSW, and filtered, compressed, or noise-superimposed speech tasks. The auditory system may handle pure tone or simple speech stimuli quite efficiently when there is a central dysfunction, but the demand of these distorted speech tests will result in unusually poor performance when a central lesion is present. Often PI-PB functions are used to probe for this breakdown.

Also of value in central assessment is the monitoring of brain waves in response to auditory stimuli. This procedure, called *electroencephalic response audiometry* (ERA), requires very expensive, specialized equipment that only a few audiologists have available to them. Another procedure requiring specialized instrumentation is *electronystagmography* (ENG). This procedure helps in locating both central and peripheral auditory lesions. It is an extension of the

Table 6-3. Classical findings in special test battery for various sites of auditory lesion

Test	Conductive	Cochlear	Neural
SISI	Low scores (0–20%)	High scores (60–100%)	Low scores (0–20%)
Tone decay	0–10 dB	10–30 dB	35 + dB
Bekesy	Type I	Type II	Type III, IV
Loudness balance	No recruitment	Recruitment	No recruitment

physician's simple caloric test procedure wherein hot and cold water are introduced into the ear canal of a patient. With ENG more extensive equipment is used and a graphic record is produced for detailed analysis. With either caloric tests or ENG, the purpose is to assess the integrity of the vestibular or balance system at the peripheral and central level. Since the vestibular and auditory systems are so closely interrelated, audiologists often administer this procedure upon the referral of a physician.

Functional Test Battery If the audiologist suspects that the patient does not, in fact, have an organic hearing loss, there are several tests he can use to discover if the responses are falsified. When results show a 20 dB or greater difference between ears, the audiologist can use the *Stenger Test* to determine the accuracy of the patient's responses. With this test, a tone or speech signal is presented to both ears, but the patient will only be able to perceive it in the ear in which it is loudest. If the patient is not honestly reporting what he hears, this will produce inconsistencies in test results.

In the *delayed auditory feedback* (*DAF*) *test,* the patient is asked to tap a pattern or read a paragraph. While he is doing this a slight delay is introduced in what he hears of the tapping pattern or of his own speech as he reads. This monitoring of the signal is presented via earphones at a level below his admitted threshold. If he can hear the delayed sound, it will interfere with his performance, and either the pattern will be disrupted or the reading rate will be reduced.

In the *galvanic skin response* (*GSR*) *test*, equipment is used that allows measurement of skin resistance and simultaneously presents a slight shock to some location on the body. Patients are conditioned to expect a shock when they hear certain sounds and then these sounds are presented at low levels and increased until an anticipatory, emotional response is observed through a change in skin resistance. It can be assumed that the patient heard the sound when such a response occurs.

A type V Bekesy tracing or certain types of impedance (reflex) results also pinpoint a functional loss. All of these tests are valuable when the patient is malingering or faking a hearing loss. This often occurs in compensation cases, and the audiologic test results are helpful to a physician who must make judgments in such situations.

Other Audiometric Tests There are, of course, other auditory assessment procedures used in evaluating infants and children.

However, because of the focus on the elderly in this text these procedures are not described here.

NONAUDIOMETRIC ASSESSMENT OF THE ELDERLY

Case History

In most case history interviews with the elderly the purposes and procedures are the same as in younger patients. The reason for evaluation, the symptoms, and the history of hearing problems need to be determined. Sometimes older patients will discuss extraneous aspects of their medical history at length. It is often a challenge to use the right blend of patience and tact to move the interview forward. Hardick (1977) stressed the need to express a genuine interest in the elderly person and their hearing problem as it affects employment, family relations, social interaction, religious activity, and so forth. He urges that clinicians not force the interview by a rigid authoritarian approach. "Tell me about your hearing problem" is the way he starts his interviews, and he claims this open approach yields benefits in clients who respond favorably in such a relationship. Occasionally, an older patient will report that he came for evaluation only at the insistence of friends or relatives (who sometimes bring the oldster in tow). The older patient will not usually acknowledge symptoms or difficulties in these cases, and a more realistic report may be obtained from the relative or friend. Such a secondary source may also be helpful in interviews where the patient has difficulty reporting symptoms and history because of memory lapse or communication problems because of advanced intellectual deterioration or stroke. Occasionally, in an institutional setting, patients will not remember their name or age. They may report an age or other information which is inaccurate, and so it is wise to double check this information with another source.

Self-Evaluation of Hearing Handicap

The HHS or other self-evaluating tools may be used with most elderly subjects. In fact, the HHS may be used informally to alert persons to a need for clinical auditory testing. Shenoy, Tannahill, and Schow (1975) suggested that this form may be administered in senior citizen centers, doctors' and dentists' offices, and in other places where older persons congregate. This can serve to inform the patient with hearing disability that his problem need not be ignored and that help is available to him beginning with a full audiologic assessment. Shenoy et al. found that, among 50 subjects age 60 and over, those who had pure tone loss (26 dB HTL+) or poor speech discrimination (<80%) could generally be identified by HHS scores of 30% or poorer. Only three out of 21 subjects needing referral based on these criteria would not have been referred using HHS and a 30% cutoff score. Only two subjects with good hearing scored poorer than 30%, so over-referral was not a problem. McCartney, Sorenson, and Maurer (1974) also found a 30% HHS score to effectively identify elderly subjects with hearing problems needing aural rehabilitation. Use of HHS in this fashion should not, however, be a basis for discouraging formal audiologic evaluation of those who suspect they have a loss.

Use of the HHS with a relative or friend of the aged person will provide additional insight concerning the patient's hearing handicap. While an assessment by a relative may be more objective, it should not cause one to ignore the report by the patient. There will be times when the older person has such limited activity that, despite a hearing loss, he will not require extensive rehabilitation. For example, a telephone amplifier may be the only need of a person who lives alone and who has very minimal social interaction. Full time hearing aid use would probably be an unrealistic recommendation for such a person unless he desires it, regardless of the feelings a relative might have. When the HHS is used, the scores may be interpreted as shown in Table 6-1. Schow and Tannahill (1977) have reported that adjustment of score interpretation is not indicated with the noninstitutionalized elderly. Berkowitz and Hochberg (1971) and Ewertsen and Nielson (1973) have also shown that such scale scores are influenced very little as a function of age so long as the patient is alert and able to respond to the questions.

With the institutionalized patient it is a different matter. The items in the HHS are not appropriate to activities of a nursing home patient, and the wording is often too involved for easy understanding. Schow and Nerbonne (1977) have developed a modified self-evaluation tool for nursing home use called the Nursing Home Hearing Handicap Index (NHHI). Two forms of this index are available, one for use with the patient and another with similar items on which a staff member may report his perception of the patient's hearing handicap (see Appendix B). With the NHHI it is possible to evaluate the seriousness of a given hearing loss as it effects an institutionalized patient. Schow and Nerbonne found, for example, that a 40-dB loss produces roughly the same handicap in an institutionalized setting as a 25-dB loss does in a noninstitutional patient. This simply reflects that hearing demands in normal society are usually greater and require better hearing than in a nursing home. Zarnoch and Alpiner (1977) have recently made a preliminary report on another assessment scale for use in extended care facilities. When completed, this scale, which is more ambitious in its design than the NHHI, should be useful in evaluating communicative function in the nursing home population.

AUDIOMETRIC ASSESSMENT OF THE ELDERLY

Pure Tone Audiometry

Pure tone testing by air and bone conduction can generally be performed on the older patient without special modification, but Hull and Traynor (1975) suggested that collapsed canals may occur in the aged due to earphone pressure on the soft tissue of the pinna. Zucker and Williams (1977) report finding a high incidence of collapsed canals in an extended care facility. If AC findings are poorer than BC results, this possibility should be considered. In the experience of the present authors, however, rigid pinnas and large canals are often found in this population. Furthermore, the incidence of hearing loss in the Williams and Zucker data where precautions were taken for collapsed canals is similar to that found in a sample where ear canal inserts were not used (Schow and Nerbonne, 1976).

It should be noted that, given actual hearing function of equal levels, the older patient will tend to show poorer thresholds than younger subjects because of a conservative response criterion. This is thought to be true for all sensory thresholds because of caution by the older patient in responding at levels softer than those where the stimulus is clearly present (Rees and Botwinick, 1971; Botwinick, 1973). Despite the need for caution in the interpretation of pure tone findings from the elderly, this tendency does make older patients very consistent, reliable responders. Therefore, they are often relatively easy to test. Some older subjects, however, have unusually long reaction times which slow down the test procedure (Willeford, 1971; also see Chapter 3). Testing can be a very difficult process with some stroke patients, with persons having other neurologic illness or extreme senility, or with many institutionalized people.

In a nursing home, one difficulty often encountered is finding a quiet test environment, since most of these residents are unable to go to a clinical facility for elaborate testing. Sound level meters may be used to determine the threshold level above which environmental noise will not interfere. Alternately, the examiner with normal hearing can determine his own thresholds within the noisy environment to roughly determine the lowest acceptable testing level.

It is often helpful to talk to the institutionalized patient during the test, asking at frequent intervals, "Did you hear that one?" Sometimes the subject cannot remember his task and the proper response but can respond to this sort of questioning. Occasionally he will give quite graphic descriptions of what he hears ("that's sharp" or "that one's far away"). Aphasic patients are challenging to test, but usually with patience some signal system can be devised through which they can communicate their responses (Ludlow and Swisher, 1971). Abbreviated testing is appropriate in most of these cases. AC thresholds at 500, 1000, 2000, and 4000 Hz, along with impedance results, will usually answer the same questions as complete air conduction and bone conduction findings, and, in a nonsound-treated environment, will provide more accurate results (Traynor and Hull, 1976). With aphasics and some others it may be necessary to divide the testing time, obtaining thresholds in two sessions.

Speech Audiometry

Routine procedures in SRT and speech discrimination testing may be used with most elderly patients, but recorded speech materials can present difficulty to the aged because of slow reaction times. Live voice presentation allows ample time for a slow response and is therefore preferable in some cases. The speech discrimination performance of the elderly has been studied by several investigators. Since people generally exhibit increasing sensorineural loss with advancing age, it is expected that mean discrimination scores will systematically decrease in groups of older persons (Table 4-2). Whether or not this decrease is a function of age, as well as sensorineural loss, has been a matter of dispute (see Chapters 8 and 9 for a full treatment of this issue). Investigations by Punch and McConnell (1969), Harbert, Young, and Menduke (1966), and Kasden (1970), would indicate, however, that speech discrimination is more closely related to the extent of hearing loss than to age. Poorer discrimination scores, therefore, can be expected when more sensorineural loss is present. Nevertheless, the Punch and McConnell and the Jerger (1973) data indicate that age has some effect on discrimination even when the elderly subject has normal hearing. Also, there will be some elderly patients who will exhibit much poorer discrimination than expected in view of the pure tone findings. This is termed "phonemic regression" (Gaeth, 1948), and some authors refer to it as a frequent characteristic of presbycusis (Yarington, 1976). The difficulty that some subjects have with even simple, 50-word, single-syllable discrimination tasks has motivated use of shorter, simpler discrimination tests of varying difficulty with this population (Schow, 1977). (See Chapter 18 for further details.)

Performance of gerontologic subjects on filtered or distorted speech tests is not only poorer than that seen in younger subjects but shows a decrement of greater magnitude when compared to scores on undistorted tests. For example, a comparison of the difference between W-22 and Rush-Hughes recordings shows that with advancing age there is an increasing tendency to exceed the normal cutoff difference of 20 dB, as shown in group data of Table 9-1 (Goetzinger et al., 1961). Other pronounced defects have been noted in the ability of elderly subjects to perform difficult speech discrimination tasks even when they perform normally on regular speech discrimination tests (Bocca, 1958; Harbert et al., 1966; Schon, 1970; Jerger, 1973; Bergman, Blumenfeld, Cascardo, Dash, Levitt, and Marguiles, 1976).

Impedance Audiometry

The use of impedance testing is valuable with the elderly, not only as an additional test but also as an alternative to routine bone conduction testing. Informal otoscopy is an important preliminary to placing the probe in the ear. If cerumen (ear wax) is extensive and near the entrance to the ear canal it can clog the probe. Also, impedance cannot be done if the canal is completely occluded as is sometimes found, particularly in the institutionalized elderly (Traynor and Hull, 1976).

A great challenge in impedance testing of the elderly is in obtaining a tight seal in the entrance to the canal, with the unusually large pinnas often found in this population. Rubber, foam, and inflatable cuffs provided with impedance equipment have been unsatisfactory in many cases, but the use of glycerin or Vaseline as a coating on the outside of these cuffs has generally produced the desired seal. Others have reported success with silicone putty (Purvis, 1974; Hull and Traynor, 1975).

There has been some controversy as to whether different normative impedance values should be used with the elderly (Jerger et al. 1972; Alberti and Kristensen, 1972; Beattie and Leamy, 1975; Thompson, Sills, and Bui, 1976a; Blood and Greenberg, 1977; Nerbonne, Bliss, and Schow, 1977). It would appear from the more recent data that no special values are needed for absolute compliance up to at least age 80. Thompson, Sills, and Bui (1976b) also examined acoustic reflex in aging ears and found no significant difference from younger subjects.

Special Site of Lesion Test Batteries

The supplementary auditory tests used to confirm sensory, neural, central, or functional disorders may generally be used with the elderly as well as with younger subjects. The findings from SISI, tone decay, Bekesy, and loudness balance testing, however, have been quite unpredictable in the case of presbycusic hearing losses.

Jerger, Shedd, and Harford (1959) found that SISI scores could be low, intermediate, or high in elderly subjects with hearing loss. Bekesy findings were reported by Jerger (1960) in 44 presbycusic cases. He found 24 type I tracings, 15 type II, 2 type III, and 3 that were questionable and therefore not classified. Harbert et al. (1966) found mainly type II tracings in 50 older subjects. They also did loudness balance testing on these patients. Using monaural loudness balance they found only 30% of their subjects showed recruitment. Goetzinger et al. (1961) also tested for recruitment in 90 elderly subjects. Of 120 ears tested there were 29 with no recruitment and many with only partial recruitment.

Harbert et al. and Goetzinger et al. also tested tone decay on their subjects. In both studies most cases showed minimal (0–10 dB) decay, but a few showed as much as 20–30 dB of decay. It would appear from these findings that, although SISI, Bekesy, and recruitment findings are quite variable in the elderly, tone decay tends to be uniformly moderate to minimal. Willeford (1971), however, has presented data on eight presbycusic subjects, and four of them exhibited 35 dB or greater tone decay. He emphasized that the Harbert et al. (1966) study employed a modified tone decay procedure that would minimize the decay found.

It is apparent, therefore, that precise special test results from this battery cannot be expected in the elderly. When these special test findings suggest neural or central involvement in the elderly patient, however, it is possible to separate presbycusis from life-threatening lesions like VIIIth nerve tumors, since loss attributable to old age will manifest itself bilaterally whereas hearing loss because of tumor will be unilateral.

A battery of central auditory tests may be used with the aged, including distorted speech testing and electroencephalic response audiometry (ERA). As previously mentioned, the elderly will definitely exhibit decreased performance on difficult speech tests; this is suggestive of the central deterioration found in many cases of presbycusis. Kolman and Shimizu (1972) have used ERA to monitor recovery from stroke in the geriatric patient. Functional tests are seldom needed with the gerontologic subject but may be used when required.

INTERPRETING ASSESSMENT FINDINGS AND RECOMMENDATIONS FOR THE ELDERLY

The preceding discussion has indicated that several kinds of information are needed to assess hearing loss in the elderly and make meaningful recommendations. Ideally this will include a medical examination of the ear as well as many of the above described nonaudiometric and audiometric procedures. The results are used to determine if the hearing loss can be medically or audiologically remediated. If the loss does not involve active pathology and is simply a consequence of aging, very little can be done medically. In considering aural rehabilitation, it must be remembered that there is a complex relation between the results of audiometric findings and the effect of these hearing problems on a person's communicative ability. This must be considered if good management is to occur. The case history interview and the self-evaluation tools are used to assess how various communication needs interact with hearing problems and therefore how great the need for rehabilitation is.

Pure tone audiometric findings will indicate the frequencies where there is hearing loss. As indicated in Chapter 4, aging tends to first cause a loss in the high frequencies and later affects the low frequencies as well, but to a lesser extent. An audiogram will also show the degree of loss whether slight, mild, moderate, severe, or profound. With age there will likely be a slow steady progression in impairment, as seen in Figure 4-1. The greater the degree of loss, the greater will be the need for remediation. This gradual progression of hearing difficulty in the elderly will contribute to a tendency of these patients not to recognize that their hearing is impaired.

Speech audiometric measures can be used along with the pure tone findings to analyze the effect of hearing loss on the reception of conversation. Useful information in this regard is the SRT and the pure tone average (average threshold of 500, 1000, and 2000 Hz) for the better ear. These values may be compared with the 45-dB audiogram level, which is the average speech loudness when sitting 3–4 feet from someone speaking at a normal intensity. It may be assumed that as the SRT approaches 45 dB, there will be a corresponding difficulty with normal conversation. When the SRT exceeds 45 dB then conversation will be heard only when it is unusually loud. The elderly, therefore, can experience decreased hearing function from the 0 dB level down to 25, 30, or 35 dB before they begin to have difficulty with speech. The aged may have even 40 to 45 dB of loss and not admit handicap if compensation is made by persons talking louder or if the subjects have minimal social interaction.

When considering the everyday influence of hearing loss, speech discrimination scores must be carefully interpreted since in the routine examination these scores represent the clarity of a person's hearing when he is listening at a comfortable listening level rather than at a normal conversational level. Another important factor in analyzing speech discrimination findings for the elderly patient is the relative importance of vowels and consonants in understanding speech stimuli. The vowels in speech are generally louder than the consonants and thus easier to hear. Also the vowels tend to be low pitched sounds, while many consonants are higher in frequency. For most elderly persons, hearing is best in the low frequencies and poorest in the high. Thus they hear the vowels better and the consonants less well.

This is illustrated by Figure 6-8, in which a typical set of pure tone thresholds from an elderly male is plotted. The area outlined in the middle of the audiogram represents the intensity and frequency distribution of ordinary conversational speech. The vowels generally will be located on the left side of this outline in the low to mid pitch region and lower on the chart since they are more intense. The consonants are found primarily on the upper and righthand side of this outline because they tend to be less intense and higher in frequency. From the circles on this audiogram the level can be determined where this person just begins to hear. He will not hear sounds

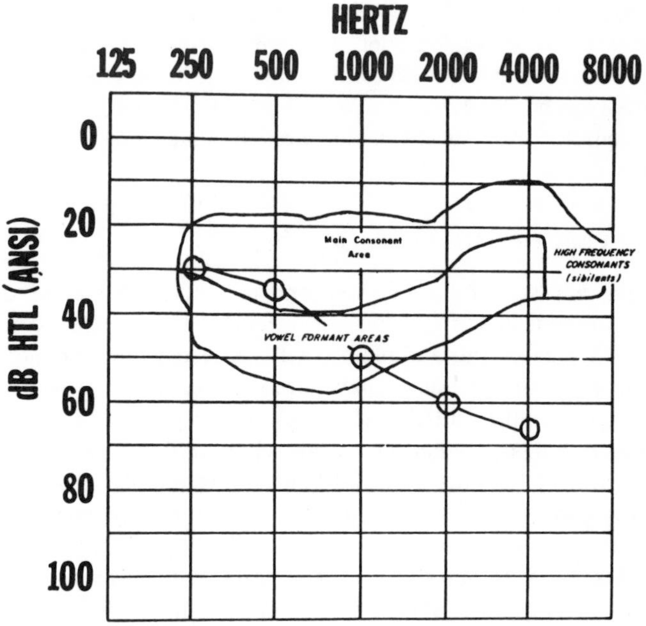

Figure 6-8. Audiogram with superimposed outline of conversational speech area. Typical air conduction thresholds for an elderly male are shown. (Source: Adapted from Fletcher, 1970.)

softer (higher on the chart) than the threshold marks. Thus this typical oldster will hear some of the vowel sounds but very few of the consonant sounds. Unfortunately, it is far more important to hear the consonants in the discrimination of speech. Early research on this question by Fletcher (1929) indicated that if the sounds below 500 Hz are not heard, about 98% of the speech signal can still be understood. However, if the information above 1500 Hz is removed then only 65% of the signal will be understood.

Most of the loudness of speech, therefore, is in the low frequencies with the vowels, but the clarity of speech is in the upper frequencies because of the consonants. This is one reason older patients will do poorly on a speech discrimination task presented at a comfortable level and have even more difficulty in daily life than the discrimination score would indicate. It is why they often report, "Oh, I hear all right; it's just that so many people mumble when they talk." Also, of course, the elderly sometimes have poor care of their outer and middle ears, causing conductive hearing loss. Furthermore, they tend to have deterioration at the sensory, neural, and central levels as shown by poor results on distorted speech tests and diverse findings on other special auditory tests like SISI, Bekesy, tone decay, and loudness balance. Further aspects of conductive, sensorineural, and central losses are discussed in the following chapters.

COUNSELING OF THE ELDERLY

An important step following assessment is the counseling of the patient. In medical settings this will often be done by the physician, and in other cases the audiologist will be responsible. If medically treatable forms of pathology have been excluded, it is urgent that the physician or the audiologist convey to the patient that help can be rendered in the form of aural rehabilitation. Far too many patients are told at this point, "Well, you're simply growing older and there isn't much we can do for you." Family members are sometimes counseled to talk louder and the rehabilitation ends there. Hearing aids can help in many cases of presbycusis, contrary to what has been said about there being no help for "nerve deafness." Most persons wearing hearing aids these days do have sensorineural loss (nerve deafness), since conductive losses can usually be medically treated. Many patients do need help in adjusting to a hearing aid, and in this and in many other ways aural rehabilitation can provide a great service to the elderly patient. The nature of this service is described in detail in Chapter 18.

SUGGESTED READINGS

Goetzinger, C. P., Proud, G. O., Dirks, D., and Embrey, J. A study of hearing in advanced age. Archives of Otolaryngology, 73, 662–674 (1961).

Martin, F. N. Introduction to Audiology. Englewood Cliffs, N.J.: Prentice-Hall, 1975.

Newby, H. A. Audiology (3rd Ed.). New York: Appleton-Century-Crofts, 1972.

Rupp, R. R. Understanding the problems of presbycusis. Geriatrics, 25, 100–107 (1970).

Willeford, J. A. The geriatric patient. In D. E. Rose (ed.), Audiological Assessment. Englewood Cliffs, N.J.: Prentice-Hall, 1971.

REFERENCES

Alberti, P., and Kristensen, R. The compliance of the middle ear: Its accuracy in routine clinical practice. In D. Rose and L. Keating (eds.),

Mayo Foundation Impedance Symposium. Rochester, Minn.: Mayo Clinic Foundation, 1972.
Alpiner, J., Chevrette, W., Glascoe, G., Metz, M., and Olsen, B. The Denver Scale of Communication Function. Denver, Col.: University of Denver, 1974.
American Academy of Ophthalomogy and Otolaryngology (AAOO). Guide for the Classification and Evaluation of Hearing Handicap. Committee on Conservation of Hearing, Transactions AAOO, 69, 740–751 (1965).
Beasley, D. S., and Maki, J. E. Time- and frequency-altered speech. In N. J. Lass (ed.), Experimental Phonetics. New York: Academic Press, 1976.
Beattie, R., and Leamy, D. Otoadmittance: Normative values, procedural variables, and reliability. Journal of the American Audiological Society, 1, 21–27 (1975).
Bergman, M., Blumenfeld, V. G., Cascardo, D., Dash, B., Levitt, H., and Marguilies, M. K. Age-related decrement in hearing for speech. Journal of Gerontology, 31, 533–538 (1976).
Berkowitz, A. O., and Hochberg, I. Self-assessment of hearing handicap in the aged. Archives of Otolaryngology, 93, 25–33 (1971).
Blood, E. and Greenberg, H. Acoustic admittance of the ear in the geriatric person. Journal of the American Audiological Society, 1, 185–187 (1977).
Bocca, E. Clinical aspects of cortical deafness. Laryngoscope, 68, 301–309 (1958).
Botwinick, J. Aging and Behavior. New York: Springer, 1973.
Brunt, M. The Staggered Spondaic Word (SSW) Test. In J. Katz (ed.), Handbook of Clinical Audiology. Baltimore: Williams & Wilkins, 1972.
Ewertsen, H., and Nielson, B. Social hearing handicap index; social handicap in relation to hearing impairment. Audiology, 12, 180–187 (1973).
Fletcher, H. Speech and Hearing. New York: Van Nostrand, 1929.
Fletcher, S. G. Acoustic phonetics. In F. S. Berg and S. G. Fletcher (eds.), The Hard of Hearing Child. New York: Grune & Stratton, 1970.
Gaeth, J. H. A study of phonemic regression associated with hearing loss. Unpublished doctoral dissertation, Northwestern University, Evanston, Ill., 1948.
Goetzinger, C. P., and Angell, S. Audiological assessment in acoustic tumors and cortical lesions. Eye, Ear, Nose and Throat Monthly, 44, 39–49 (1965).
Goetzinger, C. P., Proud, G. O., Dirks, D., and Embrey, J. A study of hearing in advanced age. Archives of Otolaryngology, 73, 662–674 (1961).
Goetzinger, C. P., and Rousey, C. L. Hearing problems in later life. Medical Times, 87, 771–780 (1959).
Harbert, F., Young, I. M., and Menduke, H. Audiologic findings in presbycusis. The Journal of Auditory Research, 6, 297–312 (1966).
Hardick, E. J. Aural rehabilitational programs for the aged can be successful. The Journal of the Academy of Rehabilitative Audiology, 10, 51–67 (1977).
High, W., Fairbanks, G., and Glorig., A. A scale for self assessment of hearing handicap. Journal of Speech and Hearing Disorders, 12, 215–230 (1964).
Hull, R. H., and Traynor, R. M. The pathologic and audiologic manifesta-

tions of presbycusis. Short course presented at the Annual Convention of the American Speech and Hearing Convention, Washington, D.C., 1975.
Jerger, J. Bekesy audiometry in analysis of auditory disorders. Journal of Speech and Hearing Research, 3, 275–287 (1960).
Jerger, J. Audiological findings in aging. Advances in Otorhinolaryngology, 20, 115 (1973).
Jerger, J., Jerger, S., and Mauldin, L. Studies in impedance audiometry. I. Normal and sensorineural ears. Archives of Otolaryngology, 96, 513–523 (1972).
Jerger, J., Shedd, J., and Harford, E. On the detection of extremely small changes in sound intensity. Archives of Otolaryngology, 69, 200–211 (1959).
Jerger. J., Speaks, C., and Trammell, J. L. An approach to speech audiometry. Journal of Speech and Hearing Disorders, 33, 318–328 (1968).
Kasden, S. D. Speech discrimination in two age groups matched for hearing loss. Journal of Auditory Research, 10, 210–212 (1970).
Kolman, I., and Shimizu, H. Recovery from aphasia as monitored by AER audiometry. Journal of Speech and Hearing Disorders, 37, 414–420 (1972).
Ludlow, C. L., and Swisher, L. P. The audiometric evaluation of adult aphasics. Journal of Speech and Hearing Research, 14, 535–543 (1971).
McCartney, J., Sorenson, F., and Maurer, J. A comparison of a self assessment scale of hearing impairment and selected audiometric data on a geriatric population. Paper presented at American Speech and Hearing Association Convention, Las Vegas, 1974.
Nerbonne, M. A., Bliss, A. T., and Schow, R. L. Acoustic impedance values in the elderly. Paper presented at the Annual Convention of the American Speech and Hearing Association, Chicago, 1977.
Olsen, W. O., and Carhart, R. Development of test procedures for evaluation of binaural hearing aids. Bulletin of Prosthetic Research, 10, 22–49 (1967).
Punch, J. L., and McConnell, F. The speech discrimination function of elderly adults. Journal of Auditory Research, 9, 159–166 (1969).
Purvis, G. The use of silicone putty for impedance audiometry. Paper presented at the Annual Convention of the American Speech and Hearing Association, Las Vegas, 1974.
Rees, J., and Botwinick, J. Detection and decision factors in auditory behavior of the elderly. Journal of Gerontology, 26, 133–136 (1971).
Sanders, D. A. Hearing aid orientation and counseling. In M. C. Pollack (ed.), Amplification for the Hearing-Impaired. New York: Grune and Stratton, 1975.
Schon, T. D. The effects on speech intelligibility of time-compression and expansion on normal-hearing, hard of hearing, and aged males. Journal of Auditory Research, 10, 263–268 (1970).
Schow, R. L. How to promote and provide speech and hearing help in nursing homes: Experiences in a state-wide program. Paper presented at the Annual Convention of the California Speech and Hearing Association, San Francisco, 1977.

Schow, R., and Nerbonne, M. Hearing levels in nursing home residents. Research Laboratory Report 1, pp. 1–10, Department of Speech Pathology and Audiology, Idaho State University, Pocatello, 1976.

Schow, R. L., and Nerbonne, M. A. Assessment of hearing handicap by nursing home residents and staff. The Journal of the Academy of Rehabilitative Audiology, 10, 2–12 (1977).

Schow, R. L., and Tannahill, J. C. Hearing handicap scores and categories for subjects with normal and impaired hearing sensitivity. Journal of the American Audiology Society, 3, 134–139 (1977).

Shenoy, M., Tannahill, C., and Schow, R. Self assessment of hearing in a geriatric population. Paper presented at Annual Meeting of the Illinois Speech and Hearing Association, Chicago, 1975.

Thompson, D., Sills, J., and Bui, D. Acoustic admittance in aging ears. Paper presented at the Annual Convention of the American Speech and Hearing Association, Houston, 1976a.

Thompson, D. J., Sills, J. A., and Bui, D. M. Acoustic reflex growth in aging ears. Paper presented at the Annual Convention of the American Speech and Hearing Association, Houston, 1976b.

Traynor, R. M., and Hull, R. H. A method of audiological assessment for the nonambulatory geriatric patient. Paper presented at the Annual Convention of the American Speech and Hearing Association, Houston, 1976.

Willeford, J. A. The geriatric patient. In D. E. Rose (ed.), Audiological Assessment. Englewood Cliffs: Prentice-Hall, 1971.

Yarington, C. T., Jr. Presbycusis. In J. L. Northern (ed.), Hearing Disorders. Boston: Little, Brown, 1976.

Zarnoch, J., and Alpiner, J. The Denver scale of communication function for senior citizens living in retirement centers: A preliminary report. Paper presented at the Annual American Speech and Hearing Association Convention, Chicago, 1977.

Zucker, K., and Williams, P. Audiological services in an extended care facility. Paper presented at the Annual Convention of the American Speech and Hearing Association, Chicago, 1977.

APPENDIX A: HEARING HANDICAP SCALE

Name ____________________ SCORE:
Age ____________ Raw score______
Date ____________________ −20
Form (A or B) ____________ ______ × 1.25 = ______%[a]

FORM A	Practically always		As often as not		Almost never
1. If you are 6–12 feet from the loudspeaker of a radio do you understand speech well?	1	2	3	4	5
2. Can you carry on a telephone conversation without difficulty?	1	2	3	4	5
3. If you are 6–12 feet away from a television set, do you understand most of what is said?	1	2	3	4	5
4. Can you carry on a conversation with one other person when you are on a noisy street corner?	1	2	3	4	5
5. Do you hear all right when you are in a street car, airplane, bus, or train?	1	2	3	4	5
6. If there are noises from other voices, typewriters, traffic, music, etc., can you understand when someone speaks to you?	1	2	3	4	5

[a] See Table 6-1 for interpretation of scores.

	Practically always		As often as not		Almost never
7. Can you understand a person when you are seated beside him and cannot see his face?	1	2	3	4	5
8. Can you understand if someone speaks to you while chewing crisp foods, such as potato chips or celery?	1	2	3	4	5
9. Can you carry on a conversation with one other person when you are in a noisy place, such as a restaurant or at a party?	1	2	3	4	5
10. Can you understand if someone speaks to you in a whisper and you can't see his face?	1	2	3	4	5
11. When you talk with a bus driver, waiter, ticket salesman, etc., can you understand all right?	1	2	3	4	5
12. Can you carry on a conversation if you are seated across the room from someone who speaks in a normal tone of voice?	1	2	3	4	5
13. Can you understand women when they talk?	1	2	3	4	5

	Practically always		As often as not		Almost never
14. Can you carry on a conversation with one other person when you are out-of-doors and it is reasonably quiet?	1	2	3	4	5
15. When you are in a meeting or at a large dinner table, would you know the speaker was talking if you could not see his lips moving?	1	2	3	4	5
16. Can you follow the conversation when you are at a large dinner table or in a meeting with a small group?	1	2	3	4	5
17. If you are seated under the balcony of a theater or auditorium, can you hear well enough to follow what is going on?	1	2	3	4	5
18. When you are in a large formal gathering (a church, lodge, lecture hall, etc.) can you hear what is said when the speaker *does not* use a microphone?	1	2	3	4	5
19. Can you hear the telephone ring when you are in the room where it is located?	1	2	3	4	5
20. Can you hear warning signals, such as automobile horns, railway crossing bells, or emergency vehicle sirens?	1	2	3	4	5

FORM B	Practically always		As often as not		Almost never
1. When you are listening to the radio or watching television, can you hear adequately when the volume is comfortable for most other people?	1	2	3	4	5
2. Can you carry on a conversation with one other person when you are riding in an automobile with the windows *closed*?	1	2	3	4	5
3. Can you carry on a conversation with one other person when you are riding in an automobile with the windows *open*?	1	2	3	4	5
4. Can you carry on a conversation with one other person if there is a radio or television in the same room playing at normal loudness?	1	2	3	4	5
5. Can you hear when someone calls to you from another room?	1	2	3	4	5
6. Can you understand when someone speaks to you from another room?	1	2	3	4	5
7. When you buy something in a store, do you easily understand the clerk?	1	2	3	4	5
8. Can you carry on a conversation with someone who does not speak as loudly as most people?	1	2	3	4	5

	Practically always		As often as not		Almost never
9. Can you tell if a person is talking when you are seated beside him and cannot see his face?	1	2	3	4	5
10. When you ask someone for directions, do you understand what he says?	1	2	3	4	5
11. If you are within 3 or 4 feet of a person who speaks in a normal tone of voice (assume you are facing each other), can you hear everything he says?	1	2	3	4	5
12. Do you recognize the voices of speakers when you don't see them?	1	2	3	4	5
13. When you are introduced to someone, can you understand the name the first time it is spoken?	1	2	3	4	5
14. Can you hear adequately when you are conversing with more than one person?	1	2	3	4	5
15. If you are in an audience, such as in a church or theater and you are seated near the *front*, can you understand most of what is said?	1	2	3	4	5
16. Can you carry on everyday conversations with members of your family without difficulty?	1	2	3	4	5

	Practically always		As often as not		Almost never
17. If you are in an audience, such as in a church or theater and you are seated near the *rear*, can you understand most of what is said?	1	2	3	4	5
18. When you are in a large formal gathering (a church, lodge, lecture hall, etc.) can you hear what is said when the speaker *does* use a microphone?	1	2	3	4	5
19. Can you hear the telephone ring when you are in the next room?	1	2	3	4	5
20. Can you hear night sounds, such as distant trains, bells, dogs barking, trucks passing, and so forth?	1	2	3	4	5

APPENDIX B: NURSING HOME HEARING HANDICAP INDEX (NHHI)

Self Version for Resident[a]

	Very often				Almost never
1. When you are with other people do you wish you could hear better?	5	4	3	2	1
2. Do other people feel you have a hearing problem (when they try to talk to you)?	5	4	3	2	1
3. Do you have trouble hearing another person if there is a radio or TV playing (in the same room)?	5	4	3	2	1
4. Do you have trouble hearing the radio or TV?	5	4	3	2	1
5. (How often) do you feel life would be better if you could hear better?	5	4	3	2	1
6. How often are you embarrassed because you don't hear well?	5	4	3	2	1
7. When you are alone do you wish you could hear better?	5	4	3	2	1
8. Do people (tend to) leave you out of conversations because you don't hear well?	5	4	3	2	1

[a] Words in parentheses are optional when items are read to the resident.
[b] See Table 6-1 for interpretation of scores.

	Very often				Almost never
9. (How often) do you withdraw from social activities (in which you ought to participate) because you don't hear well?	5	4	3	2	1
10. Do you say "what" or "pardon me" when people first speak to you?	5	4	3	2	1

TOTAL______ × 2 = ____
−20
____ × 1.25 = ____%[b]

Staff Version

	Very often				Almost never
1. When this person is with other people does he/she need to hear better?	5	4	3	2	1
2. Do members of the staff, family, and friends make negative comments about this person's hearing problem?	5	4	3	2	1
3. Do they have trouble hearing another person if there is a radio or TV playing in the same room?	5	4	3	2	1
4. When this person is listening to radio or TV do they have trouble hearing?	5	4	3	2	1

	Very often				Almost never
5. How often do you feel life would be better for this person if they could hear better?	5	4	3	2	1
6. How often are they embarrassed because they don't hear well?	5	4	3	2	1
7. When they are alone do they need to hear the everyday sounds of life better?	5	4	3	2	1
8. Do people tend to leave them out of conversations because they don't hear well?	5	4	3	2	1
9. How often do they withdraw from social activities in which they ought to participate because they don't hear well?	5	4	3	2	1
10. Do they say "what" or "pardon me" when people first speak to them?	5	4	3	2	1

TOTAL______ × 2 = ____

−20

____ × 1.25 = ____%[b]

Chapter 7
Conductive Auditory Disorders

A conductive hearing disorder is one that occurs in the outer or middle ear. A number of hearing impairments of this type are identified and discussed. Also included is a summary of the audiometric characteristics generally associated with conductive disorders. Emphasis is placed on conductive disorders commonly observed in the elderly.

Preceding chapters have presented material regarding the structures and functions of the normal auditory mechanism, as well as information relating to the changes that can occur within the auditory system as a consequence of aging. In each instance this material has been systematically presented for each of the major divisions of the auditory channel, beginning with the outer and middle ears, and concluding with the inner ear, VIIIth nerve, and brain stem-cortical divisions. The next three chapters use this same type of classification system to first discuss the various types of auditory disorders that occur in the general population and then to present disorders of specific concern among the elderly.

This chapter is confined to disorders of the outer and/or middle ear, which are termed conductive hearing disorders. This general form of auditory impairment is characterized by some degree of difficulty in the conduction of sound to the inner ear mechanism by the components of the outer and middle ear. The incidence of conductive disorders is surprisingly high, especially in preschool and early elementary-age youngsters, where it can approach 25 percent (Brooks, 1974). In adults the incidence is dramatically reduced, although investigations with nursing home residents (Grossman, 1955; Nerbonne, Schow, Goset, and Bliss, 1976; Nerbonne, Bliss, and Schow, 1977) suggest the need to be alert for outer and middle ear impairments in persons in this age range as well.

MAJOR TYPES OF CONDUCTIVE DISORDERS IN THE GENERAL POPULATION

Outer Ear

Perhaps the most frequently observed form of conductive disorder can be attributed to the accumulation of an excess amount of cerumen, or ear wax, in the external auditory meatus. If cerumen is produced in excessive amounts, a plug can form that will impede the transmission of sound waves to the eardrum, resulting in a mild hearing impairment (see Figure 7-1). If the wax comes in contact with the eardrum itself, it can also reduce the mobility of the drum, resulting in a loss of hearing. A similar problem can arise from the intrusion of foreign objects, such as pencil erasers or paper wads, into the canal. Careful removal of the obstruction by qualified personnel will usually restore hearing to normal once the condition has been detected.

Individuals may be born with an absence or malformation of the pinna and occlusion of the ear canal. This condition is termed congenital agenesis of the pinna and atresia of the canal, and is accompanied by a substantial loss of hearing if complete occlusion of the canal occurs. In many such cases structural abnormalities within the middle and inner ears may also be present, making the prognosis for reconstructive surgery an uncertainty.

Occasionally infections of the external ear canal, called external otitis, will result from a variety of causes, including various forms of bacteria and fungi. The chief symptom is generally acute pain, but most individuals do not experience any appreciable auditory deficit as a direct result of this condition.

Middle Ear

The term "otitis media" is a general term used to indicate an inflammatory condition located within the middle ear cavity. A number of different types of otitis media exist. They are distinguishable on the basis of several factors, including the presence or absence of fluid in the middle ear, the composition of the fluid (if present), and the duration of the infection.

The onset of otitis media can often be associated with the emergence of an upper respiratory infection or an allergic condition. The inflammation of the tissues of the nasopharyngeal area of the throat that usually accompanies a cold can impair the functioning of the Eustachian tube. If the tube, which is normally closed, cannot

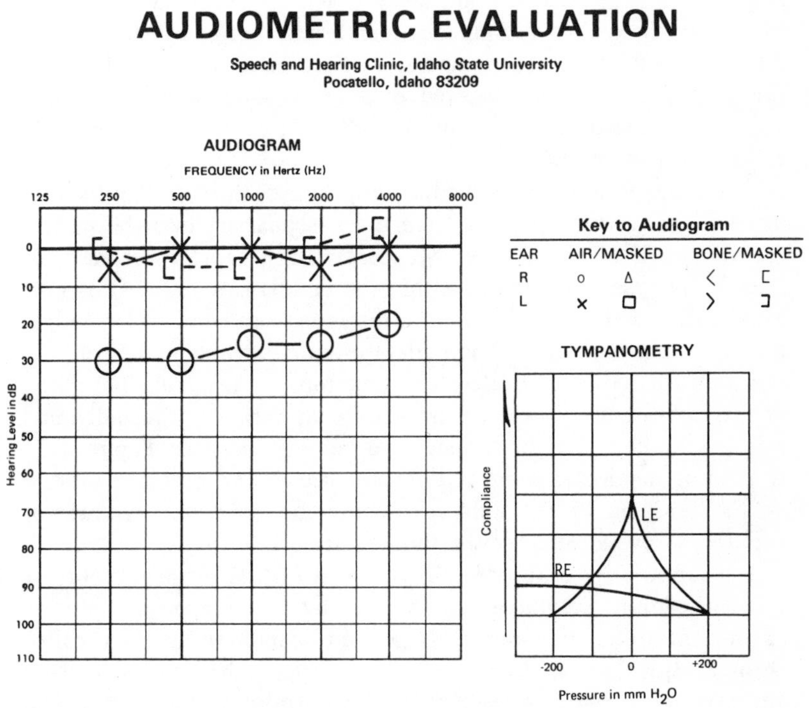

Figure 7-1. Impacted cerumen in a 10-year-old child. *History:* History of excessive cerumen, requiring periodic removal; feeling of fullness in right ear. *Audiometric results:* Mild air conduction pure tone hearing loss in the right ear, with normal bone conduction thresholds. Type B tympanogram.

open periodically to allow for the exchange of air to and from the middle ear cavity, then a condition of negative air pressure will soon occur within the middle ear because of the absorption of the remaining air by the tissues of the cavity. This will result in a retracted eardrum, with the membrane being pushed into the middle ear space by the positive pressure being applied to it in the outer ear. A retracted drum will be less able to move in response to stimulation from sound waves, resulting in a very slight hearing loss. Persistent negative pressure of the middle ear is felt to cause the suction of thin, clear fluid from its mucous membrane lining, causing a condition termed serous otitis media. A fluid line and/or bubbles in the fluid can often be observed during an otoscopic examination. Figure 7-2 illustrates the typical audiometric results observed in cases with this condition.

Another form of otitis media, suppurative, involves the invasion of bacterial or viral infection from the nasopharynx into the middle ear via the Eustachian tube. Mucousal tissue rapidly becomes inflamed and pus accumulates within the middle ear space. Otoscopic examination will generally reveal a distended eardrum, which bulges into the outer ear canal. The patient often complains of severe pain and will usually have an elevated temperature. Although the effects of this condition on hearing are somewhat variable, the individual will usually have a mild to moderate hearing loss (see Figure 7-3). If prompt medical treatment does not occur, the pressure exerted on the eardrum by the fluid may cause the drum to perforate or rupture, allowing much of the fluid to drain into the ear canal.

If suppurative otitis media is not dealt with effectively, recurring episodes of fluid accumulation, followed by a spontaneous rupturing of the eardrum, may occur. If so, this condition is then called chronic otitis media. The fluid can eventually become very thick and take on adhesive properties, with the erosion of the ossicles and other middle ear structures a likely possibility. The frequent perforation or rupture of the eardrum, followed by a spontaneous healing, can lead to an accumulation of scar tissue on the eardrum. The presence of large amounts of scar tissue on the drum can, because of the different properties associated with scarring, make the membrane less able to transduce the acoustic energy it receives. In some cases of chronic otitis media, the cells of the mastoid process of the temporal bone may become infected as well, creating a serious condition termed mastoiditis.

Medical treatment for otitis media takes a variety of forms.

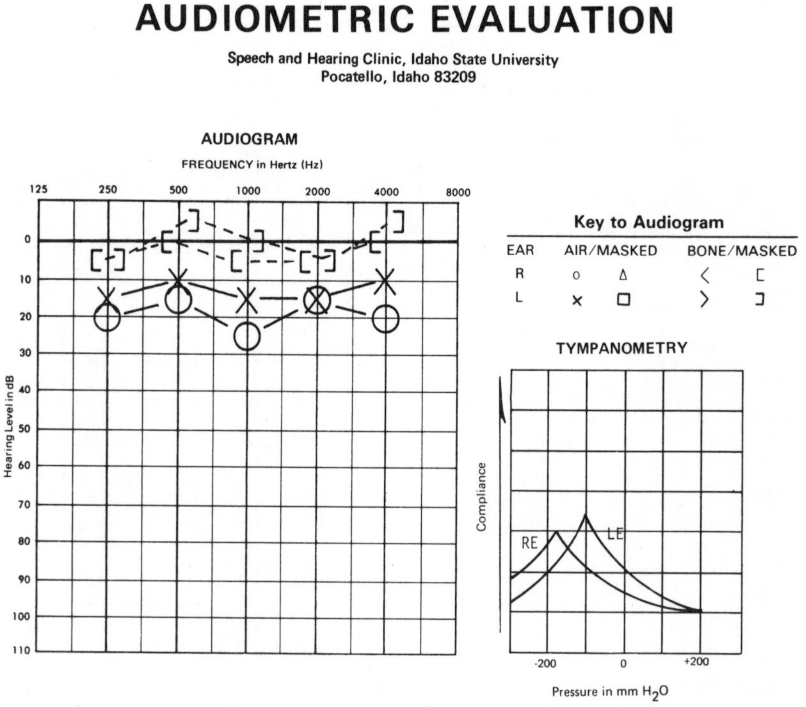

Figure 7-2. Serous otitis media in a 3-year-old child. *History:* Recent upper respiratory infection. No pain or hearing loss noted. *Audiometric results:* Borderline normal hearing bilaterally for air conduction pure tones, with normal bone conduction thresholds. Type C tympanograms in each ear.

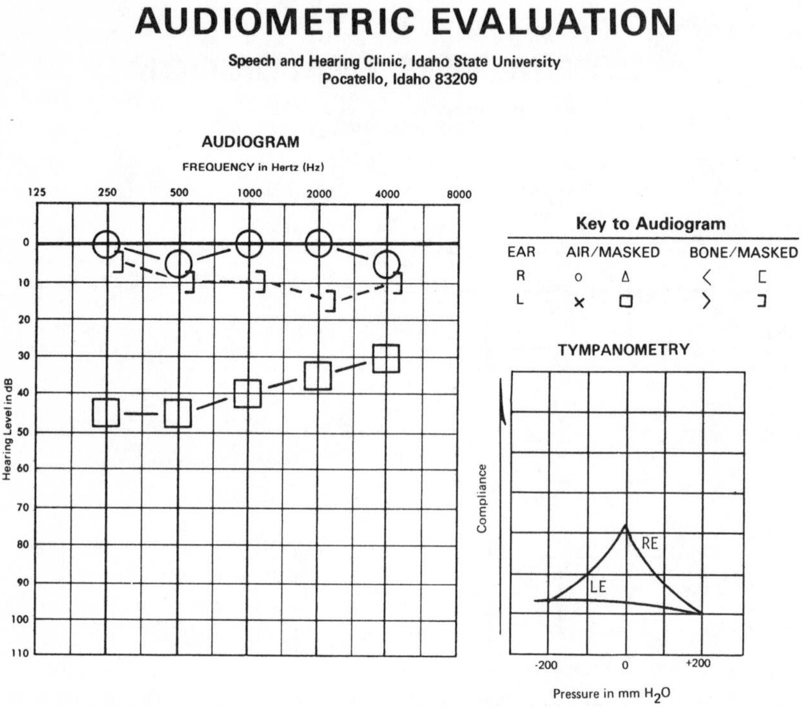

Figure 7-3. Suppurative otitis media in a 24-year-old male. *History:* Occasional ear infections; recent fullness in left ear, along with noticeable hearing loss in that ear. Some pain noted. *Audiometric results:* Mild air conduction pure tone loss in left ear, with slightly depressed but normal bone conduction thresholds. Type B tympanogram for left ear.

Numerous forms of antibiotics are employed to attack the bacterial or viral infections associated with suppurative otitis media. A procedure called a myringotomy is also used frequently in the case where fluid or pus is present. A small incision is made in the tympanic membrane and the fluid is removed with the aid of suction devices. To facilitate the recovery from an ear infection and to restore proper ventilation of the middle ear, the physician will often insert a small plastic tube through the eardrum which is designed to remain in the drum for an extended period of time. The inserted tube then temporarily supplies the functions normally provided by the Eustachian tube until this structure is again able to function normally. Decongestants and/or antihistamines are prescribed in the treatment of otitis media as well.

A sac-like pseudotumor called cholesteatoma can develop whenever skin is introduced into the middle ear. This may occur in a variety of ways, including a perforation of the tympanic membrane. Cholesteatomas can grow quite large, occupying the entire middle ear cavity. They are very erosive and may create extensive destruction of bone and other tissue. Surgery is usually necessary to remove the cholesteatomatous material.

One other conductive auditory disorder worthy of mention is that of otosclerosis. This is a condition unique to the temporal bone in which normally hard bone changes composition, becoming soft and spongy, and grows intermittently. This is followed by a return to a hard, or sclerotic, status once again. One of the more frequent sites for this to occur is at or near the oval window, which can result in the fixation of the stapes, thereby seriously limiting its movement in the oval window. The end result is a mild to moderate hearing loss, as seen in Figure 7-4. A surgical procedure called a stapedectomy can be carried out to correct the otosclerotic condition. This involves the removal of the stapes, which is replaced with a prosthetic device that is fit into the oval window. The amount of improvement in hearing provided by the surgical technique is excellent, with the restoration of normal hearing occurring in a high percentage of cases.

CONDUCTIVE DISORDERS IN THE ELDERLY

Even though the preponderance of auditory dysfunction observed in the elderly can be directly linked with abnormalities of the cochlea, VIIIth nerve, or central portions of the auditory system, the fact

AUDIOMETRIC EVALUATION

Speech and Hearing Clinic, Idaho State University
Pocatello, Idaho 83209

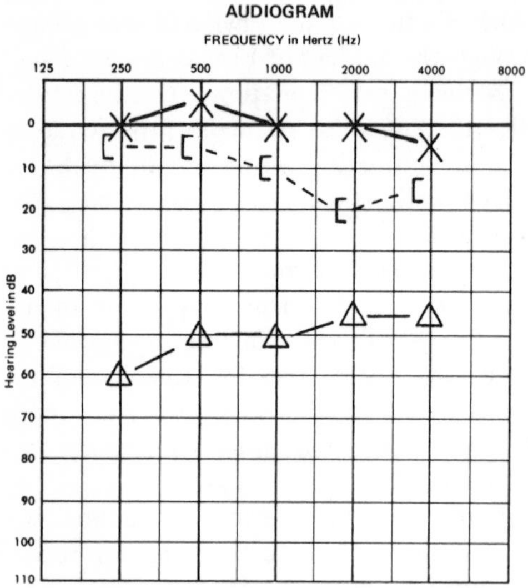

Key to Audiogram

EAR	AIR/MASKED		BONE/MASKED	
R	o	Δ	<	[
L	x	□	>	]

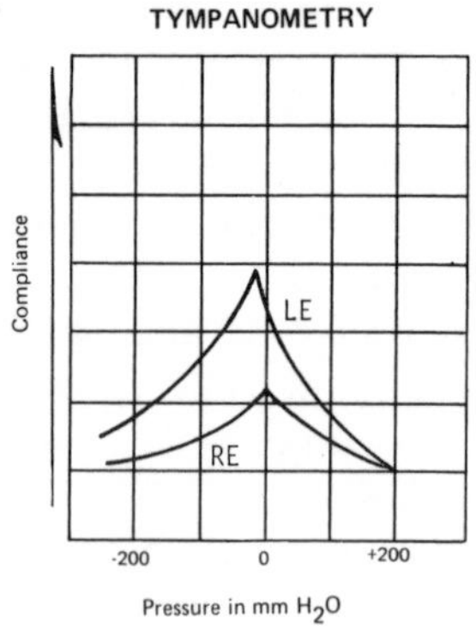

Speech Audiometry

EAR	Pure Tones: P T AVG 500-2000	Speech Thresholds: SRT ~~SAT~~	Speech Thresholds: dB RE / type	Speech Discrim.: dB HL / %	Speech Discrim.: dB RE / type
RIGHT		50		80 / 94 %	
LEFT				%	
BIN.				%	
		Spondees □ Numbers □ ______ □ MLV □ Rec. □	masking in opposite ear	W22 □ PBK □ PB50 □ ______ □ MLV □ Rec. □	masking in opposite ear

Figure 7-4. Otosclerosis in a 34-year-old female. *History:* Progressive air conduction hearing loss in right ear. Some sensation of fullness and a buzzing tinnitus. No history of middle ear infections. Family history of hearing loss. *Audiometric results:* Moderate air conduction hearing loss in right ear, with notched bone conduction thresholds within normal limits. Type A_s tympanogram. Good discrimination in right ear at sufficient presentation level.

remains that conductive disorders within the outer or middle ear can and do occur in this particular age group. Previous discussion regarding the structural changes that can take place during senescence revealed that important anatomic alterations within the outer and middle ears may produce some degree of conductive hearing impairment. While these senescent factors are felt to account for a portion of the conductive hearing loss seen in the elderly, it also is important to realize that age does not serve as a barrier to isolate this group from the other forms of outer and middle ear disorders commonly seen in the general population, such as otitis media and otosclerosis. It is obvious that any comprehensive discussion of hearing disorders in the aged will be incomplete if reference is not made to the existence of abnormalities of the outer and middle ear.

Outer Ear

Although numerous changes associated with aging do occur in the pinna, such as an increase in its size and flexibility, these modifications have not been linked with any significant decrements in hearing. A number of diseases involving the pinna may also be observed in the aged, including seborrheic dermatitis (Sutton, 1956), osteatosis or dry ear (Senturia, 1957), and simple pruritis (Senturia, 1957). These conditions also do not result in any degree of hearing loss. The health professional should, nonetheless, be alert for the onset of diseases such as these for at least three reasons: 1) to minimize the extent of any discomfort associated with the abnormality, 2) to prevent the condition from evolving into something more severe and difficult to treat, and 3) to become aware of the possible existence of an underlying life-threatening disease (Keim, 1977).

As with the pinna, few disorders of the external auditory meatus will result in hearing loss in the elderly. Diseases such as external otitis do occur in older individuals, but there appears to be a somewhat lower incidence of this disorder in persons in the sixth decade of life or older. Senturia and Carr, as reported in Senturia (1957), found the greatest incidence of external otitis in 30- to 40-year-old individuals, with the incidence in females being somewhat higher (56%) than for males (44%). Itching and dry, scaly skin often accompany chronic diffuse otitis media. According to Keim (1977), relief for the itching can be provided most patients by the insertion of only a few drops of mineral oil on a daily or weekly basis, while other topical medications are usually effective in treating any bacterial infection of the skin of the canal.

Some research has been carried out which suggests that impacted cerumen may be present in relatively high numbers of the residents of nursing homes. Grossman (1955) evaluated the hearing of 181 residents of a single nursing home and noted a high incidence of excess ear wax. Otoscopic evaluation led to the removal of cerumen in 36 of the 181 persons seen in the study. Likewise, McCartney and Alexander (1976) conducted otoscopic examinations on 616 ears of elderly residents living in three types of extended care facilities. They found that approximately 33 percent of the ears examined had an excessive accumulation of cerumen. Studies by Nerbonne et al. (1976) and Nerbonne et al. (1977) also revealed similar findings. Further research is needed to determine if the high incidence found in these investigations is attributable to the production of excess cerumen in the elderly or the lack of consistent otologic health care. Regardless of the cause, the evidence available strongly indicates the need for periodic otoscopic and/or tympanometric examinations for the elderly, particularly those residing within institutionalized settings.

Middle Ear

Although a number of degenerative modifications associated with presbycusis do occur within the middle ear, little in the way of specific information is available concerning the effect these senescent changes may have on hearing. Politzer (1926) was one of the first investigators to express the notion that an unspecified amount of the hearing loss seen in presbycusis can be, in many instances, attributed to alterations of critical structures of the middle ear. This contention was not widely accepted. For example, Pestalozza and Shore (1955) carried out a study of typical audiometric results obtained with presbycusic patients, and, in their selection of subjects, ruled out all elderly persons found to have air-bone gaps. This was apparently done on the assumption that pure presbycusic hearing impairments will not contain any conductive element.

In 1961 Glorig and Davis published findings in support of a conductive component in presbycusis. They obtained air and bone conduction pure tone thresholds on 164 men between 25 and 80 years of age with no history of excessive noise exposure. Analysis of their data revealed the presence of significant air-bone gaps above 1000 Hz in the older subjects. The gaps were especially evident at

4000 Hz, a finding that Glorig and Davis attributed to an unknown form of conductive disorder within the middle ear (see Figure 7-5). They concluded that a portion of the high frequency hearing decrement observed in a presbycusic hearing loss could be attributed to conductive involvement. This was followed by an investigation by Nixon, Glorig, and High (1962), who used data from 124 subjects previously included in the Glorig and Davis study. In these subjects, whose ages ranged from 25 to 59 years, an average air-bone gap of 8 dB was found at 4000 Hz. The authors suggested that this might be the result of a conductive element in presbycusis.

Sataloff, Vassallo, and Menduke (1965) also reported on a similar study, utilizing 55 male and female subjects from 62 to 86 years. Individuals with otologic disease or history of excessive noise exposure were not included in the study sample. The authors found no significant air-bone gaps at either 2000 or 4000 Hz, supporting the presence of a pure sensorineural impairment in presbycusis.

While strong evidence exists to support the existence of structural changes in the middle ear that stem from the process of aging, no conclusive evidence exists to substantiate that a portion of the hearing loss associated with presbycusis is conductive in nature. Apparently, the senescent changes within the middle ear are, for the most part, not sufficient to significantly affect the proper functioning

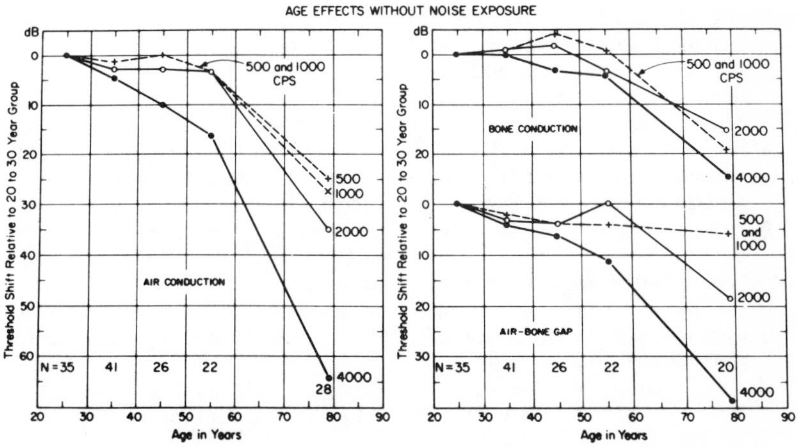

Figure 7-5. Comparison of air conduction and bone conduction thresholds in 164 men between 25 and 80 years of age with a history of no noise exposure. Note the air-bone gap as a function of age and frequency. (Source: Glorig and Davis, 1961.)

of the structures of this portion of the auditory system. However, further research appears warranted.

The elderly do experience many of the diseases of the middle ear commonly seen in the general population. Various forms of otitis media are found in older patients (Keim, 1977), and the discussion presented earlier in Chapter 4 pertaining to possible Eustachian tube dysfunction in the elderly may be of relevance here. In addition, Farrior (1963) has presented evidence to demonstrate that the elderly, as well as younger individuals, may suffer from otosclerosis. In over one-third of the 125 otosclerosis cases he presented, sclerotic fixation of the stapes occurred after 50 years of age.

SUGGESTED READINGS

Glorig, A., and Gerwin, D. (eds.). Otitis Media. Springfield, Ill: Charles C Thomas, 1972.

Schuknecht, H. Pathology of the Ear. Cambridge, Mass.: Harvard University Press, 1974.

Senturia, B. Diseases of the External Ear. Springfield, Ill: Charles C Thomas, 1957.

REFERENCES

Brooks, D. Impedance measurement in screening for auditory disorders in children. Hearing Instruments, 25, 20–21, 36 (1974).

Farrior, J. Stapes surgery in geriatrics. Surgery in the nerve-deaf otosclerotic. Laryngoscope, 73, 1084–1098 (1963).

Glorig, A., and Davis, H. Age, noise, and hearing loss. Annals of Otology, Rhinology and Laryngology, 70, 556–571 (1961).

Grossman, B. Hard of hearing persons in the house for the aged. Hearing News, 23, 11 (1955).

Keim, R. How aging affects the ear. Geriatrics, 32, 97–99 (1977).

McCartney, J., and Alexander, D. Geriatric audiology nursing home project: First year evaluation. Paper presented at the Annual Convention of the American Speech and Hearing Association, Houston. 1976.

Nerbonne, M., Bliss, A., and Schow, R. Acoustic impedance values in the elderly. Paper presented at the Annual Convention of the American Speech and Hearing Association, Chicago, 1977.

Nerbonne, M., Schow, R., Goset, F., and Bliss, A. Prevalence of conductive pathology in a nursing home population. Unpublished study, Idaho State University, Pocatello, 1976.

Nixon, J., Glorig, A., and High, W. Changes in air and bone conduction thresholds as a function of age. Journal of Laryngology and Otology, 74, 288–298 (1962).

Pestalozza, G., and Shore, I. Clinical evaluation of presbycusis on the basis of different tests of auditory function. Laryngoscope, 65, 1136–63 (1955).

Politzer, A. Diseases of the Ear. Philadelphia: Lea & Febiger, 1926.
Sataloff, J., Vassallo, L., and Menduke, H. Presbycusis: Air and bone conduction thresholds. Laryngoscope, 75, 889–901 (1965).
Senturia, B. Diseases of the External Ear. Springfield, Ill: Charles C Thomas (1957).
Sutton, R., Jr. Diseases of the Skin, Philadelphia: Lea & Febiger, 1956.

Chapter 8
Sensorineural Auditory Disorders

The major types of sensorineural disorders seen in the general population and in the elderly are identified and discussed. Audiometric procedures used in the evaluation of these auditory impairments are reviewed, as are the typical results obtained.

The term "sensorineural hearing loss" is used to refer to an auditory impairment in which pathology is located within the inner ear or along the pathway of the VIIIth nerve as it courses to the brain stem from the inner ear. Most sensorineural auditory disorders result from abnormalities within the inner ear; disorders involving the auditory nerve are relatively infrequent. This type of impairment will, of course, result in some diminution in auditory acuity, as seen in conductive disorders, but may also cause difficulty in speech discrimination. In addition, persons having sensorineural hearing disorders often will experience a condition called recruitment, which is an abnormal growth or increase in the perception of loudness as the intensity of an auditory signal is increased. Recruitment is linked directly with inner ear pathology and is not considered to be characteristic of disorders that exclusively involve the VIIIth nerve. Many sensorineural disorders are also often accompanied by a persistent high pitched tinnitus.

MAJOR TYPES OF SENSORINEURAL DISORDERS IN THE GENERAL POPULATION

Congenital Causes

Some types of sensorineural hearing impairments stem from abnormalities associated with the development of structures within the inner ear prior to birth. Numerous causes have been identified for these congenital disorders. Certain types of hearing loss can be directly related to hereditary factors, with genetic defects in the parents resulting in developmental abnormalities within the auditory mechanism of the offspring (see Figure 8-1). Rh incompatibility between the mother and the fetus can also result in a sensorineural disorder, especially in the mother's second or third pregnancy.

Certain viral diseases contracted by the mother can also cause damage to the sensorineural auditory structures, resulting in hearing loss. Rubella, or German measles, is perhaps the most feared of these. Figure 8-2 shows a typical audiogram for a hearing loss caused by rubella. Other factors which may result in congenital hearing impairment include the intake of harmful drugs by the mother during pregnancy and the presence of a syphilitic condition in the mother. A more detailed discussion regarding these congenital disorders is contained in Northern and Downs (1974) and in Jaffe (1977).

Acquired Causes

A number of viral infections experienced by an individual, particularly during childhood, can result in sensorineural hearing disorders. These include chicken pox, measles, mumps, and meningitis.

Ironically enough, a few of the drugs that have been found to be so effective in the treatment of disease have also been found to have serious side effects on hearing. These drugs, including streptomycin, neomycin, and kanamycin, can have an ototoxic effect on the delicate structures on the inner ear and cause a substantial amount of hearing loss. Even aspirin can have such an effect if large amounts are consumed on a daily basis.

Exposure to intense noise ranks along with presbycusis as a major cause of sensorineural hearing disorders. Millions of people currently have a noise-related hearing loss acquired during employment or recreational activities or while serving in the armed forces. Figure 8-3 shows an example of the hearing loss which can result from exposure to intense noise over time.

Many unilateral sensorineural impairments can be attributed to Ménière's disease. No definite cause for the disorder has been identified, although many experts feel that it stems from an overabundant production of endolymph within the organ of Corti (Sataloff, 1966). Persons with Ménière's disease often experience hearing loss, equilibrium difficulties, a feeling of fullness in the ear, and a loud, low pitched tinnitus. The balance problem, in particular, can incapacitate an individual for short periods of time. Speech discrimination is often very poor in the affected ear. Typical audiometric results for a case with Ménière's disease are seen in Figure 8-4.

AUDIOMETRIC EVALUATION

Speech and Hearing Clinic, Idaho State University
Pocatello, Idaho 83209

AUDIOGRAM

FREQUENCY in Hertz (Hz)

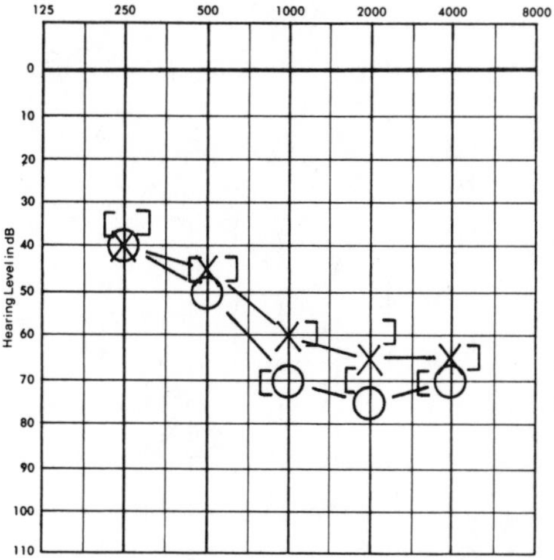

Key to Audiogram

EAR	AIR/MASKED		BONE/MASKED	
R	o	Δ	<	[
L	×	□	>	]

TYMPANOMETRY

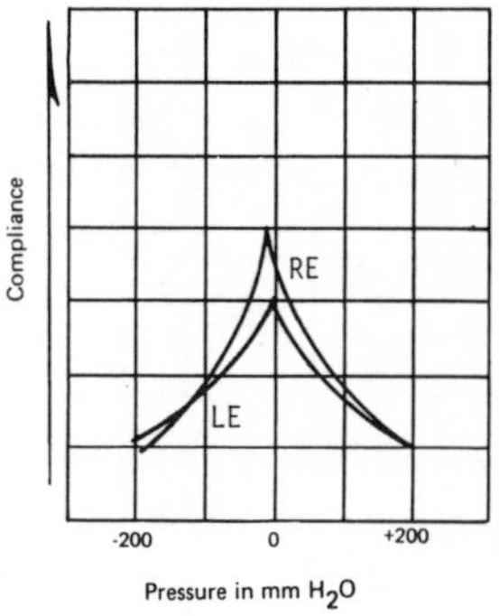

Speech Audiometry

	Pure Tones	Speech Thresholds		Speech Discrim.	
EAR	P T AVG 500-2000	SRT ~~SAT~~	dB RE / type	dB HL / %	dB RE / type
RIGHT		66		96 / 70 %	
LEFT		60		90 / 78 %	
BIN.				%	
		Spondees ☑ Numbers ☐ ______ ☐ MLV ☑ Rec. ☐	masking in opposite ear	W22 ☐ PBK ☑ PB50 ☐ ______ ☐ MLV ☑ Rec. ☐	masking in opposite ear

Figure 8-1. Hereditary auditory disorder in a 5-year-old child. *History*: Apparent hearing difficulties observed by parents at 6 months. Significant delay in speech and language development. No history of excessive conductive pathology. Hearing loss reported in father and uncle. *Audiometric results*: Moderate to severe hearing loss bilaterally, with no significant air-bone gaps. Type A tympanograms.

AUDIOMETRIC EVALUATION

Speech and Hearing Clinic, Idaho State University
Pocatello, Idaho 83209

AUDIOGRAM

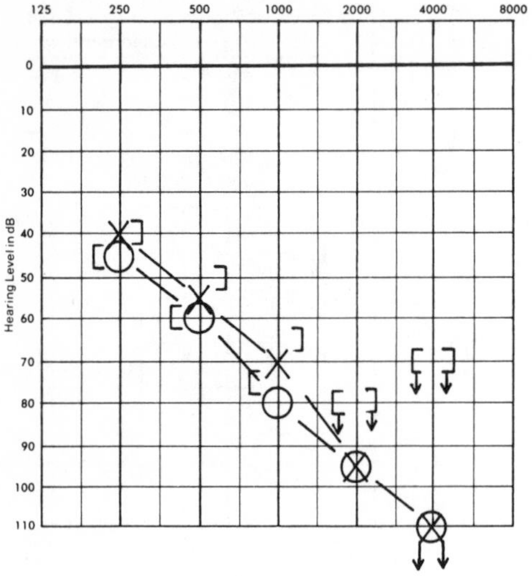

Key to Audiogram

EAR	AIR/MASKED		BONE/MASKED	
R	o	Δ	<	[
L	x	□	>	]

TYMPANOMETRY

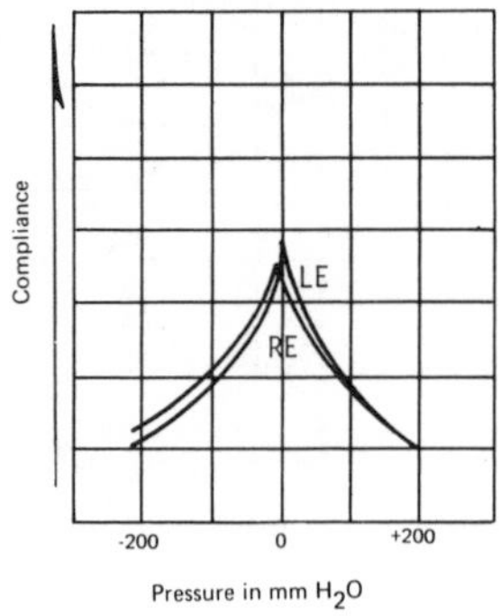

Speech Audiometry

	Pure Tones	Speech Thresholds		Speech Discrim.	
EAR	P T AVG 500-2000	~~SRT~~ SAT	dB RE / type	dB HL / %	dB RE / type
RIGHT		60		%	
LEFT		50		%	
BIN.				%	
		Spondees ☐ Numbers ☐ ________ ☐ MLV ☑ Rec. ☐	masking in opposite ear	W22 ☐ PBK ☐ PB50 ☐ ________ ☐ MLV ☐ Rec. ☐	masking in opposite ear

Figure 8-2. Hearing loss attributed to rubella in a 4-year-old child. *History*: Mother noted exposure to German measles during second month of pregnancy. Hearing loss noted at birth. No history of middle ear pathology. *Audiometric results*: Moderate to profound loss of hearing in each ear, with no significant air-bone gaps. Type A tympanograms bilaterally.

AUDIOMETRIC EVALUATION

Speech and Hearing Clinic, Idaho State University
Pocatello, Idaho 83209

AUDIOGRAM

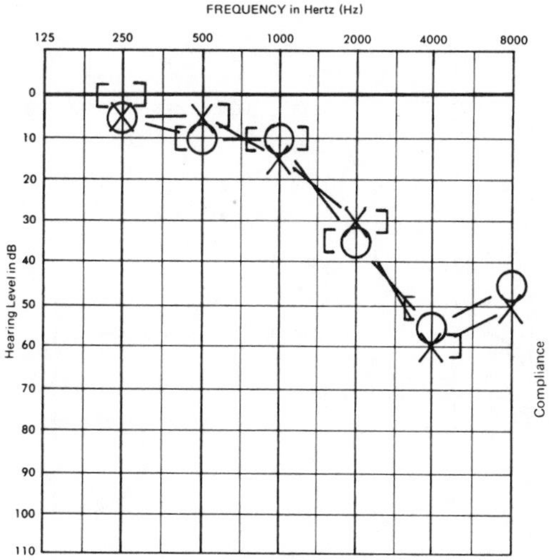

Key to Audiogram

EAR	AIR/MASKED		BONE/MASKED	
R	o	Δ	<	[
L	×	□	>	]

TYMPANOMETRY

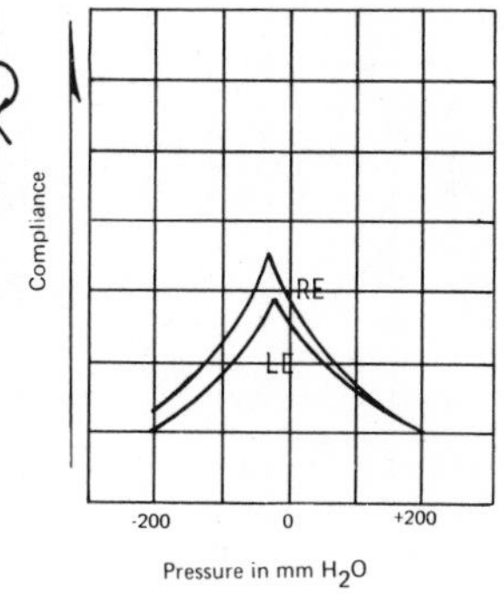

Speech Audiometry

	Pure Tones	Speech Thresholds		Speech Discrim.	
EAR	P T AVG 500-2000	SRT ~~SAT~~	dB RE type	dB HL %	dB RE type
RIGHT		10		40 84 %	
LEFT		8		38 88 %	
BIN.				%	
		Spondees ☑ Numbers ☐ ______ ☐ MLV ☐ Rec. ☑	masking in opposite ear	W22 ☑ PBK ☐ PB50 ☐ ______ ☐ MLV ☐ Rec. ☑	masking in opposite ear

Figure 8-3. Noise-induced hearing loss in a 40-year-old male. *History*: Patient reported employment in noisy plant for the past 5 years; no ear protection utilized. A considerable amount of high pitched tinnitus noted. Some difficulty in hearing speech. *Audiometric results*: Mild to moderate high frequency hearing loss bilaterally. No air-bone gaps. Type A tympanograms in each ear. Mild discrimination difficulties noted in right ear.

AUDIOMETRIC EVALUATION

Speech and Hearing Clinic, Idaho State University
Pocatello, Idaho 83209

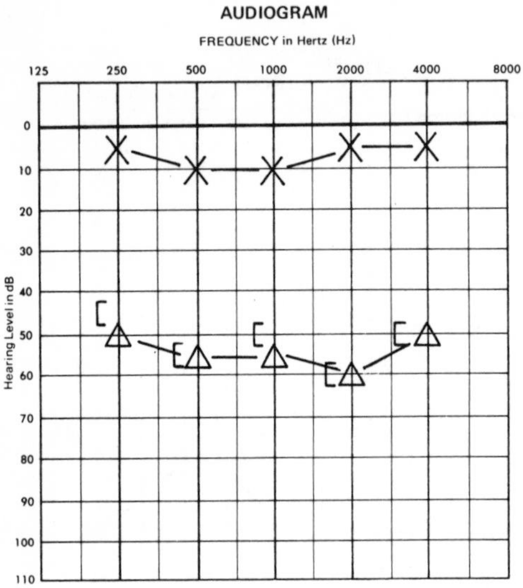

Key to Audiogram

EAR	AIR/MASKED		BONE/MASKED	
R	o	Δ	<	[
L	×	□	>	]

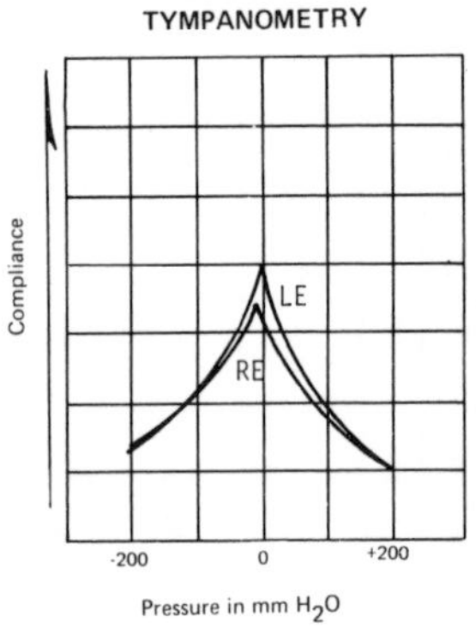

Speech Audiometry

	Pure Tones	Speech Thresholds		Speech Discrim.	
EAR	P T AVG 500-2000	SRT ~~SAT~~	dB RE / type	dB HL / %	dB RE / type
RIGHT		50	90	80 / 60 %	
LEFT		8		38 / 98 %	
BIN.				%	
		Spondees ☑ Numbers ☐ _____ ☐ MLV ☐ Rec. ☑	masking in opposite ear	W22 ☑ PBK ☐ PB50 ☐ _____ ☐ MLV ☐ Rec. ☑	masking in opposite ear

Figure 8-4. Audiometric results obtained in a patient with Ménière's disease. *History*: Patient initially experienced episodes of vertigo approximately 4 years ago. Feeling of fullness in right ear along with "buzzing" sound and progressive hearing loss. *Audiometric results*: Moderate loss of hearing in right ear, with hearing within normal limits in left ear. No air-bone gaps. Type A tympanograms. Significant speech discrimination difficulties in right ear.

Although relatively rare, tumors can appear along the pathway of the VIIIth nerve from the inner ear to the brain stem, usually within the internal auditory meatus or the cerebellopontine angle. These growths, conventionally termed acoustic neuromas, are generally benign and must be surgically removed. Hearing loss is usually present in the affected ear, with speech discrimination often being greatly disturbed (see Figure 8-5).

Other causes of sensorineural disorders seen in the general population include cochlear otosclerosis, labyrinthitis (infection within the inner ear), head trauma, and acoustic neuritis. The reader is referred to the suggested readings at the end of this chapter for a more in-depth discussion of these and other sensorineural impairments.

SENSORINEURAL DISORDERS IN THE ELDERLY

Presbycusis

Schuknecht's classification of presbycusis types (1955, 1964) serves as an effective means of discussing the manner in which the aging process manifests itself in sensorineural auditory disorders.

Sensory presbycusis is characterized by atrophy of the structures within the organ of Corti and, in some cases, degeneration of the auditory nerve in the basal end of the cochlea. According to Schuknecht (1964), the degenerative changes usually start in middle age but progress in a very gradual fashion in subsequent years. Figure 8-6 illustrates the nature of the atrophy of hair cells and spiral ganglion cells, as well as the associated pure tone audiometric results, for a 70-year-old patient identified by Schuknecht as having sensory presbycusis.

Schuknecht's second category, *neural presbycusis*, involves a loss of neurons in the auditory pathways and cochlea. Although neuronal degeneration begins relatively early in life, no significant loss of hearing results until much later, when the number of functional neurons is dramatically reduced. Unlike sensory presbycusis, neural degeneration may not manifest itself in a marked loss of auditory acuity. Rather, the chief feature of this form of presbycusis is sharply reduced speech discrimination abilities. Figure 8-7 shows the results of a histologic examination of a 70-year-old patient with neural presbycusis.

Metabolic presbycusis is felt to be the result of defects in the

AUDIOMETRIC EVALUATION

Speech and Hearing Clinic, Idaho State University
Pocatello, Idaho 83209

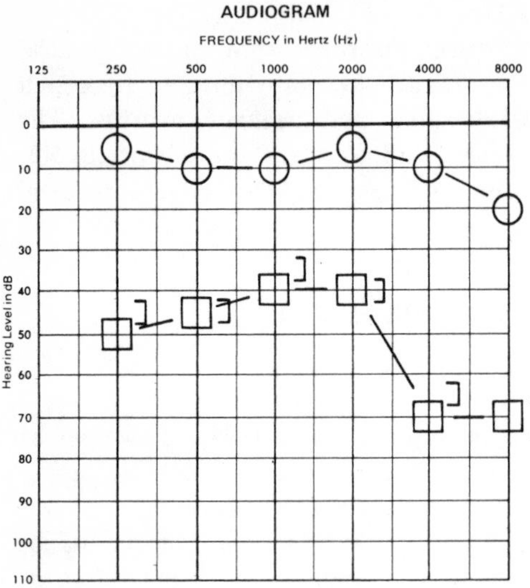

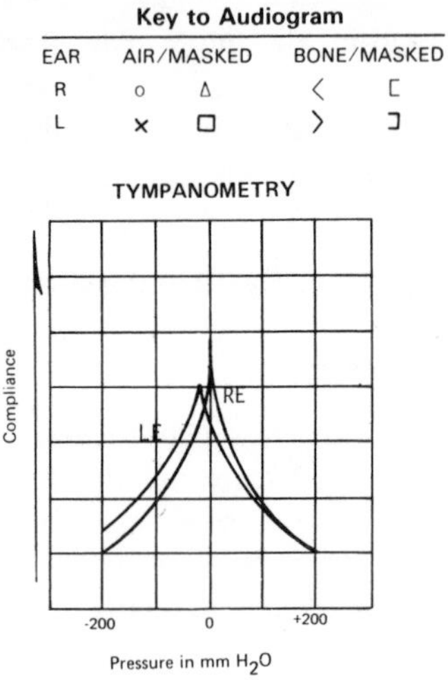

Speech Audiometry

	Pure Tones	Speech Thresholds		Speech Discrim.	
EAR	P T AVG 500-2000	SRT ~~SAT~~	dB RE / type	dB HL / %	dB RE / type
RIGHT		10		50 / 98 %	
LEFT		40	90	80 / 26 %	
BIN.				%	
		Spondees ☑ Numbers ☐ ______ ☐ MLV ☐ Rec. ☑	masking in opposite ear	W22 ☑ PBK ☐ PB50 ☐ ______ ☐ MLV ☐ Rec. ☑	masking in opposite ear

Figure 8-5. Audiometric results in a patient with an VIIIth nerve tumor. *History*: Patient noted a hearing loss in the left ear and excessive tinnitus. Some dizziness was also reported. Onset of loss apparently occurred within the last 6 weeks. *Audiometric results*: Moderate to severe hearing loss in the left ear with no air-bone gaps. Type A tympanograms bilaterally. Poor speech discrimination in the left ear only.

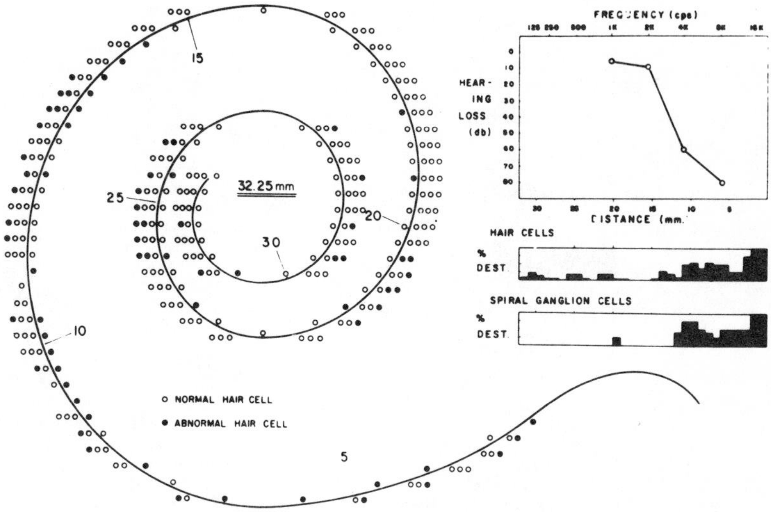

Figure 8-6. *Sensory presbycusis.* In the graphic reconstruction of the organ of Corti the black dots represent abnormal appearing hair cells and the open circles represent normal hair cells. In the audiogram frequency is arranged on the anatomic frequency scale (in accordance with their location along the basilar membrane). The barograms show the percentage of hair cell and ganglion cell loss in the cochlea as a function of distance along the basilar membrane. Thus, the audiometric data and pathology can be compared on parallel coordinates. In this case there is an atrophic change in the organ of Corti, most severe in the basal 11 mm accompanied by secondary nerve degeneration. (Source: Schuknecht, 1964.)

physical and chemical processes of production of the energy needed by the cochlea. It was Schuknecht's contention that atrophy of the stria vascularis is closely linked with this type of presbycusis. The audiometric and histologic results for an 89-year-old patient with metabolic presbycusis are shown in Figure 8-8. A flat configuration for the pure tone audiogram is thought to be characteristic of this form of presbycusis.

The last type identified by Schuknecht was *mechanical presbycusis*, which he attributed to abnormalities in the motion properties of the cochlear duct. Mechanical presbycusis is characterized by a sloping, high frequency hearing loss (see Figure 8-9).

A fifth form of presbycusis has recently been proposed by Johnson and Hawkins (1972), termed "vascular presbycusis." It involves the closure of small blood vessels supplying the spiral ligament and stria vascularis. Vascular presbycusis may actually be linked with metabolic presbycusis.

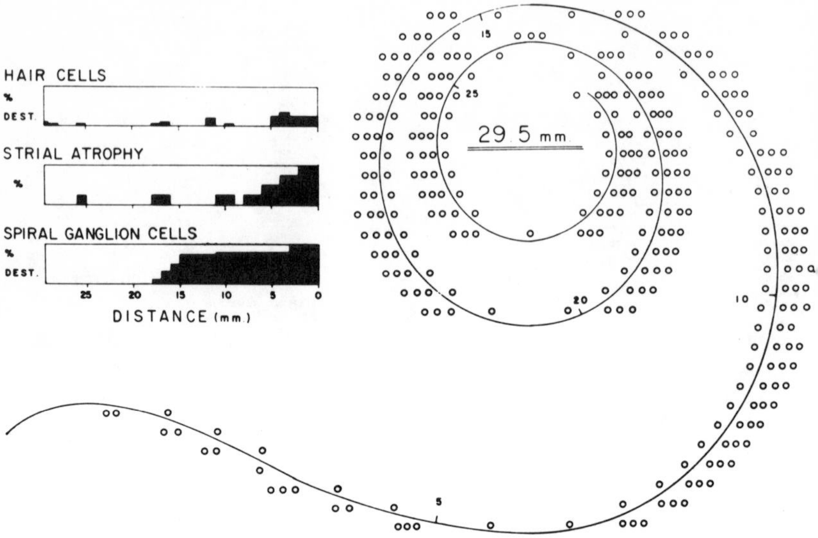

Figure 8-7. *Neural presbycusis.* There is very slight loss of hair cells in the organ of Corti mainly in the back region of the cochlear duct. There is also strial atrophy in the lower basal turn. The most striking finding, however, is severe loss of spiral ganglion cells in the basal 17 mm of the cochlea, a finding which probably is the cause for the severe loss in speech discrimination which this patient experienced during the terminal months of his life. (Source: Schuknecht, 1964.)

Each of these types of presbycusic hearing impairments involves some degree of degeneration within what has been referred to as the sensorineural mechanism. However, Schuknecht (1964) has pointed out that neural presbycusis is the result of neuron atrophy throughout the entire central nervous system. This implies the involvement of the neural pathways and centers of the brain stem and auditory cortex as well. For this reason, neural presbycusis is discussed further as a part of material associated with central auditory disorders in the elderly (Chapter 9).

Presbycusis and Speech Discrimination

The assessment of speech discrimination, in addition to pure tone and site of lesion audiometry, plays an important role in the audiometric assessment of the various forms of presbycusis. Discrimination abilities are impaired by all of the types of presbycusis, but the degree of impairment appears to be greatest with neural presbycusis (Schuknecht, 1964). Some concern has been raised in the literature regarding whether this decreased discrimination in most of the types

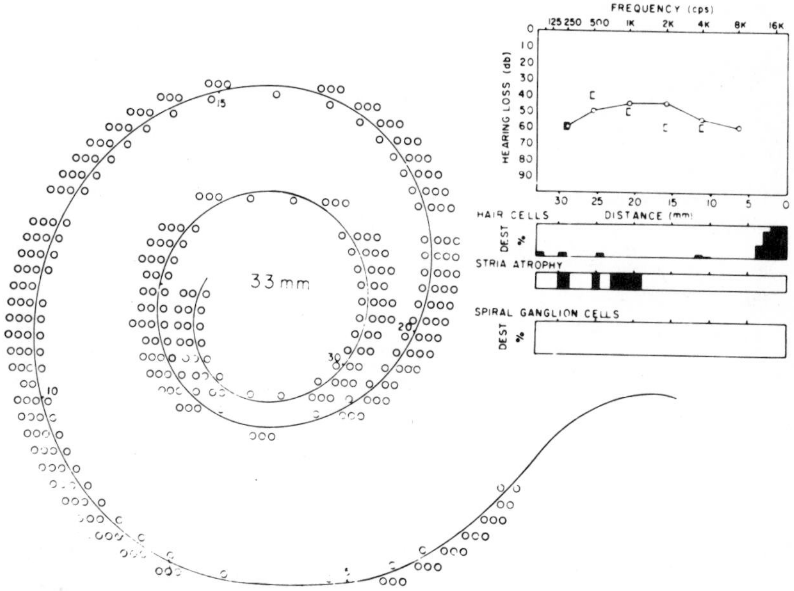

Figure 8-8. *Metabolic presbycusis.* There is hearing loss characterized by a flat audiometric curve. There is a loss of hair cells in the basal 4 mm of the cochlea representing a mild sensory presbycusis which is of no functional significance. The most striking finding is areas of atrophy of the stria vascularis in the apical half of the cochlea. (Source: Schuknecht, 1964.)

of presbycusis can be attributed to the age of the individual or the degree of sensorineural hearing loss. Gaeth (1948) found unusually poor discrimination in some elderly subjects which was unexpected on the basis of pure tone findings. Schuknecht (1955, 1964) and Hinchcliffe (1962) have suggested that a discrepancy between pure tone audiometry and speech discrimination results is evidence of brain stem or cortical involvement, but Harbert, Young, and Menduke (1966) cited evidence to show it is also present in the case of more peripheral damage. In fact, the Harbert et al. study seemed to indicate elderly subjects' discrimination is more related to speech reception threshold (degree of peripheral hearing loss) than to age and its associated neural degeneration. Kasden (1970) also presented evidence of this sort in support of the importance of the amount of acuity loss in determining discrimination abilities. He used two groups, one from 60 to 69 years of age and the other from 20 to 40 years; the groups were matched on the degree of hearing loss.

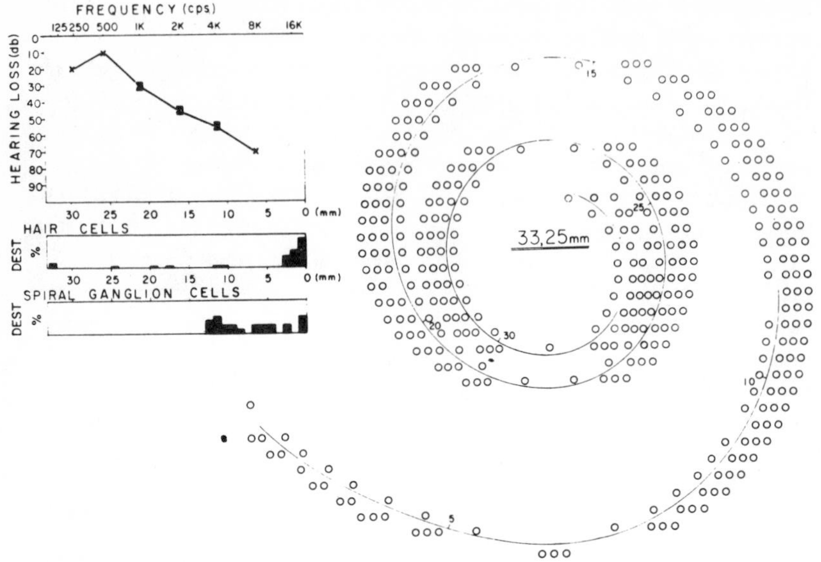

Figure 8-9. *Mechanical presbycusis.* A descending audiometric curve exists in the presence of a very small hair cell loss in the extreme basal end of the cochlea and a moderate ganglion cell loss in the basal 13.5 mm of the cochlea. These pathologic changes do not account for the functional loss. (Source: Schuknecht, 1964.)

He found no differences in speech discrimination scores between the two groups. Punch and McConnell (1969) found evidence to suggest that both age and degree of hearing loss can significantly influence speech discrimination.

No clear resolution has emerged concerning the degree to which age and amount of hearing loss influence speech discrimination. What is apparent is that both factors can and do produce decrements in speech discrimination in the elderly. The importance of each factor varies from case to case, although in instances where sharp discrepancies exist between acuity and speech discrimination measures, the likelihood of extensive neural atrophy within the auditory system appears more probable. Essentially all people with presbycusic hearing loss will have some degree of difficulty in speech discrimination, with the amount of difficulty being determined by the degree and location of the atrophy associated with aging.

The test procedures and material routinely employed in the assessment of speech discrimination with the general population may be useful in demonstrating deficiencies in speech discrimination with cases having presbycusis. This generally involves the presentation of monosyllabic word lists, such as the W-22s or NU-6s, under phones or in a sound field at a comfortable suprathreshold intensity level, usually 30–40 dB above the listener's speech reception threshold. Utilization of this testing regimen will show varying degrees of discrimination deficiencies, the precise amount dependent on factors such as degree of hearing loss, the frequencies involved in the impairment, and the specific speech discrimination list used during testing. In most sensorineural disorders, these factors will be closely associated with the discrimination score obtained. Exceptions to this include persons with Ménière's disease and acoustic neuromas. Schuknecht (1964) has stated that patients with presbycusic impairments which do not involve the auditory neural pathway will usually not have severe discrimination problems, while those with substantial neural degeneration within the auditory system will show marked difficulty. This is consistent with the research of others, including Hinchliffe (1962) and Kirikae, Sato, and Shitara (1964). In these instances, the degree of discrimination will far exceed the associated loss of acuity. Conventional auditory discrimination testing procedures may not be effective in revealing the presence of speech processing difficulties in neural presbycusis, and more specialized testing techniques are often necessary to disclose pathology of this nature. Further discussion on these methods is included in Chapter 9.

Noise-Induced Hearing Loss

As with younger age groups, the aged also may be afflicted with hearing impairment that stems directly from exposure to intense noise. Glorig (1958) has pointed out that this noise exposure may occur from two chief sources: 1) noise associated with an individual's employment (occupational hearing loss), and 2) noise connected with the activities of our modern society (sociocusis). With the older individual, the opportunity for noise exposure to occur from these two sources is increased by the factor of longevity. This will, of course, make it more likely that the elderly will have a higher incidence of noise-induced hearing loss than may be seen in younger age groups.

The existence of noise-induced hearing loss concurrently with presbycusis has resulted in considerable difficulty in isolating the amount of hearing loss that can be directly attributed to the process of aging. The potential contribution of each was alluded to in research conducted by Rosen and his co-workers (Rosen, Bergman,

Plester, El-Mofty, and Salti, 1962; Rosen, Plester, El-Mofty, and Rosen, 1964). These investigations involved the assessment of hearing acuity in the elder members of an isolated tribe living in the Sudan called the Mabaans. These studies (data shown in Figure 8-10) revealed that the Mabaans retained far superior hearing in advanced age than do the elderly in modern civilizations. This suggested the possibility that a substantial portion of the hearing loss commonly observed in the elderly in our society may be attributable to factors unrelated to aging, such as noise.

Ménière's Disease

Although Ménière's disease is thought to primarily affect persons from 30 to 60 years of age (Harken and McCabe, 1973), Mathog (Mathog, Paparella, Huff, Siegel, Lassman, and Bozarth, 1974) has stated that it is also observed in the elderly. The associated triad of symptoms—vertigo, tinnitus, and hearing impairment—can be very disturbing to a person of any age, but may be particularly distressful to the aged because of the many other adjustments they must undergo at the same time associated with growing old. Diuretics, sedatives, alterations in diet, and other procedures including surgery are often prescribed in the treatment of this disorder. Remission of symptoms related to Meniere's disease has been estimated to be in the vicinity of 60–70 percent, according to Huff (Mathog et al., 1974).

Labyrinthitis

Labyrinthitis, also termed otitis interna, involves an inflammation or infection of the labyrinth of the inner ear. According to Rossenwasser (1964), labyrinthitis can occur in the elderly, particularly in connection with the existence of chronic middle ear infection. It is Rossenwasser's contention that the incidence of chronic middle ear pathology is relatively high in the elderly, especially in those cases with accompanying diabetes. This fact makes it more likely for further complications, such as labyrinthitis, to occur in older individuals, since infection within the middle ear may reach the inner ear via the oval or round window. Severe to profound hearing loss may result in the affected ear if medicinal and/or surgical intervention is not initiated early in the progression of the disorder.

Sudden Hearing Loss

The high incidence of arteriosclerosis in the elderly makes it impor-

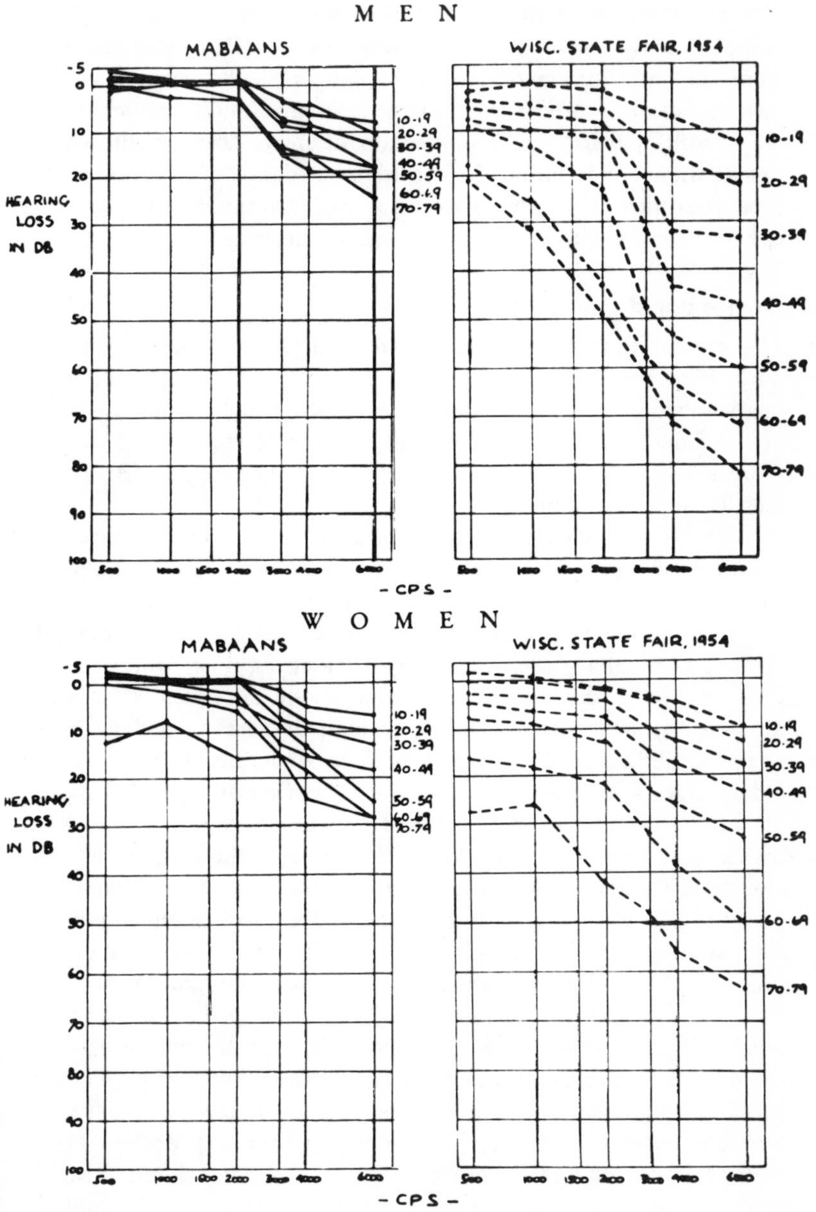

Figure 8-10. Comparison between decade audiograms (medians used) of African Mabaan and American women and men as a function of age. (Source: Rosen, et al., 1962.)

tant to be aware of the possibility of the onset of a sudden, unilateral hearing loss in this population (Snow, 1973). This can stem from the interruption of the blood supply to the cochlea via the internal auditory artery. A severe to profound auditory impairment may result, particularly if immediate intensive therapy directed at vasodilation is not initiated. The high incidence of diabetes in the aged (Bacchus, 1977), with its associated arteriosclerosis, serves to enhance the likelihood of vascular-related hearing loss.

Drug-Induced Ototoxicity

The probability of drug-induced ototoxicity in advancing age is quite high because of at least two factors: 1) the high volume of medication utilized in the treatment of acute and chronic disorders in the elderly, and 2) the possibility that older individuals may be more susceptible to ototoxicity, as reported by Finegold (Bergstrom and Thompson, 1976).

The sensorineural hearing loss which results from the intake of certain antibiotics, such as neomycin, streptomycin, and gentamycin, can be of severe proportions and is almost always permanent.

Worthy of special attention is the ototoxic effect of the salicylates, particularly aspirin. This particular form of drug normally does not have any ototoxic effect if taken infrequently in small amounts. However, if it is taken in high dosages on a daily basis, as in the treatment of arthritis, a mild to moderate hearing loss may result (Myers and Bernstein, 1965). The excessive use of aspirin usually results in a mild sensorineural impairment bilaterally. What makes this type of ototoxic loss different from those discussed previously is the fact that, except in rare instances (Jarvis, 1966), the hearing loss is reversible if the amount of medication is reduced substantially. The high incidence of arthritis in the elderly makes it probable that salicylate ototoxicity is relatively common in the aged.

It is felt that a thorough history regarding medication usage be obtained routinely with older patients whenever possible to assist in the detection of cases with ototoxicity associated with drugs. Patients for whom ototoxic medications have been prescribed should receive frequent hearing evaluations to closely monitor any decrements in auditory functioning which may occur. Attempts should also be made to reduce the use of excessive amounts of potentially ototoxic drugs, including aspirin, whenever possible.

SUGGESTED READINGS

Mathog, R., Paparella, M., Huff, J., Siegel, L., Lassman, F., and Bozarth, M. Common hearing disorders. Geriatrics, 49–88 (1974).

Willeford, J. The geriatric patient. In D. Rose (ed.), Audiological Assessment. Englewood Cliffs, N.J.: Prentice-Hall, 1971.

REFERENCES

Bacchus, H. Rational Management of Diabetes. Baltimore: University Park Press, 1977.

Bergstrom, L., and Thompson, P. Ototoxicity. In J. Northern (ed.), Hearing Disorders. Boston: Little, Brown, 1976.

Gaeth, J. A study of phonemic regression associated with hearing loss. Unpublished doctoral dissertation, Northwestern University, Evanston, Ill., 1948.

Glorig, A. Noise and Your Ear. New York: Grune & Stratton, 1958.

Harbert, F., Young, I., and Menduke, H. Audiological findings in presbycusis. Journal of Auditory Research, 6, 297–312 (1966).

Harken, L., and McCabe, B. Meniere's disease and other peripheral labyrinthine disorders. In M. Paparella and D. Shumrick (eds.), Otolaryngology (Vol. 2: The Ear). Philadelphia: W. B. Saunders, 1973.

Hinchcliffe, R. The anatomical locus of presbycusis. Journal of Speech and Hearing Disorders, 27, 301–310 (1962).

Jaffe, B. (ed.). Hearing Loss in Children. University Park Press, Baltimore, 1977.

Jarvis, J. A case of unilateral permanent deafness following acetylsalicylic acid. Journal of Laryngology, 318 (1966).

Johnson, L., and Hawkins, J. Sensory and neural degeneration with aging seen in micro-dissections of the human inner ear. Annals of Otology, Rhinology and Laryngology, 81, 179–193 (1972).

Kasden, S. Speech discrimination in two age groups matched for hearing loss. Journal of Auditory Research, 10, 210–212 (1970).

Kirikae, I., Sato, T., and Shitara, T. A study of hearing in advanced age. Laryngoscope, 74, 205–220 (1964).

Mathog, R., Paparella, M., Huff, J., Siegel, L., Lassman, F., and Bozarth, M. Common hearing disorders. Geriatrics, 49–88 (1974).

Myers, E., and Bernstein, J. Salicylate ototoxicity—a clinical and experimental study. Archives of Otolaryngology, 82, 483–493 (1965).

Northern, J., and Downs, M. Hearing in Children. Baltimore: Williams & Wilkins, 1974.

Punch, J., and McConnell, F. The speech discrimination function of elderly adults. Journal of Auditory Research, 9, 159–166 (1969).

Rosen, S., Bergman, M., Plester, D., El-Mofty, A., and Salti, M. Presbycusis study of a relatively noise-free population in the Sudan. Annals of Otology, Rhinology and Laryngology, 71, 727–743 (1962).

Rosen, S., Plester, D., El-Mofty, A., and Rosen, H. High frequency audiometry in presbycusis. Archives of Otolaryngology, 79, 18–32 (1964).
Rossenwasser, H. Otitic problems in the aged. Geriatrics, 19, 11–17 (1964).
Sataloff, J. Hearing Loss. Philadelphia: J. B. Lippincott, 1966.
Schuknecht, H. Presbycusis. Laryngoscope, 65, 402–419 (1955).
Schuknecht, H. Further observations on the pathology of presbycusis. Archives of Otolaryngology, 80, 369–382 (1964).
Snow, J. Sudden deafness. In M. Paparella and D. Shumrick (eds.), Otolaryngology (Vol. 2: The Ear). Philadelphia: W. B. Saunders, 1973.

Chapter 9
Central Auditory Disorders

The major types of central auditory disorders are reviewed for both the general population and the aged. Many of the tests which have been proposed for assessment of central impairments are also discussed.

MAJOR TYPES OF CENTRAL AUDITORY DISORDERS IN THE GENERAL POPULATION

Auditory impairments stemming from lesions located within the brain stem or auditory cortex are referred to as central auditory disorders. According to Jerger (1973a), the two principal loci of auditory disorders within the central nervous system are: 1) the brain stem pathway in the lateral lemniscus, and 2) the primary auditory projection area (Heschl's gyrus) on the superior convolution of the temporal lobe of the brain. Most of these disorders stem from one of the following conditions: congenital factors, physical trauma and tumors, vascular abnormalities, and neural abnormalities.

Congenital Factors

Numerous congenital factors may be associated with the existence of central auditory disorders. Northern and Downs (1974) described both genetic and nongenetic conditions which may result in central nervous system damage, including the auditory neural structures. This includes maternal rubella, where central deafness may occur along with both conductive and sensorineural auditory disorders. Improper or lack of development of certain critical structures of the central auditory system during embryologic development may also occur. Rh incompatibility has also been discussed in connection with central auditory deafness. Papparella and Capps (1973) cited evidence by Goodhill (1967) to the effect that cochlear pathology is minimal or absent in cases of kernicterus deafness. Because mental retardation and cerebral palsy are associated with this type of deafness,

Papparella and Capps concluded that a lesion therefore probably occurs in the central nervous system to explain the auditory deficit. Carhart (1967) suggested that the hearing loss observed in cases with Rh incompatibility may be attributable to involvement within the cochlear nuclei rather than the cochlea. Northern and Downs (1974) indicated that conflicting reports concerning the precise location of the lesion associated with this disorder suggest that its location is as yet unresolved, with evidence available which suggests the possible involvement of the cochlea, cochlear nuclei, and the central nervous system. Further research on this matter is clearly warranted.

Other congenital factors discussed as potential causes of central auditory disorders include physical trauma and anoxia, which may occur during the birth process (Martin, 1975).

Trauma and Tumors

Head trauma has been singled out by Mathog (1973) as a definite cause of central hearing impairments. Direct insults to the skull can result in substantial neural damage at the level of the brain stem and the auditory cortex. Tumors within the brain stem or the temporal lobe may also precipitate central auditory dysfunctions. Jerger (1973a) and Lynn and Gilroy (1976), among others, have thoroughly described the audiometric results generally observed in patients with a wide variety of tumors within the central nervous system through a presentation of case studies. Surgical removal of the tumor will inevitably result in some degree of central auditory impairment, with the extent and nature of the dysfunction dependent on variables such as the location and size of the tumor and the degree of trauma which occurs as a consequence of its removal.

Vascular Abnormalities

The inability of the vascular system to supply oxygen to the central nervous system, including those neurologic structures critical for the process of audition, can lead to severe damage. Disturbances of this type within the vascular system can take one of a number of forms. Among these are blood clots, which can occur as a consequence of embolisms or thromboses. Clotting can lead to a disruption in the flow of blood and/or a rupture of the wall of the blood vessel involved. When such a rupture occurs, this is termed a vascular accident. A cerebrovascular accident, or stroke, occurs exclusively within the brain, resulting in specific damage to those tissues normally supplied by the ruptured vessel. Closely associated with vascular accidents is arteriosclerosis, a disorder which manifests itself in increased rigidity of the walls of blood vessels and a thickening and narrowing of their inner walls, caused by an accumulation of fatty deposits. The increased rigidity and narrowing of these vessels can result in disruption of the flow of blood from clogging and rupturing of the vessel walls. Cerebral arteriosclerosis, of course, poses a direct threat to the normal functioning of the cortical areas of the auditory system.

Neural Abnormalities

As discussed previously in Chapter 4 in connection with the auditory structures of the central nervous system, degeneration of neural tissue within the central nervous system does occur as a direct consequence of the process of aging (Brody, 1955; Schuknecht, 1955, 1964; Hinchcliffe, 1962; Kirikae, Sato, and Shitara, 1964). Their research, however, has suggested that the process of degeneration may actually start in mid-life and progress rather steadily throughout the latter stages of life. Other types of neural degeneration may also occur with certain disorders, such as multiple sclerosis and syphilis, which can also have a devastating effect on central auditory processing (Pinsker, 1972).

CENTRAL AUDITORY DISORDERS IN THE ELDERLY

As expected, all of the conditions discussed previously may serve to explain the presence of central auditory disorders in the elderly. However, certain of these conditions are more frequently involved with this specific age group because of factors associated with aging. Among these are cerebrovascular accidents (CVA or stroke) and neural presbycusis. The high incidence of cerebrovascular accidents in the aged can be primarily attributed to the preponderance of arteriosclerosis in persons of advanced age. According to Busse (1959), patients displaying symptoms of a brain disorder stemming from cerebral arteriosclerosis have an average age of 66 years, although numerous cases of the disease have occurred far earlier in life. It also appears that arteriosclerotic disease is much more common in males than in females (Malamud, 1972). According to Schuknecht (1955), neural degeneration occurs independently of cerebral arteriosclerosis, but may exist simultaneously in varying degrees. These two conditions, then, appear to contribute significantly toward the high incidence of central auditory pathology in the elderly.

ASSESSMENT OF CENTRAL FUNCTION

Detection of disorders within the central portion of the auditory system with the conventional audiometric battery of tests has, until recent years, been a relatively difficult task. Conventional tests were developed exclusively for the assessment of peripheral auditory dysfunctions. A listing of the effects of central auditory pathology, provided by Hodgson (1972, p. 313) serves to explain, in part, why these tests have not been effective. These are:

1. Little or no change in threshold for pure tones or speech
2. Little or no change in performance on suprathreshold pure tone tests
3. Reduction in speech discrimination ability on the ear contralateral to the lesion, particularly when the speech is made more difficult by distortion
4. Reduced discrimination of binaural messages when part of the information is presented to one ear and part to the other
5. Reduced discrimination of monaural messages in the presence of a competing signal in the other ear

The normal administration of pure tone audiometry and site of lesion tests, such as the SISI, ABLB-MLB, Bekesy, and tone decay, with a person having central pathology generally will result in normal or near normal findings, making an accurate diagnosis based on these tests virtually impossible. The standard speech discrimination test, while effective in some cases with central disorders, will usually not provide diagnostically relevant information either.

An obvious need existed for some time for the development of tests which would be effective in revealing the presence of central auditory disorders. This need was partially met by the early work of two Italians, Bocca and Calearo. Their investigations (Bocca, Calearo and Cassinari, 1954; Bocca, 1955; Bocca, Calearo, Cassinari, and Miglivacca, 1955; Calearo, 1957; Bocca and Calearo, 1963) served to establish that temporal lobe lesions would manifest themselves in significantly depressed speech discrimination scores in the ear opposite the hemisphere of the brain having the disorder. They found that this was particularly true if one of a variety of modifications was made in the speech material presented to make it a more difficult perceptual task for the listener. Subsequent contributions by a host of investigators (Goetzinger and Rousey, 1959; Matzger, 1959; Katz, 1962, 1968; Jerger and Jerger, 1971; and many others) resulted in refinements in the basic procedures brought forth by the Italians, as well as the introduction of new approaches to the assessment of central auditory disorders. The next portion of this discussion reviews several of the currently utilized tests which have been designed for this purpose.

CENTRAL AUDITORY TESTS

Rh Difference Test

The Rh Difference Test was first suggested by Goetzinger and Roussey (1959). It involves the use of the Rush-Hughes recordings of the PB-50s, along with the W-22s. When these two tests are administered to an individual, a relatively large difference is observed in the discrimination scores obtained. This is the result of the increased difficulty of the Rush-Hughes Test, which is, in part, the result of distortion in the material stemming from poor recording quality. Goetzinger and Roussey found this difference in the scores between these two tests to be in the vicinity of 20% for subjects without central disorders. When the difference score exceeded 30%, the likelihood of central auditory pathology is increased. The abnormally large difference score is always observed in the ear contralateral to the involved temporal lobe. Table 9-1 contains the mean scores for the W-22 and Rush-Hughes tests, as well as the difference score, for a large group of listeners as a function of age, as reported by Goetzinger (1972). Note the sharp increase in the magnitude of the difference score for the group with a mean age of 84 years. According to Goetzinger, this is a strong suggestion of central auditory dysfunction.

The Rush-Hughes Difference Score Test is easily administered. The W-22s and Rush-Hughes Tests are simply administered via earphones in a monaural listening condition at quite high sensation levels (40 dB SL for the W-22s and approximately 50 dB SL for the Rush-Hughes Test) and percentage scores calculated for each. The score for the Rush-Hughes Test is then subtracted from the W-22 score, resulting in the difference score.

Performance-Intensity Function for Phonetically Balanced Words

The performance-intensity function for PB words, generally referred to as the PI-PB function, was developed by Jerger and Jerger (1971). In this test PB discrimination lists are presented in each ear at four

Table 9-1. Means and standard deviations for recorded W-22 and Rush-Hughes tests as well as for the difference scores (D/S) of normal hearing subjects with reference to age

			W-22		Rush-Hughes			
Number of ears	Chronologic age (mean)	SRT mean	Mean	SD	Mean	SD	D/S	D/S SD
	yrs							
30	11½	normal	94.3	1.8	75.1	5.2	19.2	4.7
40	27	5.0	97.0	2.1	81.0	4.6	16.3	4.5
10	46	1.2	97.8	1.7	81.6	4.4	16.6	4.8
64	66	12.8	88.0	10.2	67.8	12.0	20.0	7.0
64	74	15.9	81.2	12.7	58.0	14.9	22.8	9.3
64	84	26.5	78.1	8.5	43.8	14.5	33.2	10.8
			Sensorineurals[a]					
18	56	39.9	86.7	10.8	62.6	16.1	24.0	8.5

Source: Goetzinger and Rousey (1959).

[a] Data are shown also for subjects with sensorineural hearing loss.

to five different sensation levels ranging from 10 to 50 dB. The resulting discrimination scores are plotted as a function of intensity, as seen in Figure 9-1. Individuals with normal hearing or having a conductive or cochlear auditory disorder usually will display a PI-PB function that rises gradually as the intensity of the speech material is increased until a maximum performance level is reached. This is followed by a leveling off or a slight decrease in the function as the intensity is increased further. According to Jerger (1973a), a person showing a consistent ear difference in the PI-PB function, with no corresponding difference in the results of pure tone testing, should be suspected of having a central auditory disorder. A feature Jerger termed rollover in the PI-PB function is also considered to be indicative of central dysfunction. Here the PI-PB function does not remain relatively level as intensity of the speech material is increased beyond the maximum discrimination score obtained. Rather, there is a sharp decrease in the performance of the listener, resulting in a rollover in the PI-PB function. This is shown in Figure 9-2. Any case in which rollover in the PI-PB function occurs, or where significant asymmetry exists in the PI-PB functions of the two ears even though pure tone results are similar, should be suspected of having some type of central auditory pathology on the side opposite the affected ear (Jerger, 1973a). Gang (1976) has found similar rollover results in cases with suspected neural presbycusis. According to Gang, this may limit the

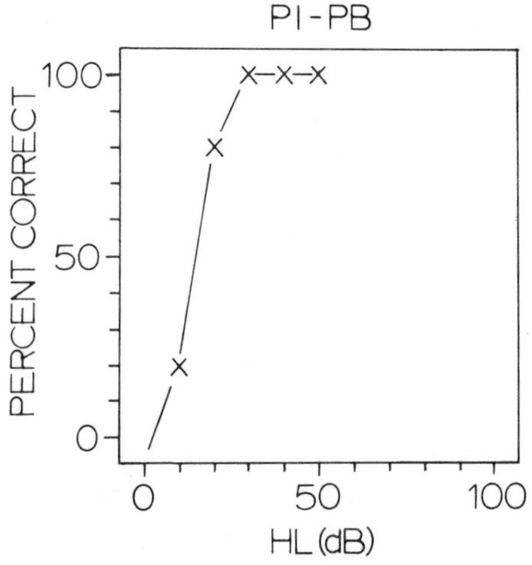

Figure 9-1. Example of normal PI-PB function.

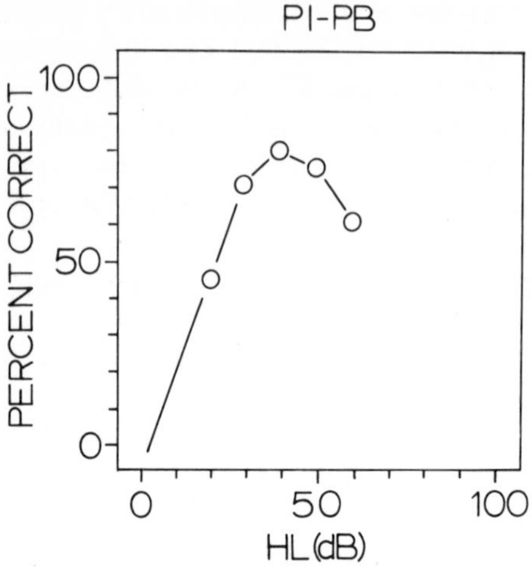

Figure 9-2. Example of rollover in the PI-PB function.

applicability of the rollover phenomenon in the PI-PB function with the elderly. This procedure appears, however, to show promise in identifying persons with substantial neural degeneration within the central auditory system.

Filtered Speech Tests

The use of filtered speech material in the assessment of central auditory disorders was substantiated by the research of Bocca et al. (1954). In their investigation PB disyllabic word lists were distorted by being passed through a low pass filter, which eliminated a majority of the acoustic energy contained in the frequencies above 800 Hz. When this material was presented monaurally, the authors found that patients with temporal lobe tumors demonstrated substantially reduced discrimination scores in the ear contralateral to the tumor when compared to the scores obtained from the other ear. However, no substantial ear differences were noted when unfiltered speech stimuli were presented under similar circumstances.

In 1960 Jerger used a similar approach with PB-50 lists, filtering out frequencies above 500 Hz. Using subjects with normal hearing sensitivity and good speech discrimination scores with unfiltered speech, Jerger found about 30% poorer discrimination on the ear contralateral to the temporal lobe lesion when the filtered PBs were utilized. Other investigations (Jerger, 1964; Goetzinger and Angell, 1965; Hodgson, 1967) revealed similar findings with filtered speech presented monaurally.

Filtered speech material can also be effective in the detection of central auditory pathology when presented binaurally in a dichotic manner. The basic procedure calls for speech material to be filtered into two separate frequency bands, for example, 300–600 Hz and 1800–2400 Hz. One band is presented to one ear while the other is simultaneously presented to the other ear. Persons having a normal central auditory system will be capable of fusing the material into an intelligible whole, while those with central pathology, particularly brain stem disorders, will not be able to do so with any degree of effectiveness. The findings of Matzger (1959) and Smith and Resnick (1969) and others have lended further support to the use of this form of test in the assessment of central lesions.

The Staggered Spondaic Word Test

The Staggered Spondaic Word Test, developed by Katz (1962, 1968), involves the presentation of two spondee words, one to each ear, in an overlapping fashion. The first syllable of one spondee is presented to one ear with no competing signal in the other ear. Just as the second syllable of the spondee in that ear is being presented, the first syllable of the second spondee is presented simultaneously in the opposite ear; each signal thus serves as a competing message to the other. The last syllable of the second word is produced without any competing signal in the opposite ear. An example of the sequencing involved in the presentation of two spondees for the Staggered Spondaic Word Test (SSW) is shown in Figure 9-3.

It is possible to record one's own test material for the SSW, but a recorded version of the test is available.[1] A high quality stereo tape recorder is used in conjunction with a two-channel speech audiometer to administer the SSW. Test items are given at a 50 dB SL, and the listener is asked to repeat back both spondees. Forty spondee pairs are presented and a percentage of correct responses is calculated for each ear and for both ears combined. Significantly reduced scores suggest the presence of central auditory pathology on the side contralateral to the ear affected.

[1] Available from Hearing and Speech Department, Menorah Medical Center 4949 Rockhill Road, Kansas City, Mo. 64110.

	Time →		
	1	2	3
Right ear	OUT	SIDE	
Left ear		IN	LAW

Figure 9-3. Example of the sequencing involved in the presentation of two spondees for the SSW. (Source: Martin, 1975.)

Synthetic Sentence Identification Tests

In 1965 Speaks and Jerger developed artificial or synthetic sentences to be used for speech discrimination testing. An example of a list of 10 such sentences is shown in Table 9-2. The subject is given the list and instructed to indicate which sentence was produced after the presentation of each sentence.

Jerger (1973a) extended this basic format by also including both ipsilateral and contralateral competing messages in the form of continuous discourse. For the ipsilateral competing message procedure using the synthetic sentence identification (SSI-ICM), both the sentences and the competing message are presented via earphone to the same ear at varying intensity levels. According to Jerger, when the message (synthetic sentences) and the competition (connected discourse) are at the same intensity level, normal listeners usually perform at 100%. When the message is 10 dB less than the competition, the score for normal listeners drops to around 80%. When the message is presented at 20 and 30 dB below the compe-

Table 9-2. A list of 10 synthetic sentences: Sample message set consisting of 10 alternative synthetic sentences, constructed as third-order approximations to real sentences

Alternative sentences
1. Small boat with a picture has become
2. Built the government with the force almost
3. Go change your car color is red
4. Forward march said the boy had a
5. March around without a care in your
6. That neighbor who said business is better
7. Battle cry and be better than ever
8. Down by the time is real enough
9. Agree with him only to find out
10. Women view men with green paper should

Source: Jerger (1973a).

tition, the average scores of normal listeners drop to 55 and 20%, respectively. Jerger feels that the SSI-ICM is sensitive to brain stem auditory lesions. In such cases the ear contralateral to the deficit will perform markedly poorer than the other ear as the message-to-competition ratio is made less favorable, and will also yield scores markedly deviant from those usually obtained with normal subjects (see Figure 9-4). With presbycusic cases, Jerger (1973b) has found the SSI-ICM procedure to be effective in isolating neural involvement.

In the contralateral competing message procedure (SSI-CCM) synthetic sentence material is presented to one ear and connected discourse goes to the opposite ear. As with the SSI-ICM, the message-to-competition ratio is varied from 0 dB (message and competition having equal intensity) to –40 dB (message 40 dB less than competition). In normal listeners, performance will generally remain at or near 100% for all of these ratios. Jerger (1973a) stated that persons with temporal lobe disorders will experience substantial difficulty when the message is presented to the ear contralateral to the central lesion and the competition is sent to the other ear, as shown in Figure 9-5. Patients with brain stem disorders, according to Jerger, usually experience little difficulty with the SSI-CCM.

In summary, Jerger (1973a) has suggested that the SSI-ICM is particularly effective in detecting brain stem disorders, while the

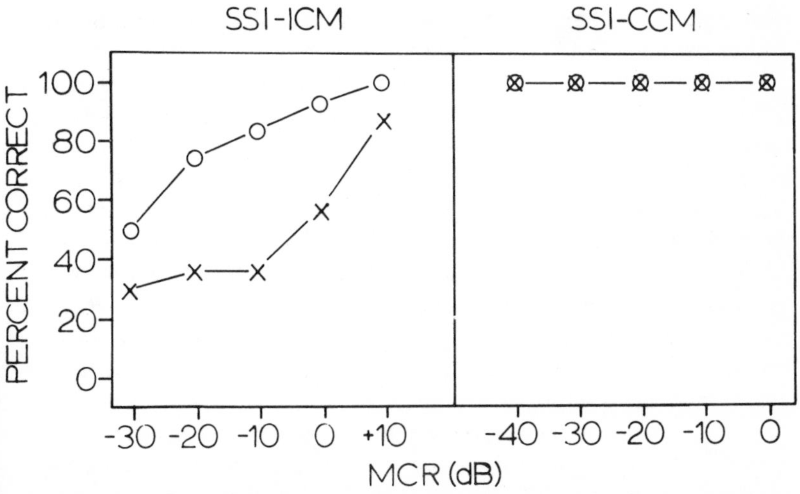

Figure 9-4. Example of abnormal SSI-ICM performance in case with brain stem pathology.

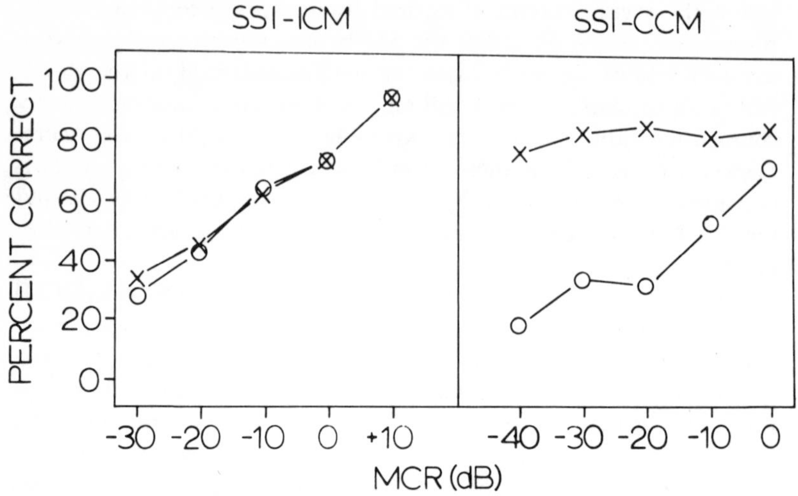

Figure 9-5. Example of abnormal SSI-CCM performance in patient with temporal lobe lesion.

SSI-CCM is able to reveal pathology within the temporal lobe of the central auditory system. Use of the SSI under these two conditions can prove beneficial in the differentiation of brain stem and temporal lobe disorders.

Temporally Distorted Speech Material

Athough not as firmly established as a test of central auditory disorders as many of the other procedures previously discussed, the use of temporal or time-distorted speech stimuli has been shown to be effective in identifying impairments of this type (Calearo and Lazzaroni, 1957; Bocca and Calearo, 1963; deQuiros, 1964). As the term implies, temporally distorted speech testing involves the assessment of speech perception skills at suprathreshold intensity levels with speech material in which the time parameter has been altered by either compressing or lengthening the duration of the utterance presented to the listener. The reader is referred to Beasley and Maki (1976) for further elaboration on time-altered speech, including discussion pertaining to the various methods of altering the temporal dimension of speech stimuli.

The effects of aging on the intelligibility of time-compressed speech have been investigated by numerous researchers. Luterman, Welsh, and Melrose (1966) presented 10 and 20% time-compressed PB word lists (W-22s) to three groups of listeners, a group of normal hearing young adults, a group of young subjects with sensorineural hearing loss, and a group of aged persons also having sensorineural impairments. The authors found that no significant difference occurred in the performance of the older subjects, relative to the two younger groups, for time-compressed speech when compared with speech discrimination results obtained with no compression. Their results are shown in Figure 9-6.

In another investigation of age and the perception of time-compressed speech, Sticht and Gray (1969) presented PB word lists time-compressed by 36, 46, and 59% to four different subject groups distinguished on the basis of age and type of hearing loss. These groups included: 1) seven normal hearing young adults, 2) seven normal hearing adults over 60 years of age, 3) seven young adults with sensorineural hearing loss, and 4) seven individuals over 60 years of age, also having a sensorineural impairment. As indicated in Figure 9-7, Sticht and Gray found that the two groups of older subjects experienced substantially greater decrements in intelligibility than the younger subjects as the rate of compression of the speech stimuli increased from 36 to 59%. These results clearly suggested an inability on the part of the older listener to adequately process time-compressed speech. The fact that the young and old

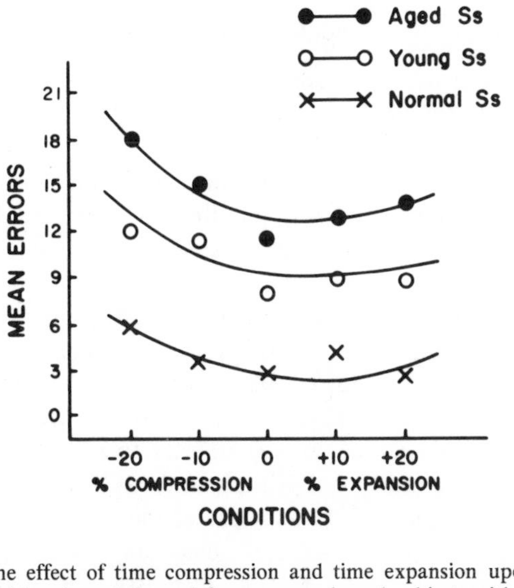

Figure 9-6. The effect of time compression and time expansion upon intelligibility scores for normal hearing adults and for young and aged subjects with high frequency hearing losses. (Source: Adapted from Luterman et al., 1966.)

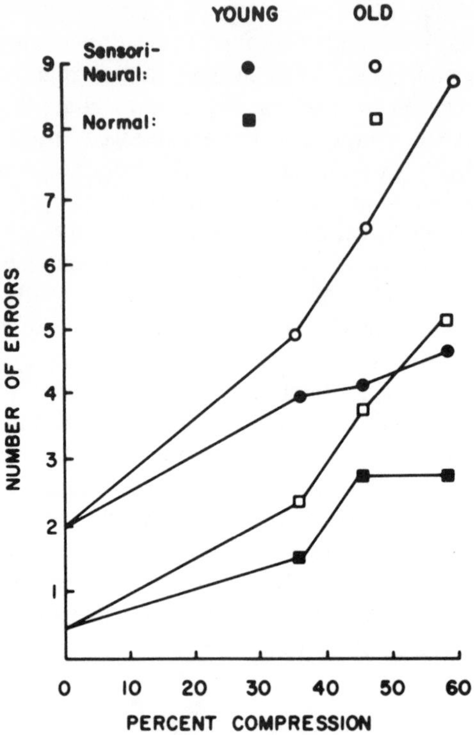

Figure 9-7. Effect of time compression on intelligibility scores of normal and sensorineural hearing-impaired young and elderly listeners. (Source: Adapted from Sticht and Gray, 1969.)

subjects were matched in regard to auditory acuity prompted Sticht and Gray to speculate that this inability to discriminate time-compressed speech resulted from involvement of the central auditory mechanism.

These findings were substantiated further by the investigation of Konkle, Beasley, and Bess (1977) with four groups of elderly subjects from 54 to 60, 61 to 67, 68 to 74, and 75 years and older. Their findings, shown in Figure 9-8, reveal a clear distinction between the performances of young subjects from previous investigations (Beasley, Foreman, and Rintelmann, 1972; Beasley, Schwimmer, and Rintelmann, 1972) and those of the older subject groups at all rates of time compression and sensation levels employed. The data also indicated a trend toward increasing intelligibility decrements for time-altered speech with increasing age within the older

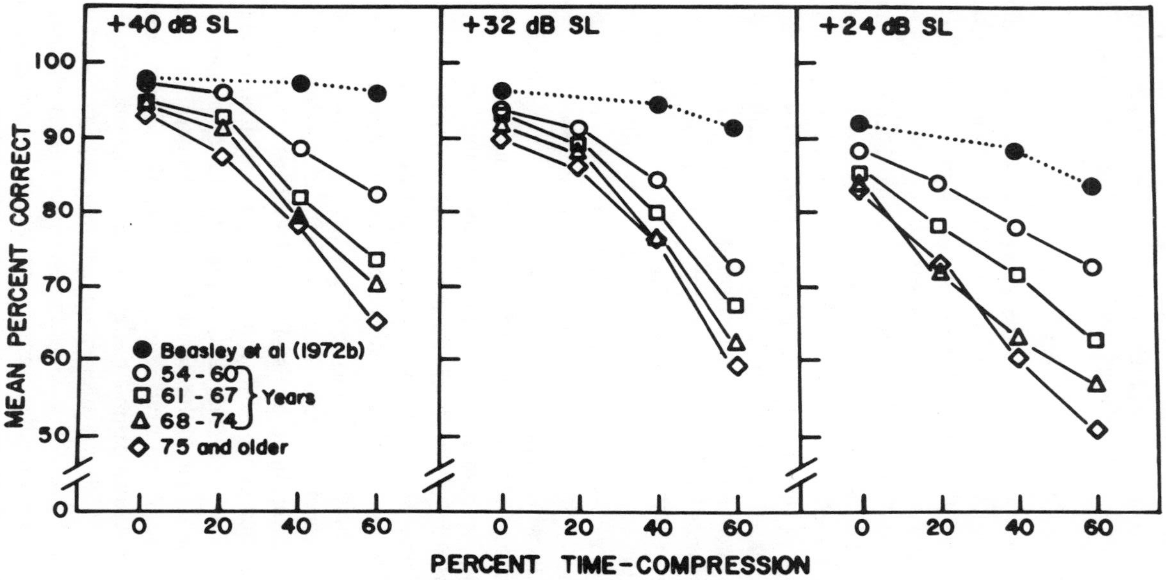

Figure 9-8. Mean percentage correct scores for the four age groups at each condition of time compression and sensation level. The Beasley et al. data for 24 and 32 dB SL and 40 dB SL are shown for comparison purposes. (Source: Konkle, Beasley, and Bess, 1977.)

subjects. The authors concluded by stating: "Consequently, it appears that time-compressed speech may be used as a part of a test battery to assist the audiologist in effectively delineating peripheral and central processing problems as a function of aging" (p. 114). This conclusion is reinforced by the findings of Jerger (1973b).

Other Tests of Central Auditory Disorders

Although not widely used at the present time, other audiometric tests have been cited as useful in the identification of central auditory disorders. The Short Increment Sensitivity Index (SISI), for example, has been shown by Hodgson (1967) and Jerger, Weikers, Sharbrough, and Jerger (1969) to be somewhat effective in the diagnosis of central disorders. The procedure suggested calls for the presentation of 1 dB increments above the intensity level of a steady tone at regular intervals as the sensation level of the test is systematically increased. Markedly reduced intensity discrimination may be present in the ear opposite the affected side of the brain. Greisen and Rasmussen (1970) have also reported that the acoustic reflex may be absent in brain stem lesions, primarily in the ear contralateral to the central dysfunction. Other tests within the peripheral auditory battery, such as Bekesy audiometry and other measures of adaptation, as well as the loudness balance procedures, tend to reveal results which are usually consistent with those associated with normal hearing. Berlin, Chase, Dill, and Hogepanos (1965) did note the tendency for patients with some temporal lobe lesions to exhibit excursion widths of 25–30 dB during Bekesy audiometry.

Other nonspeech stimuli have been used during the audiometric evaluation of central hearing disorders. The measurement of auditory reaction time (ART) has been promoted by Chocholle (in Calearo and Antonelli, 1973). This involves the presentation of tone pulses at suprathreshold levels and the determination of the subject's auditory reaction time. ART results are considered abnormal if the ART in one ear is 10–20% longer than in the other ear. Such an outcome would suggest the possibility of a temporal lobe lesion in the hemisphere of the brain contralateral to the affected ear. Aged individuals may also exhibit prolonged ARTs in both ears.

Matzger (1959) has also suggested that assessment of lateralization may be beneficial in identifying central auditory impairments. His procedure calls for the presentation of auditory clicks at variable intensity levels binaurally via earphones. The patient must indicate the intracranial location of the stimuli as the stimulus parameters are varied systematically. Evidence gathered thus far suggests that persons with central lesions may not be capable of localizing the signal as successfully as normals. Walsh (1957) has also utilized a similar procedure for assessment of localization abilities for diagnostic purposes with cases suspected of central auditory disorders.

Berlin (1976) recently presented a review of tests for the evaluation of central auditory machanisms, and focused on what he described as "...five of the most promising procedures available to clarify central auditory mechanisms." These procedures are (p. 833):

1. The masking level difference (MLD)
2. Stapedial reflex recordings (both ipsilateral and contralateral elicited)
3. Electrocochleography
4. Brain stem potentials (1 to 12 msec)
5. Dichotic listening

In the MLD procedure, a test tone is presented to a particular ear and a masking signal is also presented to the same ear at a level just sufficient to mask the tone. The same type of masker is then presented to the opposite ear exactly 180° out of phase with the noise in the outer ear, which will suddenly make the tone audible. With normal hearing subjects there is about an 11–15 dB release from masking, or improvement in threshold of the test signal. This shift is termed the masking level difference. Cullen and Thompson (1974) have found a similar degree of MLD in cases with cortical lesions, while Olsen, Noffsinger, and Carhart (1976) found a markedly reduced MLD in patients with multiple sclerosis. This has prompted Berlin (1976) to suggest that a reduced MLD may be observed in cases having lesions of the IVth ventricle, as well as the trapezoid and olivary bodies of the brain stem.

The utility of stapedial reflex testing in assessment of central function is based on the inclusion of brain stem structures in the reflex arc necessary to elicit the reflex. As described by Berlin (1976), a patient with central involvement near the IVth ventricle will not have a stapedial reflex when an attempt is made to stimulate one contralaterally with an auditory signal. Ipsilateral stimulation will, however, result in the observance of a reflex.

In Berlin's battery of tests, electrocochleography is utilized primarily to allow for an objective assessment of the peripheral auditory system. Its importance is especially enhanced in cases where the ability of the patient to participate in the test is doubtful. Normal results from electrocochleography imply an intact peripheral mechanism and make it more likely that brain stem and/or cortical dysfunction is present.

Brain stem potential measurement is an electrophysiologic means of assessing the status of the major nuclei of the brain stem. The nature of the brain stem responses obtained presumably can allow for a specific determination of the point of dysfunction within this portion of the central mechanism.

The last procedure advocated by Berlin is that of dichotic testing, where two different speech stimuli are presented simultaneously, one to each ear. In patients with temporal lobe lesions, perception of the material presented in the ear contralateral to the affected lobe will be sharply reduced relative to that of the outer ear.

These five procedures, according to Berlin (1976), can prove very effective in the identification of central auditory disorders, particularly if used together as a battery of tests with a given patient.

Summary

It is obvious that large numbers of audiometric tests are now available for assessing central auditory function, making the detection of lesions within the brain stem and cortical structures of the auditory system somewhat more possible than in the past. However, the application of many of these tests in the assessment of central processing in the elderly has not taken place. While some may prove to be effective, it is conceivable that a portion of these tests may not be of use with the aged because of the complexity of the tasks involved for the listener and other similar factors. Caution is therefore advised in both the selection and administration of these instruments in a clinical setting. It may be advisable to employ some of the less complex procedures, such as the Rush-Hughes Difference Test, for this reason. It should also be pointed out that none of the tests discussed in this chapter will allow for a differential diagnosis of neural degeneration associated with the aging process, as opposed to the other forms of central disorder. Each will merely provide information concerning the presence of central pathology, and may also supply some information concerning its possible location within the central system.

SUGGESTED READINGS

Berlin, C., and Lowe, S. Temporal and dichotic factors in central auditory testing. In J. Katz (ed.), Handbook of Clinical Audiology. Baltimore: Williams & Wilkins, 1972.

Bocca, E., and Calearo, C. Central hearing process. In J. Jerger (ed.), Modern Developments in Audiology (1st ed.). New York: Academic Press, 1963.

Jerger, J. Diagnostic audiometry. In J. Jerger (ed.). Modern Developments in Audiology (2nd ed.). New York: Academic Press, 1973.

REFERENCES

Beasley, D., Forman, B., and Rintelmann, R. Perception of time-compressed CNC monosyllables. Journal of Auditory Research, 12, 71–75 (1972a).

Beasley, D., and Maki, J. Time- and frequency-altered speech. In N. Lass (ed.), Contemporary Issues in Experimental Phonetics. New York: Academic Press, 1976.

Beasley, D., Schwimmer, S., and Rintelmann, R. Intelligibility of time-compressed CNC monosyllables. Journal of Speech and Hearing Research, 15, 340–350 (1972b).

Berlin, C. New developments in evaluating central auditory mechanisms. Annals of Otology, Rhinology and Laryngology, 85, 833–841 (1976).

Berlin, C., Chase, R., Dill, A., and Hogepanos, T. Auditory findings in patients with temporal lobectomies. Paper presented at the Annual Convention of the American Speech and Hearing Association, Chicago, 1965.

Bocca, E. Binaural hearing: Another approach. Laryngoscope, 1164 (1955).

Bocca, E., and Calearo, C. Central hearing processes. In J. Jerger (ed.), Modern Developments in Audiology. New York: Academic Press, 1963.

Bocca, E., Calearo, C., and Cassinari, V. A new method for testing hearing in temporal lobe tumors; preliminary report. Acta Otolaryngologica, 44, 219–221 (1954).

Bocca, E., Calearo, C., Cassinari, V., and Miglivacca, F. Testing cortical hearing in temporal lobe tumors. Acta Otolaryngologica, 45, 289–304 (1955).

Brusse, E. W. Psychopathology. In J. E. Birren (ed.), Handbook of Aging and the Individual. Chicago: University of Chicago Press, 1959.

Brody, H. Organization of cerebral cortex: III. A study of aging in the human auditory cortex. Journal of Comparative Neurology, 102, 511–556 (1955).

Calearo, C. Binaural summation in lesions of the temporal lobes. Acta Otolaryngologica, 392–395 (1957).

Calearo, C., and Antonelli, A. Disorders of the central auditory nervous system. In M. Paparella and D. Shumrick (eds.), Otolaryngology (Vol. 2: The Ear). Philadelphia: W. B. Saunders, 1973.

Calearo, C., and Lazzaroni, A. Speech intelligibility in relation to the speed of message. Laryngoscope, 67, 410–419 (1957).

Carhart, R. Audiologic tests: Questions and speculation. In F. McConnell and P. Ward (eds.), Deafness in Childhood. Nashville, Tenn.: Vanderbilt University Press, 1967.

Cullen, J., and Thompson, C. Masking release for speech in subjects with temporal lobe resections. Archives of Otolaryngology, 100, 113–116 (1974).

deQuiros, J. Accelerated speech audiometry, and examination of test results. Translations of the Beltone Institute of Hearing Research, No. 17, Chicago, 1964.

Gang, R. The effects of age on the diagnostic utility of the rollover phenomenon. Journal of Speech and Hearing Disorders, 41, 63–69 (1976).

Goetzinger, C. The Rush Hughes Test in auditory diagnosis. In J. Katz (ed.), Handbook of Clinical Audiology. Baltimore: Williams & Wilkins, 1972.

Goetzinger, C., and Angell, S. Audiological assessment in acoustic tumors and cortical lesions. Eye, Ear, Nose, and Throat Monthly, 44, 39–49 (1965).

Goetzinger, C., and Rousey, D. Hearing problems in later life. Medical Times, 87, 771–780 (1959).

Goodhill, V. Auditory pathway lesions resulting from Rh incompatibility. In F. McConnel and P. Ward (eds.), Deafness in Childhood. Nashville, Tenn.: Vanderbilt University Press, 1967.

Greisen, O., and Rasmussen, P. Stapedius muscle reflexes and otoneurological examinations in brain stem tumors. Acta Otolaryngologica, 70, 366–370 (1970).

Hinchcliffe, R. The anatomical locus of presbycusis. Journal of Speech and Hearing Disorders, 27, 301–310 (1962).

Hodgson, W. Audiological report of a patient with left hemispherectomy. Journal of Speech and Hearing Disorders, 32, 39–45 (1967).

Hodgson, W. Filtered speech tests. In J. Katz, (ed.), Handbook of Clinical Audiology. Baltimore: Williams & Wilkins, 1972.

Jerger, J. Observations on auditory behavior in lesions of the central auditory pathways. Archives of Otolaryngology, 71, 797-806 (1960).

Jerger, J. Auditory tests for disorders of the central auditory mechanism. In W. Fields and B. Alford (eds.), Neurological Aspects of Auditory and Vestibular Disorders. Springfield, Ill.: Charles C Thomas, 1964.

Jerger, J., Weikers, N., Sharbrough, F., and Jerger, S. Bilateral lesions of the temporal lobe: A case study. Acta Otolaryngologica, Supplement 258 (1969).

Jerger, J. Diagnostic audiometry. In J. Jerger (ed.) Modern Developments in Audiology. New York: Academic Press, 1973a.

Jerger, J. Audiological findings in aging. Advances in Oto-Rhino-Laryngology, 20, 115–124 (1973b).

Jerger, J., and Jerger, S. Diagnostic significance of PB word functions. Archives of Otolaryngology, 93, 573–580 (1971).

Katz, J. The use of staggered spondaic words for assessing the integrity of the central auditory system. Journal of Auditory Research, 2, 327–337 (1962).

Katz, J. The SSW Test: an interim report. Journal of Speech and Hearing Disorders, 33, 132–146 (1968).

Kirikae, I., Sato, R., and Shitara, T. A study of hearing in advanced age. Laryngoscope, 74, 205–220 (1964).

Konkle, D., Beasley, D., and Bess, F. Intelligibility of time-altered speech in relation to chronological aging. Journal of Speech and Hearing Research, 20 108–115 (1977).

Luterman, D., Welsh, O., and Melrose, J. Responses of aged males to time-altered speech stimuli. Journal of Speech and Hearing Research, 9, 226–230 (1966).

Lynn, G., and Gilroy, J. Central aspects of audition. In J. Northern (ed.), Hearing Disorders. Boston: Little, Brown, 1976.

Martin, F. Introduction to Audiology. Englewood Cliffs, New Jersey: Prentice-Hall, 1975.

Malamud, N. Neuropathology of organic brain syndromes associated with aging. In C. Gaitz (ed.), Aging and the Brain. New York: Plenum Press, 1972.

Mathog, R. Otologic manifestations of retrocochlear disease. In M. Papparella and D. Shumrick (eds.), Otolaryngology (Vol. 2: The Ear). Philadelphia: W. B. Saunders, 1973.

Matzger, J. Two new methods for the assessment of central auditory functions in cases of brain disease. Annals of Otology, Rhinology, and Laryngology, 68, 1185–1197 (1959).

Northern, J., and Downs, M. Hearing in Children. Baltimore: Williams & Wilkins, 1974.

Olsen, W., Noffsinger, D., and Carhart, R. Masking level differences encountered in clinical populations. Audiology, 15, 287–301 (1976).

Papparella, M., and Capps, M. Sensorineural deafness in children—nongenetic. In M. Papparella and D. Shumrick (eds.), Otolaryngology (Vol. 2: The Ear). Philadelphia: W. B. Saunders, 1973.

Pinsker, O. The Otological correlates of audiology. In J. Katz (ed.), Handbook of Clinical Audiology. Baltimore: Williams & Wilkins, 1972.

Schuknecht, H. Presbycusis. Laryngoscope, 65, 402–419 (1955).

Schuknecht, H. Further observations on the pathology of presbycusis. Archives of Otolaryngology, 80, 369–382 (1964).

Smith, B., and Resnick, D. An auditory test for assessing brain stem integrity: Preliminary report. Paper presented at the Annual Convention of the American Speech and Hearing Association, Chicago, 1969.

Speaks, C., and Jerger, J. Method for measurement of speech identification. Journal of Speech and Hearing Research, 8, 179–193 (1965).

Sticht, T., and Gray, B. The intelligibility of time-compressed words as a function of age and hearing loss. Journal of Speech and Hearing Research, 12, 443–448 (1969).

Walsh, E. An investigation of sound localization in patients with neurological abnormalities. Brain, 8C, 222–250 (1957).

Section III
DISORDERS OF SPEECH AND LANGUAGE

Chapter 10
Agnosia

This chapter considers agnosia, or those nonlanguage disorders of perception that affect vision, hearing, and touch. Specific types of agnosia are discussed, and the effect of such disorders on the communication process.

DEFINITION

The term "agnosia" is generally recognized as referring to disorders characterized by failure to recognize the nature of an incoming stimulus (Nielsen, 1946). Thus, agnosia is usually regarded as a disturbance in perceiving the nature of sensations while the ability to receive and experience sensations is unaffected. Inherent in this definition of agnosia is the concept that the disorder is specific to a given sensory modality such as touch, vision, or hearing (Perkins, 1977). However, the disorder does not include primary sensory defects such as impaired visual acuity, intellectual degeneration, or lack of familiarity with a given object. Although the term "agnosia" was originally used to describe recognition problems, it has since been extended to include failures in recognizing one's body parts, faces, and spatial relationships (Brain, 1965).

The word itself provides some further understanding as to its intended meaning: *a*, without; *gnosia*, knowing. Early physicians were aware of the clinical manifestations of this type of disorder and referred to it by names such as "asymbolia" and "imperception." The latter term was used by Jackson (1879) to describe the failure of some patients in recognizing objects. Recently, the term "imperception" has begun to appear in the literature again. For example, Merifield, Hall, and Merrell (1976) discussed the problems of "auditory imperception" in children and preferred the use of this term to auditory agnosia and a variety of other labels. It was Freud (1891) who first proposed the use of the term "agnosia" as an appropriate name for disorders of perception and it has since come into general use.

TYPES OF AGNOSIA

Although the literature discusses agnosia in terms of visual, tactile, and auditory imperceptions, it rarely mentions such disorders relative to taste or smell. Nielsen (1946) suggested that olfactory (smell) and gustatory (taste) agnosias are not definitely known entities. Most of the agnosia studies have concentrated on the visual modality. Some work has been completed with regard to tactile agnosias. However, only a limited amount of research exists relative to auditory agnosia.

The evidence from the literature suggests that agnosic disorders are modality bound. That is, a particular agnosia is associated with only one sensory channel. For the purposes of this book, a classification of the agnosias based on modality and general clinical observations will probably best serve the needs of the reader. The classification presented here is limited to agnosias of vision, hearing, and touch and synthesizes schemes used by Brain (1965), Brown (1972), and Frederiks (1969).

Visual Agnosia

There are a fairly large number of visual agnosias that have been discussed in the literature. The more important ones are listed in Table 10-1.

Auditory Agnosia

Auditory agnosias are unusual and are hard to differentiate from aphasia. Three forms of this agnosia are commonly recognized. Each of these forms reveals the same fundamental deficit, namely, the patient knows he is hearing something but cannot recognize what it is. Table 10-2 lists the major types of auditory agnosia.

Tactile Agnosia

The patient having tactile agnosia fails to recognize objects by touch even though the ability to distinguish size, shape, and texture is well preserved. This disorder does not include difficulties with tactile recognition of objects caused by sensory loss.

REALITY OF THE CLASSICAL DEFINITION OF AGNOSIA

When trying to understand the nature and characteristics of the various agnosias that may result from brain injury, there are a few problems which deserve attention and of which the reader should be aware. One major problem which has not been completely resolved

Table 10-1. Types of visual agnosia

Type	Characteristic
Agnosias for environmental properties	
Visual object agnosia Associative visual agnosia	The inability to recognize objects visually, particularly small ones; visual defects are common
Simultanagnosia Apperceptive visual agnosia Psychic blindness	The patient is unable to fuse into whole objects the separate parts of a picture; details may be identified but the meaning or intent of the whole is not; matching abilities are impaired; visual attention is narrowed to a single object or configuration
Color agnosia	The inability to match or sort colors by shade or intensity; does not include color naming
Agnosias for body parts	
Prosopagnosia	The inability to recognize faces; patients are unable to identify human faces that are familiar or even their own face
Autotopagnosia Asomatognosia	The inability to recognize parts of the body; the patient has difficulty matching his own body parts to others, pictures, or one side of the body to the other; he may even deny any knowledge of named body parts or mislocate them; Gerstmann's syndrome (finger agnosia) is part of this disorder
Anosognosia	A failure to recognize one's illness or paralysis; confabulation is typical
Agnosias for spatial relationships	
Visual-spatial agnosia Apractagnosia Optic apraxia Constructional apraxia	The inability to localize objects in space or construct dimensional relationships; depth and distance perception are impaired as well as left-right relations
Topographical agnosia Topographagnosia	The inability to recognize geographical relationships, read maps or find routes

is establishing a definitive relationship between agnosia symptoms and their neurologic substrates. That is, researchers are not entirely sure if the agnosias do indeed represent a type of neurologic injury separate and apart from the apraxias and aphasia (Fredericks, 1969). In this regard, several investigators have expressed their doubts that the classical notion of agnosia is correct (Bay, 1953; Critchley, 1964;

Table 10-2. Types of auditory agnosia

Type	Characteristic
Auditory agnosia	The inability to recognize nonlinguistic or environmental sounds
Verbal agnosia Verbal deafness Word deafness	The inability to recognize letter sounds, words, phrases, or sentences (speech); is accompanied by a slower temporal sequencing ability for such stimuli
Amusia Sensory amusia	A failure to recognize music

Geschwind, 1965; Teuber, 1965; Luria, 1966). For example, Geschwind (1965) has proposed that most of the classical agnosias are really "modality-specific naming defects resulting from isolation (disconnection) of the primary cortex from the speech area and associated with marked confabulatory responses." He cited the example of a patient who had difficulty naming objects placed in his left hand but could draw the object afterward or select it by touch or visually from a group of objects. This patient could correctly identify objects via nonverbal means, but he could not name them verbally. Bay (1965) recently concluded that the agnosias appear to consist of a number of sensory and nonsensory disorders that have been arbitrarily grouped together because of superficial similarities. Furthermore, Alajuanine and Lhermitte (1973) observed that what is called agnosia really constitutes a set of behavior patterns evoked by the tests given to the patient. Apparently, what was originally thought to be a fairly easy problem to define and understand has proved to be a complicated clinical syndrome, the true nature of which will require more extensive clinical and neurologic research.

AGNOSIA AND AGING

The problem of agnosia relative to aging is much the same as for aphasia. Since agnosia is produced by neurologic damage primarily attributable to stroke or tumors, it is probably safe to say that the elderly are more than well represented among those having agnosic deficits. In most instances these deficits are associated with the more severe forms of aphasia. For example, the patients identified by Schuell (1964) as having aphasia and visual recognition deficits (group 2) or who suffer from aphasia plus reduced sensory information and impaired auditory and proprioceptive feedback processes (group 3) would be representative. For this reason, specific incidence data for the agnosias are rarely available in the literature.

SUGGESTED READINGS

Brain, W. R. Speech Disorders: Aphasia, Apraxia and Agnosia (2nd Ed.). Washington, D.C.: Butterworths, 1965.

Brown, J. W. Aphasia, Apraxia and Agnosia: Clinical and Theoretical Aspects. Springfield, Ill.: Charles C Thomas, 1972.

REFERENCES

Alajuanine, T., and Lhermitte, F. Some problems concerning the agnosias, apraxias, and aphasia. In L. Halpern (ed.), Problems of Dynamic Neurology. Jerusalem, Hebrew University Hadassa Medical School, 1973.

Bay, E. Disturbances of visual perception and their examination. Brain, 76, 515–550 (1953).

Bay, E. Disturbances of agnosia, apraxia and aphasia after a history of a hundred years. Journal of Mount Sinai Hospital, 32, 637–650 (1965).

Brain, W. R. Speech Disorders: Aphasia, Apraxia and Agnosia (2nd Ed.). Washington, D.C.: Butterworths, 1965.

Brown, J. W. Aphasia, Apraxia and Agnosia: Clinical and Theoretical Aspects. Springfield, Ill.: Charles C Thomas, 1972.

Critchley, M. The problem of visual agnosia. Journal of Neurological Science, 1, 274–290 (1964).

Fredericks, J. A. M. The agnosias: Disorders of perceptual recognition. In P. J. Vinken and G. W. Bruyn (eds.), Handbook of Clinical Neurology (Vol. 4.). Amsterdam: North-Holland, 1969.

Freud, S. On Aphasia (Trans. by E. Stengel). New York: International Universities Press, 1953. First published in Germany, 1891.

Geschwind, N. Deconnection syndromes in animals and man. Brain, 88, 237–294; 585–644 (1965).

Jackson, J. H. On affections of speech from disease of the brain. Brain, 1, 304–330 (1879).

Luria, A. R. Higher Cortical Functions in Man. New York: Basic Books, 1966.

Merifield, D. O., Hall, C. M., and Merrell, H. B. Auditory imperception. Annals of Otolaryngology, 85, 225–260 (1976).

Nielsen, J. M. Agnosia, Apraxia and Aphasia. New York: Harper, 1946.

Perkins, W. H. Speech Pathology, An Applied Behavior Science (2nd Ed.). St. Louis: C. V. Mosby, 1977.

Schuell, H., Jenkins, J. J., and Jimenez-Pabon, E. Aphasia in Adults. New York: Harper & Row, 1964.

Teuber, H. L. Postscript: Some needed revisions of the classical views of agnosia. Neuropsychology, 3, 371–378 (1965).

Chapter 11
Apraxia of Speech

This chapter explores the disorder of apraxia of speech, defined as a disturbance in phonologic programming in the absence of aphasia or dysarthria. Three issues are discussed: terminology problems, clinical manifestations, and apraxia among the aging.

THE TERMINOLOGY PROBLEM

Before discussing the clinical manifestations of a distinctive disorder now commonly labeled "apraxia," the reader should be aware of the considerable controversy and divergence of terms used to describe this problem. Very briefly, patients who have sustained damage to the base of the third frontal convolution (Broca's area) of the dominant (usually left) hemisphere display a rather typical set of behaviors. A partial list of these includes variable articulatory patterns, disturbed prosody, oral struggle behavior, and inappropriate phonemic sequencing (Darley, Aronson, and Brown, 1975).

Historically, Broca has been credited with the first description of this disorder, and he considered it quite separate from the more generalized language impairment known as aphasia. Broca first used the term "aphemia," and later the terms "Broca's aphasia," "motor aphasia," and "subcortical motor aphasia" emerged as synonyms (Johns and Darley, 1970). The term "apraxia" to designate this problem was suggested by Liepmann (1900, 1913). Since then, many other terms have been proposed, including "apraxic dysarthria" (Nathan, 1947), "peripheral motor aphasia" (Goldstein, 1948), "cortical dysarthria" (Bay, 1962), "phonemic paraphasia" (Lecours and Lhermitte, 1969), "articulatory apraxia" (Critchley, 1970), and "aphasic phonological impairment" (Martin, 1974).

For purposes of this chapter, the term "apraxia of speech" (or more conveniently, "apraxia") is used, and there is adherence to the definition provided most recently by Darley et al. (1975):

> Apraxia of speech is a distinct motor speech disorder distinguishable from the dysarthrias (speech disorders due to impaired innervation of speech musculature) and aphasia (a language disorder due to impair-

> ment of the brain mechanism of decoding and encoding the symbol system used in spoken and written communication). Apraxia of speech is a disorder of motor speech programming manifested primarily by errors in articulation and secondarily by compensatory alterations in prosody. The speaker shows reduced proficiency in accomplishing the oral postures necessary for phoneme production and the sequences of those postures for productions of words. (p. 267)

It should be noted that Martin (1974) registered rather strong opposition to the term "apraxia" and his reasoning warrants brief review. A fundamental issue raised in Martin's paper relates to the fact that apraxia may be connoted as the output aspect of a rather archaic model of language functioning. This outdated model compartmentalizes language operations in a dichotomous fashion such that "language" and "speech" processing are separate events. It is Martin's contention that these two operations cannot be viewed as separate. Rather, he has argued that the very act of language formulation involves a motor programming component:

> Even with a postulated separate mechanism for the motor production of speech, its operation depends upon its interlocking relationship with the language system....The same operations necessary for the processing of linguistic units, the impairments of which may be classified as aphasia, operate in programming the movements that produce the linguistic event—the phoneme. (p. 56)

Obviously such a criticism rather seriously challenges the definition employed in this chapter and the partitioning of language encoding into four stages, as proposed in Chapter 2. Furthermore, Martin has marshalled several good arguments illustrating the strong interrelationships between motor speech programming and other aspects of language processing. The response of the present authors to these contentions is one of agreement. From our readings of the literature, however, Darley and his various associates at the Mayo Clinic never intended to isolate apraxias as wholly independent from other language operations. In Darley et al. (1975), the following lines of reason are proposed to illustrate this point:

> The central language processor is believed to select the words and proper sequences of words to transform meaningful internal content into language for externalization. Having accomplished this selection, it converts the word sequences into a neural code of directions for the motor speech programmer....Patients with apraxia may exhibit alterations of language....There are several possible reasons for such occurrences. First, the lesion damaging the anterior speech area may extend posteriorly and also damage the posterior language area. It is also possible

> that damage to the anterior (Broca's) area impairs the operational efficiency of the posterior area....Damage to Broca's area may disturb the balance between the two hemispheres, leading to interference by the non-dominant one. Again, the posterior area may not have sole direction of word and syntax choice, leaving limited freedom in word and syntax choice to Broca's area. (pp. 258–259)

Furthermore, Darley et al. documented that isolated infarcts of Broca's area produce apraxia of speech with little or no difficulty in language interpretation or written expression. In summary, it is agreed that simplistic division of language processing and motor speech programming is irresponsible. However, conceptualizing language encoding with reference to interdependent stages or operations is judged both appropriate and convenient.

CLINICAL MANIFESTATIONS

Variability of Error

Until recently, very little formal experimentation was undertaken to document the exact nature of symptoms associated with apraxia of speech. However, a growing body of research has added substantially to our understanding of the features of this disorder. This section directs attention to the principal clinical dimensions of apraxia, and, where appropriate, reviews the experimental literature to provide insight regarding specific aspects of symptomatology.

As mentioned in the earlier definition of apraxia, the disorder is fundamentally one of articulation. Perhaps its central characteristic is variability or inconsistency of error. A transcribed error pattern of an apractic patient uttering the word "merthiolate" appears as follows:

> *moo*-uh-*mer*tholate-uh-*me*thiolit-uh
> *mor*thiolite-uh-*mer*tholiolate-uh
> *mer*tholate

It is apparent by examination of the first syllable of each attempt that the sequence "mer" was variably produced as "moo," "mer," and "mor." In three of the six attempts, the syllable was correctly produced.

As Martin (1974) pointed out, variability in phonetic output does not necessarily imply a random or haphazard error pattern. Indeed, there is experimental evidence to support this contention. Shankweiler and Harris (1966) sought to describe the nature of phonetic substitutions in five patients with vascular damage to the anterior portion of the left cerebral hemisphere. These subjects were asked to produce 200 real-word monosyllables with even distribution of singleton consonants and consonant clusters. Broad phonetic transcription was completed and it was discovered that consonants were more difficult than vowels. Fricatives and affricates were the most difficult consonants, and consonant clusters precipitated the least accurate productions.

Further insight regarding the nature of these errors was provided by Johns and Darley (1970), who examined patterns of misarticulation in 30 adults (10 normal, 10 apraxic, 10 dysarthric). A variety of experimental tasks was devised to evaluate integrity and consistency of phoneme production. In one task, 60 words (30 real, 30 nonsense) were presented to the subject visually (printed), auditorily, and audiovisually, and he was asked to repeat the word. All subjects performed better on real words and with the audiovisual mode of presentation. The apraxics were inferior to the normals but superior to the dysarthrics. In another task, the subjects were asked to produce progressively longer words with the same root (e.g., thick, thicker, thickening). The apraxics and dysarthrics had increasing difficulty with longer words. In a third task, the subjects were asked to read a prose passage at a faster than normal rate. The apraxic subjects made fewer errors and gained intelligibility with increased rate. Several other tasks were evaluated but these three illustrated rather important features of the apraxia of speech. The disorder can often be alleviated by providing an audiovisual model, by reducing word length and complexity, and by focusing on speed rather than accuracy of production.

In follow-up study, Deal and Darley (1972) discovered with 12 apraxic patients that the frequency of phonemic errors can be greatly increased when multisyllabic nouns, verbs, adjectives, and adverbs are attempted. Enforcing a response delay, introducing masking noise while responding, and self-monitoring in a mirror while responding had no significant impact on error rate for these subjects.

Finally, at least three sources (LeCours and Lhermitte, 1969; Martin, 1974; Trost and Canter, 1974) have documented that substitution errors in apraxia approximate the desired response with respect to distinctive feature patterns. According to Trost and Canter, place of articulation is most commonly disturbed, followed by manner of production and voicing errors.

Struggle Behavior

It has been rather consistently observed that apraxic patients exhibit struggle when speaking. They approximate articulatory targets effortfully and hesitantly. Johns and Darley (1970) described it as "tiptoeing through their words" (p. 581), while Darley et al. (1975) reported than an apraxic patient "effortfully gropes to find the correct articulatory postures and sequences of them" (p. 263). This was reflected experimentally in the study by Deal and Darley (1972), where it was noted that:

> The apraxic subjects would often require three or four seconds, and occasionally more, to make a response but this latency apparently occurred randomly. There was some relationship between latency and severity. . ." (p. 651)

Automatic versus Volitional Speech

As noted earlier, speeding the speech response of apraxic subjects greatly increases intelligibility and reduces errors. It is possible that such a task increases the automatic nature of articulatory sequencing and gesturing and thereby mitigates the aforementioned set to grope and struggle for precision of articulation. If this is true, it would lend credence to historic observations that automatic or reflexive speech acts (e.g., counting, reciting a common jingle, saying the Lord's Prayer, etc.) are typically uttered fluently by patients with apraxia of speech (Darley et al., 1975).

Auditory and Oral Perceptual Skills

Because of the frequent speculations regarding the role of oral sensory and auditory feedback in articulatory production, the question has arisen as to whether or not apraxia is associated with such sensory disturbances. Several experiments have shed light on this issue. Perhaps the first was that of Shankweiler and Harris (1966), who asked four of the five patients described earlier to identify 75 real-word monosyllables using a closed response set. Two of the subjects performed at near normal levels and two exhibited depressed scores. It is significant to note that perceptual skill and articulatory performance were not highly correlated.

In a more comprehensive study, Aten, Johns, and Darley (1971) evaluated auditory perceptual skills with 10 apraxic patients and 10 matched normal subjects who listened to 190 sentences, to which they were required to respond by pointing to pictures. As a group, the apraxic subjects were inferior, but several performed within normal limits suggesting that apraxia can occur in relatively pure form without the presence of auditory perceptual deficits.

With respect to oral sensory function, Rosenbek, Wertz, and Darley (1973) administered three tests of oral sensory integrity: oral stereognosis (form discrimination), two-point discrimination, and mandibular kinesthesia. Apraxic subjects performed significantly poorer than normal or aphasic subjects on all tasks. However, some of the apraxic patients (usually those with mild deficits) evidenced normal or near normal scores. These data were interpreted as evidence of higher cortical sensory impairments in some cases of apraxia.

Oral Apraxia

Some, though not all, patients with apraxia of speech also exhibit a condition commonly called "oral apraxia." This is a disorder wherein the patient has difficulty with volitional movements of the oral structures during nonspeech tasks such as whistling, protruding the tongue, blowing, and kissing. De Renzi, Pieczuro, and Vignolo (1966) reported that aphasic subjects with severe phonemic-articulatory disorders (apraxia of speech) evidenced a number of oral apraxic problems. However, it is important to note that several patients with apraxia of speech did not exhibit oral apraxia. Therefore, the two disorders are not always present together.

APRAXIA OF SPEECH AND AGING

There are no available data on the incidence of apraxia among the elderly. Certainly much of this relates to the difficulty in diagnosing the disorder, its concomitant presence with other sequelae of brain damage, and the varying terminology used to describe it. According to Brust, Shafer, Richter, and Bruun (1976), approximately 54% of the males and 46% of the females with aphasia have a "nonfluent" form of the disorder (see Chapter 13). From this, one can assume that apraxia of speech may be a principal contributor to the nonfluent characteristic. However, beyond this general statement, incidence figures are difficult to secure. It was also suggested in Chapter 5 that some of the hesitancy behavior, reduced rate, and dysfluency patterns of the "normal" gerontologic subject might reflect subtle apraxic disturbances, but this speculation has not been documented.

SUGGESTED READING

Darley, F. L., Aronson, A., and Brown, J. R. Motor Speech Disorders. Philadelphia: W. B. Saunders, 1975.

REFERENCES

Aten, J. L., Johns, D. F., and Darley, F. L. Auditory imperception of sequenced words in apraxia of speech. Journal of Speech and Hearing Research, 14, 131–143 (1971).

Bay, E. Aphasia and non-verbal disorders of language. Brain, 85, 411–426 (1962).

Brust, J. C. M., Shafer, S. Q., Richter, R. W., and Bruun, B. Aphasia in acute stroke. Stroke, 7, 167–174 (1976).

Critchley, M. Aphasiology. London: Edward Arnold, 1970.

Darley, F. L., Aronson, A., and Brown, J. R. Motor Speech Disorders. Philadelphia: W. B. Saunders, 1975.

Deal, J. L., and Darley, F. L. The influence of linguistic and situational variables on phonemic accuracy in apraxia of speech. Journal of Speech and Hearing Research, 15, 639–653 (1972).

De Renzi, E., Pieczuro, A., and Vignolo, L. A. Oral apraxia and aphasia. Cortex, 2, 50–73 (1966).

Goldstein, K. Language and Language Disturbances. New York: Grune & Stratton, 1948.

Johns, D. F., and Darley, F. L. Phonemic variability in apraxia of speech. Journal of Speech and Hearing Research, 13, 556–583 (1970).

Lecours, A. R., and Lhermitte, F. Phonemic paraphasias: Linquistic structures and tentative hypotheses. Cortex, 5, 193–228 (1969).

Liepmann, H. Das Krankheitsbild der Apraxie. Monatsschrift Psychiatrie und Neurologie, 8, 182–197 (1900).

Liepmann, H. Motorische Aphasie und Apraxie. Monatsschrift Psychiatrie und Neurologie, 34, 485–494 (1913).

Martin, A. D. Some objections to the term "apraxia of speech." Journal of Speech and Hearing Disorders, 39, 53–64 (1974).

Nathan, P. W. Facial apraxia and apraxic dysarthria. Brain, 70, 449–478 (1947).

Rosenbek, J. C., Wertz, R. T., and Darley, F. L. Oral sensation and perception in apraxia of speech and aphasia. Journal of Speech and Hearing Research, 16, 22–36 (1973).

Shankweiler, D., and Harris, K. L. An experimental approach to the problem of articulation in aphasia. Cortex, 2, 277–292 (1966).

Trost, J. E., and Canter, G. J. Apraxia of speech in patients with Broca's aphasia: A study of phoneme production accuracy and error patterns. Brain and Language, 1, 63–79 (1974).

Chapter 12
Dysarthria

This discussion focuses on peripheral speech execution disorders resulting from neurologic disease. In accordance with the classificatory scheme developed by Darley, Aronson, and Brown (1975), six forms of dysarthria are reviewed: flaccid, ataxic, spastic, hypokinetic, hyperkinetic, and mixed. Etiologies, brief discussions of pathophysiology, and speech symptoms are presented.

A now classic definition of the term "dysarthria" was offered by Darley, Aronson, and Brown (1969a). Specifically, they considered dysarthria to be:

> . . . a collective name for a group of speech disorders resulting from disturbances in muscular control over the speech mechanism due to damage of the central or peripheral nervous system. It designates problems in oral communication due to paralysis, weakness, or incoordination of the speech musculature. It differentiates such problems from disorders of higher centers related to the faulty programming of movements and sequences of movements (apraxia of speech) and to the inefficient processing of linguistic units. (p. 246)

As has been suggested in earlier chapters, older people are more susceptible to diseases of the nervous system and it is logical to conclude that dysarthria is much more prevalent among geriatric patients.

Unfortunately, there are limited incidence data for most of the current dysarthria classifications. Spahr (1971) indicated that according to a U.S. National Health Survey, there are an estimated 90,000 people over age 65 with speech handicaps and the number is expected to exceed 148,000 by 1980. The percentage of these handicapped persons who have an isolated dysarthria or dysarthria in combination with other problems is unknown. Spahr also reported that the National Institute of Neurological Diseases and Stroke estimated that roughly 600,000 people have aphasia. It may be assumed that a large percentage of these people also have a dysarthric problem. Some general inferences can also be made from a handful of community surveys that have been conducted. For example, after reviewing several relatively small sample studies,

Bollinger (1974) estimated that between 40 and 50% of patients in extended care facilities have speech and language handicaps. Furthermore, he concluded that, "In large part the speech and language disorders are secondary to degenerative brain diseases..." (p. 217). Of course, what percentage of this general incidence figure can be ascribed to dysarthria is unknown, but one can assume that it is much greater than that of an average adult population. In addition, there are many more noninstitutionalized elderly patients with dysarthric handicaps who were not included in the surveys studied by Bollinger.

It is important for all health care professionals, particularly speech pathologists, to recognize that the incidence of dysarthria will undoubtedly increase in the future. As Foley (1975) has noted:

> ... more incurable diseases are going to be prolonged. They are going to be treated more effectively and people will live longer with them. ... The result will be that more nervous systems are going to be damaged in more people in older age groups. ... Patients who survive a manageable disease that is curable or incurable for longer than the usual then become victimized by the neurologic consequences of the disease. (p. 2)

Certainly Foley's observations are applicable to neurologic diseases that result in a dysarthric problem.

TYPES OF DYSARTHRIA

For purposes of the present discussion, the popular classification system of dysarthria offered by Darley, Aronson, and Brown (1975) will be used, and the reader is referred to their excellent book, *Motor Speech Disorders,* for a more comprehensive review of this area. This classification system is based upon the historic observation that different forms of dysarthria have different auditory perceptual characteristics depending upon the neurologic site of lesion. Consequently, they developed a six-fold classification system, which is reviewed in the following sections. Specifically, the dysarthria types to be reviewed are: flaccid, ataxic, spastic, hypokinetic, hyperkinetic, and mixed. Extensive consideration of the neurologic substrates of the various disorders is deferred to other, more comprehensive sources.

Flaccid Dysarthria

Flaccid dysarthria refers to speech problems which result from diseases or disorders of the lower motor neuron system. This system involves two principal components: 1) anterior horns of the spinal cord, and 2) motor nuclei of the cranial nerves. Of course, the peripheral extensions of these motor unit origins (motor neuron cell bodies, peripheral nerves, myoneural junction or synapse, and muscle) are also components of the system. (See Chapter 2 for a review of the anatomy associated with this system.) Damage to any component of the lower motor neuron system can result in "weakness, loss of muscle tone, and reflexes of affected muscle, producing flaccidity or paralysis" (Darley et al., 1975, p. 101).

A number of factors can result in damage to components of the lower motor neuron system, and the following is a partial list of the common problems which can typically appear in adulthood. (For a more complete listing of neuromuscular problems resulting in flaccidity, the reader is referred to Chusid, 1970.)

1. *Bulbar palsy* results from nuclear involvement of the last four or five motor cranial nerves (facial, glossopharyngeal, vagus, accessory, and hypoglossal). Since the courses of several of these nerves may be diverse, it is possible to have involvement of only one or two of the nerves. Darley, et al. (1975) suggested, therefore, that cranial nerve palsies be considered individually as facial, masticator, hypoglossal, pharyngolaryngeal, and generalized. Factors such as tumors, strokes, and trauma, congenital factors, and viral infections can produce bulbar palsy.
2. *Muscular dystrophy* is a disease which can take one of several forms and directly affects the muscles of the body. It is usually a progressive condition and is characterized by atrophy and weakness of muscles. There appears to be a hereditary component and, according to Chusid (1970), the limb-girdle and distal myopathy forms are most apt to appear in adulthood.
3. *Myasthenia gravis* is a disease affecting synaptic transmission at the myoneural junction. It is important to note Chusid's (1970) observation that myasthenia gravis has a particular "affinity for muscles innervated by the bulbar nuclei" (p. 412). It is thought that the transmitter substance in the myoneural junction is either rapidly deactivated or insufficiently produced, which results in muscular weakness and fatigability.
4. *Polymyositis* is a condition resulting in muscular atrophy or weakness secondary to inflammatory conditions. Chusid (1970) has characterized the tissue changes as involving necrosis of muscle fibers, active phagocytosis, and cellular infiltration. The

condition appears prominently in middle age and more often among women.

From a clinical speech standpoint, all of the above conditions present a similar symptom picture. If the respiratory system is involved, the driving force for speech may be reduced resulting in shortened phrases, decreased pitch and intensity variability, and a generalized intensity reduction. With respect to phonation, there may be laryngeal hypovalving resulting in a "breathy" voice quality, the presence of diplophonia (perception of two fundamental frequencies of vibration), and inhalatory stridor. Because of the direct valving control of the larynx over respiratory flow, laryngeal flaccidity can also contribute to reduce pitch and intensity variability. Finally, if flaccidity affects oral cavity musculature, the following problems may occur: 1) velopharyngeal incompetence (weakness) resulting in a hypernasal resonant quality and nasal emission; and 2) lingual, labial, and mandibular weakness resulting in reduced articulatory rate and precision as well as deteriorations in intelligibility. See Table 12-1 for a summary of these clinical manifestations.

Ataxic Dysarthria

Ataxic dysarthria commonly results when there is generalized damage to the cerebellum. The function of the cerebellum in regulating force, speed, timing, range, and direction of movements is well established (Darley et al., 1975). Consequently, lesions of the cerebellum will result in spatial orientation problems, postural difficulties, dysmetrias (problems modulating voluntary movement), intention tremors, and hypotonia.

Several agents may be responsible for cerebellar damage. A partial list would include:

1. *Cerebrovascular accidents* resulting from hemorrhage, thrombosis, embolism, or vascular malformation of the posteroinferior cerebellar artery or superior cerebellar artery may produce ataxic dysarthria.
2. *Tumors* most commonly affecting the cerebellum in adults are astrocytomas, medulloblastomas (more common in children), and metastitic tumors frequently from bronchogenic carcinomas.
3. *Multiple sclerosis* is a disease which initially involves destruction of the myelin sheath and ultimately results in the degeneration of the nerve, leaving residual sclerotic plaques or scars. Typ-

Table 12-1. Summary of clinical speech manifestations of flaccid dysarthria

Respiratory deviations	Clinical implications	Laryngeal deviations	Clinical implications	Articulatory deviations	Clinical implications
Muscle force weakness (hypotonia)	Reduced driving for speech	Muscle force weakness (hypotonia)	Breathy voice	Muscle force weakness (hypotonia)	Imprecise consonants
	Shortened phrases		Diplophonia		Hypernasal resonant quality and nasal emission
	Reduced loudness variability		Inhalatory stridor		Reduced articulatory rate
	Reduced pitch variability		Reduced loudness variability		Reduced intelligibility
	Reduced average vocal loudness		Reduced pitch variability		Reduced diadochokinetic rates

ically, multiple sclerosis has its onset between ages 20 and 40, but the survival times may be relatively long, averaging approximately 27 years (Chusid, 1970).

4. *Toxic and Metabolic* disorders may influence cerebellar functioning and alcohol toxicity is one of the chief among these.
5. *Encephalitis* or inflamation of the brain may affect cerebellar functions as a part of its generalized damage.

Clinically, several important speech functions will be affected by cerebellar disturbances. As Darley et al. (1975) noted, the contemporary literature regarding the influence of cerebellar function on respiratory control for speech is "inadequate and non-definitive" (p. 158). It has been suggested that respiratory control for speech purposes is disturbed (Luchsinger and Arnold, 1965), but no experimental support for this suggestion currently exists. With regard to laryngeal activity during phonation, more experimental data are available. Perhaps Kammermeier's (1969) dissertation is the most complete work to date on this variable. He found a slightly elevated fundamental frequency range. The subjects also exhibited reduced pitch and intensity variability and intermittant "bursts" of vocal effort. Similar findings have been reported in experiments dealing with multiple sclerosis, a disease which typically results in cerebellar damage. Zemlin (1962) and Haggard (1969) reported individual disturbances in vocal fold vibratory patterns, including extreme aperiodicity and irregularities in vibratory onset.

One of the major diagnostic clues to the presence of ataxic dysarthria, as reported by Darley, Aronson, and Brown (1969b) is irregular articulatory breakdown. To this characteristic, Darley et al. added distorted vowels and imprecise consonants, thereby forming an "articulatory inaccuracy" dimension representative of ataxic dysarthrics. In addition, oral diadochokinesis (rapid repetitive movements of the articulators) will usually be seriously affected in these patients both with respect to rate and regularity. Lehiste's (1965) spectrographic evaluation of one ataxic dysarthric revealed irregular control of velopharyngeal function such that inappropriate velar opening and closing was recorded. Because of the elegant neuromuscular control required, the generalized dysmetria characteristic of dysarthrics is particularly evident in articulatory function. Table 12-2 summarizes the clinical speech characteristics.

Spastic Dysarthria

The disorder termed "spastic dysarthria" results from damage to the

Table 12-2. Summary of clinical speech manifestations of ataxic dysarthria

Respiratory deviations	Clinical implications	Laryngeal deviations	Clinical implications	Articulatory deviations	Clinical implications
Unknown but possible asynchrony of respiratory musculature or dysmetria	Intermittant reduction in driving force	Tremors (?)	Small perturbations in pitch (?)	Dysmetria	Irregular articulatory breakdown including velopharyngeal control
		Dysmetria	"Bursts" of vocal effort		Distorted vowels
	Inappropriate modulations in pitch and loudness		Aperiodicity of vocal fold vibration		Imprecise consonants
			Irregularities in vibratory onset		Disturbances in diadochokinetic regularity
		Muscle force weakness (hypotonia)	Reduced pitch and loudness variability	Hypotonia	Imprecise consonants
					Distorted vowels
					Reduced diadochokinetic rates
			Elevated pitch (cause uncertain)		

upper motor neuron system, involving both pyramidal and extrapyramidal components. The associated clinical signs are loss of discrete movement control, spasticity (resistance to passive movement), and increased stretch reflexes. Essentially two generic terms have been used for diseases or disorders resulting in upper motor neuron disease. The first is a disease of infancy and is not discussed in detail here.

1. *Spastic cerebral palsy* results from damage to the upper motor neuron system as a result of pre-, peri-, or post-natal factors.
2. *Pseudobulbar palsy* is essentially a neuromotor syndrome which can result, in adulthood, from tumors, trauma, infections, degenerative disease, vascular disturbances, etc.

As Darley et al. (1975) have observed, very little research concerning the speech problems of pseudobulbar palsy has been forthcoming. Most of the experimental effort has focused on childhood cerebral palsy, and to extend those observations to adventitious upper motor neuron disturbances is hazardous. No research concerning respiratory function has been completed with subjects having pseudobulbar palsy. If one assumes that research on respiratory capabilities of the cerebral palsied is also generally true for those with pseudobulbar palsy, the following deviations might be expected: 1) involuntary movement (McDonald and Chance, 1964), 2) antagonistic activity of inspiratory and expiratory muscles (Hardy, 1961; McDonald and Chance, 1964), 3) reduced vital capacity (Hardy, 1961), and 4) inefficient air stream valving which is largely attributable to control problems in the laryngeal and supraglottal regions. The effect of these anomalies on speech is considerable; pitch and intensity variability suffers as does integrity of phrasing. Indeed, some support for these speculations was provided by Darley et al. (1969b).

With respect to laryngeal function, one of the most notable features of voice production by patients with pseudobulbar palsy is laryngeal hypervalving. This was represented by Darley et al. (1969a) as two perceptual dimensions of voice: "harse voice" and "strained-strangled" voice quality. Furthermore, Kammermeier (1969) reported lower fundamental frequencies and reduced pitch variability among subjects with pseudobulbar palsy. As noted earlier, laryngeal control problems may also contribute to disturbances in the valving of respiratory air flow and intensity variation.

Darley et al. (1969a) described the articulatory deviations of those with pseudobulbar palsy as an "articulatory-resonatory incompetence" characterized by the dimensions of hypernasality, imprecise consonants, and distorted vowels. Kammermeier (1969) provided laboratory support for such perceptions by reporting reduced oral reading rate, exaggerated syllable length, and increased phonatory and pause durations. Netsell (1969) discovered a number of velopharyngeal deviations in patients with spastic dysarthria including slow and inappropriate velar movement. These several clinical signs are summarized in Table 12-3.

Hypokinetic Dysarthria

The problem of hypokinetic dysarthria is the result of one neurologic disease—Parkinsonism (paralysis agitans). Since the dysarthria is associated with a unitary neurologic disease, it is possible to cite incidence figures. The American Speech and Hearing Association (1975) estimated that between 500,000 and 1 million people in the United States have Parkinson's disease. Furthermore, between 25,000 and 43,000 new cases are reported each year. This disease has a particular affinity for the aged, and this same source estimated that one of every thousand over age 50 will be afflicted with Parkinson's disease.

Patients with Parkinsonism appear to have a deficiency of dopamine, a chemical substance manufactured in the substantia nigra and released in the corpus striatum (globus pallidus and caudate) of the basal ganglia. It is thought to function as an inhibitory transmitter substance. According to Darley et al. (1975) the extrapyramidal system, of which the basal ganglia are a part, serves two functions: 1) via an ascending path, to the thalamus and cortex, it provides a checking or reducing action upon cortically generated movement commands; 2) via a descending path to the brain stem, it provides for diminution of tone and facilitation of movement. If the inhibitory activity of dopamine is lost or reduced, some cortically generated movement commands will be issued without adequate extrapyramidal governance. Alternatively, facilitation of movements will be impaired and tone will be exaggerated. The clinical manifestations of hypokinesia, therefore, are slowness of movement, limited range of movement, cogwheel rigidity, reduced automaticity of movement, resting tremor, and festination (Darley et al., 1975).

Table 12-3. Summary of clinical speech manifestations of spastic dysarthria

Respiratory deviations	Clinical implications	Laryngeal deviations	Clinical implications	Articulatory deviations	Clinical implications
Involuntary movement (probable)	Disturbances in phrasing	Hypervalving	Tension quality to the voice	Muscle control problems (strength, speed, range)	Imprecise consonants
	Problems sustaining phonation		Reduced pitch variability		Distorted vowels
	Disturbances in prosody		Reduced loudness variability		Velopharyngeal control problems
Reduced vital capacity (probable)	Reductions in sustained driving force		Low pitch (probable)		Reduced rate
	Shortened phrases				Increased phonatory and pause duration
Expiratory-inspiratory muscle antagonism (probable)	Same as above				Reduced diadochokinetic rates

There is a growing body of experimental evidence regarding the clinical speech manifestations of hypokinetic dysarthria. Some controversy exists concerning the respiratory deviations observed among patients with Parkinsonism, but several researchers have reported rapid rates of exchange (Cramer, 1940; Kim, 1968), reduced vital capacity (Laszewski, 1956; de la Torre, Mier, and Boshes, 1960), difficulties in initiating phonation (Ewanowski, 1964), and altering automatic respiration to that required for speech (Kim, 1968). The rigidity of the respiratory system described by Kim (1968) might partially explain the reduced intensity level and intensity variability discovered by Darley et al. (1969b).

Several studies have focused on an evaluation of fundamental frequency in patients with paralysis agitans. Both Canter (1963) and Kammermeier (1969) reported noticeably higher fundamental frequencies. These two studies were also consistent in documenting a markedly reduced phonational frequency range. There is difficulty in explaining the higher fundamental frequency. Possibly the increased tone of certain laryngeal muscles acts to reduce the vibrating mass of the vocal folds. To the knowledge of the present authors, however, this speculation has no experimental support. The limited range of movement characteristic of hypokinesia serves to explain the reduced pitch variability. In this context, one might anticipate vocal intensity to be reduced in accordance with the observation of Darley et al. (1969a) that loudness was judged lower among Parkinsonian patients. However, Canter (1963, 1965a) did not provide experimental evidence in support of that expectation.

In their perceptual studies, Darley, et al. (1969a, b) reported seven major deviations in judged voice quality: 1) reduced pitch variability, 2) reduced loudness variability, 3) reduction of proper stress, 4) low pitch (a finding inconsistent with research reported earlier), 5) harshness (breathiness and laryngeal tension), 6) breathiness, and 7) inappropriate silences (probably because of difficulties in voluntary initiation of phonation).

In considering the articulatory deviations characteristic of hypokinetic dysarthria, one rather common observation continually emerges in the literature. Though it has been variously labeled, perhaps Darley et al. (1975) described it best as "inadequate articulatory valving" (p. 188). Presumably, there are reduced excursions of movable articulators and diminished contact forces which result in several notable articulation problems. For example, Canter (1965b) and Lehiste (1965) reported numerous manner of articulation errors particularly in the case of fricative production. This observation was supported by the perceptual characteristic of imprecise consonants discovered in the Darley et al. (1969a, b) studies.

A rather extensive experiment involving electromyographic recordings of several labial muscles in 12 patients with Parkinsonism was undertaken by Leanderson, Meyerson, and Persson (1972). The findings may be summarized as follows. 1) The patients exhibited exaggerated background hypertonicity in all muscles that was often so great that it masked the muscle responses for articulatory activity during speech. 2) The synergistic activity of the reciprocal muscle groups was disturbed. 3) The onset of lip activity for labial sounds was much earlier among patients with Parkinsonian dysarthria. 4) Most normal speakers tended to exhibit differences in electromyographic activity for the same phoneme in varying contexts; this differential functioning tended to be diminished among the patients. 5) The electromyographic findings were sensitive to progression of the disease and showed improvements resulting from administration of L-dopa.

A final important observation concerning hypokinetic dysarthria relates to the unique pattern of behavior often elicited when a patient is asked to perform a rapid repetitive movement of the articulators (diadochokinesis). For example, the speech pathologist might ask the patient to repeat the syllable "tuh" as rapidly as possible. What commonly happens is that the patient will exhibit a rapid acceleration with reduced articulator range such that discrete productions are blurred and a continuant sound emerges (Canter, 1965b). This common clinical observation was not confirmed by Ewanowski (1964) or Kreul (1972). The clinical manifestations of hypokinetic dysarthria are summarized in Table 12-4.

Hyperkinetic Dysarthria

Adventitious hyperkinesias are relatively rare and are therefore only discussed briefly in the present chapter. The reader is referred to Darley et al. (1975) for a more comprehensive treatment. Hyperkinetic states result from damage to the extrapyramidal system (principally the corpus striatum) that in turn results in unchecked movements generated by the cerebral motor cortex. As noted in the previous section, one function of the extrapyramidal system was described as inhibition of the cerebral cortex. Hyperkinesias are thus characterized by abnormal involuntary movements which may be sustained or unsustained, typically random, and usually un-

Table 12–4. Summary of clinical speech manifestations of hypokinetic dysarthria

Respiratory deviations	Clinical implications	Laryngeal deviations	Clinical implications	Articulatory deviations	Clinical implications
Rapid rate of exchange (?)	Disturbances in phrasing	Hypertonia	Elevated pitch	Hypotonia	Limited range of articulatory movement
			Tension quality to the voice		Imprecise consonants-particularly manner of production errors
Reduced vital capacity (?)	Shortened phrases (?)	Limited range of laryngeal muscle and cartilage movement	Reduced pitch variability	Festination	Abnormally rapid or "blurred" diadochokinetic movements
Problems alternating between vegetative and speech breathing leading to problems initiating phonation	Inappropriate silences		Reduced loudness variability Reduced loudness (?)		
Hypertonia	Reduced pitch variability Reduced loudness variability	Problems initiating laryngeal movement	Inappropriate silences		

patterned (Darley et al., 1975). Hyperkinetic states and, therefore, hyperkinetic dysarthrias may be of two types: quick and slow.

Quick hyperkinetic dysarthria may be found in disorders characterized by myoclonic jerks, tics, chorea, and ballism. Darley et al. (1969a, b) discovered the most prominant perceptual correlates of this dysarthria to be: imprecise consonants, prolonged interword or intersyllable intervals, variable rate, reduced pitch variability, harsh voice quality (breathiness and laryngeal tension), inappropriate silences, distorted vowels, and sudden, uncontrolled variations in loudness. Beyond this extensive perceptual experiment, however, little or no formal research with the quick hyperkinesias has been completed.

According to Darley et al. (1975), slow hyperkinetic dysarthria may be seen in the neurologic conditions of athetosis, dyskinesia, and dystonia. Typically, patients with dystonia will exhibit imprecise consonants, distorted vowels, harsh voice quality, irregular articulatory breakdown, strained-strangled voice quality, and reduced pitch and loudness variability (Darley et al., 1969a, b). Similar descriptions exist in the literature with respect to athetoid patients (Rutherford, 1944; Palmer, 1952; Lencione, 1953; Byrne, 1959). In addition, Hardy (1964) and McDonald and Chance (1964) described reduced ventilatory capabilities and increased breathing rates among athetoid children. Of course, these respiratory disturbances would reduce the sustained driving force typically needed for speech production.

Table 12-5 summarizes the clinical speech manifestations found in patients with hyperkinetic dysarthria.

Mixed Dysarthria

As might be anticipated, the generalized nature of certain central nervous system lesions (e.g., cerebrovascular accidents, tumors, inflammation, widespread degeneration, etc.) makes possible the existence of dysarthric conditions involving characteristics of more than one of the "pure" forms heretofore described. These are not discussed in detail here and the reader is again referred to Darley et al. (1975) where an excellent discussion of three mixed forms is available. The first, amyotrophic lateral sclerosis, typically involves both upper and lower motor neuron centers, thereby resulting in a mixed flaccid-spastic dysarthria. The problem of multiple sclerosis was observed to affect primarily the cerebellum or the cerebellum and brain stem with ataxic dysarthria a prominant symptom. A good review of dysarthria associated with multiple sclerosis may be

Table 12–5. Summary of clinical speech manifestations in hyperkinetic dysarthria

Respiratory deviations	Clinical implications	Laryngeal deviations	Clinical implications	Articulatory deviations	Clinical implications
Sudden, often excessive inspiratory and expiratory exchange (Q)	Vocal arrests Pitch and loudness variations	Intermittent hypervalving (Q and S)	Tension quality to the voice	Disturbed oral motor accuracy and dysmetria (Q and S)	Imprecise consonants
			Variations in pitch and loudness		Distorted vowels
	Sighs				Disturbances in diadochokinetic regularity
Reduced vital capacity (S and perhaps Q)	Reductions in sustained driving force	Intermittent hypovalving (S and perhaps Q)	Breathy voice		Prolonged phonemes
	Reduced phrases	Intermittent, brief, and random laryngeal occlusions (Q)	Vocal arrests		
Expiratory-inspiratory muscle antagonism (S and perhaps Q)	Same as above				
Problems alternating between vegetative and speech breathing leading to problems initiating phonation (S)	Inappropriate silences	Muscle force weakness (S)	Reduced pitch and loudness variability		
			Overall prosodic disturbances result from above deviations		

[a]Q, quick form; S, slow form.

found in Darley et al. (1972). The third disorder, described in detail in Berry, Darley, Aronson, and Goldstein (1974), is Wilson's disease. Briefly, patients with this disorder will often exhibit characteristics of hypokinetic, ataxic, and spastic dysarthria.

A CLINICAL COMMENT

As can be seen from this brief review of dysarthria, the various neuromuscular patterns evidence rather unique perceptual characteristics. Accordingly, a trained speech pathologist can frequently identify the site of lesion by careful analysis of the speech samples. As noted by Aronson (1977), speech disruptions can often appear very early in certain neuromotor conditions, and the competent speech pathologist can play an important role in assisting the neurologist to diagnose a particular disorder. This point is amplified in Chapter 20.

SUGGESTED READING

Darley, F. L., Aronson, A., and Brown, J. R. Motor Speech Disorders. Philadelphia: W. B. Saunders, 1975.

REFERENCES

American Speech and Hearing Association. Resource Materials for Communicative Problems of Older Persons. Washington, D.C.: U.S. Department of Commerce, HRP-0014306, 1975.

Aronson, A. E. Motor speech disorders. Paper presented at the biannual convention of the Idaho Speech and Hearing Association, Sun Valley, 1977.

Berry, W. R., Darley, F. L., Aronson, A. E., and Goldstein, N. P. Dysarthria in Wilson's disease. Journal of Speech and Hearing Research, 17, 169–183 (1974).

Bollinger, R. L. Geriatric speech pathology. Gerontologist, 14, 217–220 (1974).

Byrne, M. C. Speech and language development of athetoid and spastic children. Journal of Speech and Hearing Disorders, 24, 231–240 (1959).

Canter, C. J. Speech characteristics of patients with Parkinson's disease: I. Intensity, pitch, and duration. Journal of Speech and Hearing Disorders, 28, 221–229 (1963).

Canter, G. J. Speech characteristics of patients with Parkinson's disease: II. Physical support for speech. Journal of Speech and Hearing Disorders, 30, 44–49 (1965a).

Canter, G. J. Speech characteristics of patients with Parkinson's disease:

III. Articulation diadochokinesis and overall speech adequacy. Journal of Speech and hearing Disorders, 30, 217–224 (1965b).

Chusid, J. G. Correlative Neuroanatomy and Functional Neurology. Los Altos, Cal.: Lange Medical Publications, 1970.

Cramer, W. De spraak bij patienten met Parkinsonism. Logopedics en Phoniatrics, 22, 17–23 (1940).

Darley, F. L., Aronson, A. E., and Brown, J. R. Differential diagnostic patterns of dysarthria. Journal of Speech and Hearing Research, 12, 246–269 (1969a).

Darley, F. L., Aronson, A. E., and Brown, J. R. Clusters of deviant speech dimensions in the dysarthrias. Journal of Speech and Hearing Research, 12, 462–496 (1969b).

Darley, F. L., Aronson, A. E., and Brown, J. R. Motor Speech Disorders. Philadelphia: W. B. Saunders, 1975.

Darley, F. L., Brown, J. R., and Goldstein, N. P. Dysarthria in multiple sclerosis. Journal of Speech and Hearing Research, 15, 229–245 (1972).

de la Torre, R., Mier, M., and Boshes, B. Studies in parkinsonism. IX. Evaluation of respiratory function, preliminary observations. Quarterly Bulletin of the Northwestern University Medical School, 34, 332–336 (1960).

Ewanowski, S. J. Selected motor-speech behavior of patients with parkinsonism. Unpublished doctoral dissertation, University of Wisconsin, Madison, 1964.

Foley, J. M. Sensation and behavior. In W. S. Fields (ed.), Neurological and Sensory Disorders in the Elderly. New York: Stratton Intercontinental Medical Book Corp., 1975.

Haggard, M. P. Speech waveform measurements in multiple sclerosis. Folia Phoniatrica, 21, 307–312 (1969).

Hardy, J. C. Lung function of athetoid and spastic quadriplegic children. Developmental Medicine and Child Neurology, 6, 378–388 (1961).

Hardy, J. C. Lung function of athetoid and spastic quadriplegic children. Developmental Medicine and Child Neurology, 6, 378–388 (1964).

Kammermeier, M. A. A comparison of phonatory phenomena among groups of neurologically impaired speakers. Unpublished doctoral dissertation, University of Minnesota, Minneapolis, 1969.

Kim, R. The chronic residual respiratory disorder in post-encephalitic parkinsonism. Journal of Neurology, Neurosurgery, and Psychiatry, 31, 393–398 (1968).

Kreul, E. J. Neuromuscular control examination (NMC) for parkinsonism: Vowel prolongations and diadochokinetic and reading rates. Journal of Speech and Hearing Research, 15, 72–83 (1972).

Laszewski, Z. Role of the Department of Rehabilitation in preoperative evaluation of Parkinsonian patients. Journal of the American Geriatric Society, 4, 1280–1284 (1956).

Leanderson, R., Meyerson, B. A., and Persson, A. Lip muscle function in parkinsonian dysarthria. Acta Otolaryngologica, 73, 1–8 (1972).

Lehiste, I. Some acoustic characteristics of dysarthric speech. Bibliotheca Phonetica, Fasc. 2, (1965).

Lencione, R. M. A study of the speech sound intelligibility status of a group of educable cerebral palsied children. Unpublished doctoral dissertation, Northwestern University, Evanston, 1953.

Luchsinger, R. E., and Arnold, G. E. Voice-Speech-Language. Belmont, Cal.: Wadsworth, 1965.

McDonald, E. T., and Chance, B. Cerebral Palsy. Englewood Cliffs, N.J.: Prentice-Hall, 1964.

Palmer, M. F. Speech therapy in cerebral palsy. Journal of Pediatrics, 40, 514–524 (1952).

Netsell, R. Evaluation of velopharyngeal function in dysarthria. Journal of Speech and Hearing Disorders, 34, 113–122 (1969).

Rutherford, D. A comparative study of loudness, pitch, rate, rhythm, and quality of the speech of children handicapped by cerebral palsy. Journal of Speech Disorders, 9, 263–271 (1944).

Spahr, F. T. White House conference on aging. 13, 14–17 (1971).

Zemlin, W. R. A comparison of the periodic function of vocal fold vibration in a multiple sclerosis and a normal population. Unpublished doctoral dissertation, University of Minnesota, Minneapolis, 1962.

Chapter 13
Aphasia

Aphasia is defined as a disorder of language resulting from damage to the central nervous system. Consideration is given to the causes and types of aphasia. A brief historical overview of aphasia is given to acquaint the reader with some of the issues in this area.

DEFINITION OF APHASIA

Aphasia is one of the more difficult and complex communication disorders encountered by the health professional working with the aged. This disorder is not a modality-specific communication impairment such as agnosia or apraxia of speech. Rather, it is a unified impairment of all language modalities: auditory processing, speech, reading, and writing, resulting from damage to the speech and language centers of the brain (Schuell, Jenkins, and Jimenez-Pabon, 1964; Smith, 1972; Duffy and Ulrich, 1976). Damage to the central language processor of the brain impairs that patient's ability to use the grammar system and lexicon as explained in the latter portion of Chapter 2. Although aphasia is usually compounded, to one degree or another, by the presence of intellectual degeneration, agnosias, and apraxias, it does not include disturbances such as psychoses, developmental speech disorders, or dysarthria.

TYPES OF APHASIA

One of the problems encountered in dealing with aphasia is describing the aphasic patient's problem in a concise and mutually understood fashion. At present, there are really no satisfactory classifications of aphasia that everyone is willing to accept. As evidence of this there have been many classification schemes devised from Wernicke's time (late 1800s) to the present.

For the purposes of this chapter an emperically oriented classification system is used. The main intent is to provide the reader with a framework to understand aphasia. The categories of aphasia used here reflect the large history of clinical descriptions and the associated anatomic evidence. For these reasons three main types of aphasia have been selected as being most representative: 1) nonfluent aphasia, 2) fluent aphasia, and 3) global aphasia (Geschwind, 1971).

Based on the results from autopsies (Geschwind, 1970, 1972), cortical excision (Milner, 1967), split-brain studies or callosal sectionings (Gazzaniga, 1967; Sperry, 1968), cortical stimulation (Penfield and Roberts, 1959), focal brain lesion studies (Luria, 1958, 1970) brain scans (Benson, 1967), and clinical observations (Jackson, 1878; Head, 1926; Schuell et al., 1964), the accumulated evidence strongly suggests that fluent aphasias are associated with posterocortical lesions whereas nonfluent aphasias are associated with more anterocortical lesions. As summarized by Darley (1977): 1) a lesion limited to Broca's area (see Figure 2-21) produces apraxia of speech; 2) a lesion involving Broca's area plus adjacent cortical tissue results in a combination of apraxia of speech and aphasia (nonfluent aphasia); 3) a lesion in Wernicke's area (see Figure 2-21) impairs the use of the grammar and lexical systems in all language modalities (fluent aphasia); 4) posterior lesions peripheral to Wernicke's area produce isolated language deficits; and 5) massive lesions of the midtemporal-anteroparietal region result in global aphasia. Table 13-1 presents these findings in a more concise form.

Language Symptoms of Aphasics

As suggested earlier, the aphasic patient has difficulty in using the grammar and lexical systems of a given language. In order to more fully appreciate the nature of these deficits, some examples from the speech of fluent and nonfluent aphasics might be instructive. A

Table 13-1. Neurologic deficits, site of lesion, and symptomology

Deficit	Site of lesion	Symptoms
Nonfluent aphasia	Broca's area and adjacent parieto-temporal areas	Apraxia of speech plus aphasia
Fluent aphasia	Wernicke's area	Aphasia: impaired language abilities as manifest in auditory processing, speech, reading, and writing
Global aphasia	Massive involvement of the midtemporal-anteroparietal cortex	Severe aphasia impairment

typical extract from the transcript of a fluent aphasic's speech is, for example:

Examiner:	"What do people wear on their heads?"
Patient:	"People work?" "Like I do?"
Examiner:	"No—"
Patient:	"Oh, where do people going out. Well, you take a girl woman where they buy things ... ah—different women ya mean? What they ... take look not we don' drink ... they drink ya know ... or we have our stuff ... just men instead of a woman. Right? They we would take clothes an' nice. Am I speaking it?"

In this speech sample the patient spoke fairly rapidly and with ease. However, the semantic and syntactic elements are disrupted. The nonfluent aphasic, on the other hand, has difficulty in putting together a connected utterance and also mispronounces the words that are said. The following example is illustrative:

Examiner:	"When did you get sick?"
Patient:	"Ah ... fie ... yera ... ah ... "
Examiner:	"What kind of work did you used to do?"
Patient:	"Ah, wal ... wal ... when ... oh ah, mishom ... yes-brokem brem. Ah ... oh! No ... ah."
Examiner:	"What are your children's names?"
Patient:	"Ah-Ma ... ah, Mer ... no, ... Mary? No! Ah,Sishy ...ah, Shuzie, ... Debb, 'un Marka."

In the case of the global aphasic little if any language output of any kind is evident. Furthermore, these patients do not seem to comprehend what is said to them and as a result are essentially noncommunicative.

Dominant Hemisphere Factors

In the overwhelming majority of cases, aphasia results from damage to the left cerebral hemisphere. This is true for most right-handers and even many left-handers (Brown and Simonson, 1957). Annett (1975) examined the question of hand preference and laterality of language functions for speech by comparing the data from five aphasia studies. A summary of these studies indicates that very few right-handers suffer aphasia from right hemisphere lesions. Bogen and Bogen (1976) have indicated that the odds are about 50 to 1 that an aphasiogenic lesion is in the left hemisphere of a right-handed person. Such a lesion only occurs in the right hemisphere of a right-handed person about 1–2% of the time. In the case of left-handedness, Annett concludes that lesions in either the left or right hemisphere may produce aphasia, with left hemisphere lesions being more frequently implicated.

SPECIFIC CAUSES AND INCIDENCE

The specific causes of aphasia in the older patient are most frequently linked to cerebrovascular disorders and their end product, stroke. According to Marks, Taylor, and Rusk (1957), 94% of all aphasic syndromes are the result of thromboses, hemorrhage, arterial compression, and arterial spasms. Brown and Simonson (1957) reported similar findings: infarct and mass lesions, 93%; all other causes, 7%. Stroke in old age is apparently the product of a lifelong exposure to conditions which contribute to the development of arteriosclerosis and coronary and hypertensive heart disease (Librach, Schadel, Seltzer, Hart and Yellin, 1977).

The incidence, symptoms, and signs of stroke have been reported for a number of large stroke populations (Gurdjian, Lindner, Hardy, and Webster, 1960; Whisnant, Fitzgibbons, Kurland, and Sayre, 1971; Matsumoto, Whisnant, Kurland, and Okazaki, 1973; Brust, Shafer, Richter, and Bruun, 1976; Librach et al., 1977). Except for the study by Brust et al., few details were given in these reports relative to language impairments. For example, neither Whisnant et al. nor Librach et al. mentioned how many of the stroke patients they studied had aphasic deficits. Matsumoto et al. did report that of the 610 stroke patients who had survived at least 6 months, 10% were aphasic. Gurdjian et al. reported that 25% of the 600 patients they studied were aphasic. Similarly, Brust et al. indicated that 21% of the 850 stroke patients in their population were aphasic. Using the latter two studies as a basis of estimation it would appear that a conservative estimate of 400,000 aphasic survivors of stroke live in the United States.

Brust et al. (1976) further categorized their aphasic subjects by type, average age, sex, presence of hemianopsia (visual field defects), and severity. Table 13-2 summarizes their findings. From this table some interesting differences become apparent between the fluent and nonfluent aphasics studied by these authors. The fluent aphasics were a bit younger on the average, mostly women, and had milder defects. Conversely, nonfluent aphasics were older, mostly men, and had more severe deficits. The aphasic age data reported by these authors are also very similar to an earlier study by Brown and Simonson (1957). These latter authors indicated that 42% of

Table 13-2. Summary of aphasia patient characteristics (N = 177)

Aphasia type	Average age (years)	Involvement by sex (%) Males	Females	Hemianopsia Present (%)	Severity (%) Mild	Moderate	Severe
Fluent	65	44	56	32	49	28	23
Nonfluent	68	54	46	55	13	28	59

Source: Adapted from Brust et al. (1976).

the aphasic patients they studied were age 60 or older at the time of their insult.

NONLANGUAGE PROBLEMS

Several nonlanguage behaviors are typically manifest as part of the syndrome called aphasia. These behaviors may be grouped under three broad categories: physical, emotional, and intellectual.

Physical

The physical symptoms associated with aphasia may include facial paresis or weakness, right hemiplegia (in most cases), sensation deficits such as visual field defects (homonymous hemianopsia) and loss of a sense of touch, and loss of balance. Any of these problems or a combination thereof may impair the patient's ability to walk, eat, get dressed, or toilet himself. Food preferences may be altered, or the aphasic patient might complain that food is tasteless and uninteresting to eat. These patients may also complain of pain in their paralyzed limbs and suffer the embarrassment of bladder and bowel incontinence.

Emotional

Emotional problems in the aphasic are probably the most difficult to deal with. Typical behaviors manifest here include inappropriate laughing or crying or, in the case of catastrophic reactions, a longer lasting, more severe disorganization accompanied by physical violence. These problems arise, in part, because of lowered defense thresholds and an inability to cope with deprivation, frustration, grief, failure, conflict, or threat. In this regard a study by Skelly (1975) as reported in Chapter 22, of the concerns of 50 aphasic patients is particularly enlightening. This study indicates that health care professionals could help relieve some of the emotional problems of the elderly aphasic patient by being more aware of their problems.

Intellectual

In the broad area of reduced intellective capacity the aphasic person faces a number of problems that are apparently part of the aphasic syndrome. These problems include a reduced attention span, not being alert, being easily distracted, tiring easily, perseveration, impaired short-term memory, reduced learning capacity, reduced ability to reason abstractly, and a loss of geographic orientation or a loss of body scheme. Other intellectualization impairments include mental retardation, senility, and psychological disorders. Since the aging are particularly susceptible to these latter problems as a function of general body deterioration, these disorders of intellectualization are more properly regarded as substrates or concomitant factors rather than as part of the aphasic syndrome.

By the time most individuals reach old age they have learned and developed strategies for responding to illnesses, incapacities, frustrations, and the influences they are subject to in everyday living. How a person responds to the effects of aphasia will largely depend on the kind of person he was before the insult. Personality will usually be modified in each instance, but almost never in the direction of improvement. However, aphasia will probably not produce a new personality that is unrelated to the person's premorbid state of behavior.

SOME COMMENTS ON THE STUDY OF APHASIA

Historical Perspective

Judging from the available evidence mankind has a long history of suffering from language impairments during adult life. Benton and Joynt (1960) and Benton (1964) have provided an exhaustive account of the history of aphasia prior to 1800. Despite the emphasis of some writers on the contributions made in the mid to late 19th century, a very substantial body of knowledge about aphasia existed before that time in the form of clinical descriptions.

According to Benton (1964), the 17th and 18th centuries were a time of profound developments in our understanding of aphasia. In particular, the contributions of Johann Gesner in 1770 are worthy of note because he was one of the first to attribute aphasic disorders to specific verbal memory impairment rather than to a general intellectual decline. Other researchers in aphasiology laid the foundation for the later developments occurring after 1850. Hence, by the time Broca and Wernicke came to the fore a great deal was already known about aphasia upon which these and other researchers could build their theories (Geschwind, 1964).

From 1850 onward, a huge corpus of literature has been accumulated on aphasia. An extensive review is well beyond the scope of this chapter. For more complete accounts interested readers should examine the works of Head (1926), Weisenberg and McBride (1935), Schuell et al. (1964), Brain (1965), and Meyer (1974).

The Localization Controversy

Since the mid-1800s two main streams of thought have dominated the literature regarding aphasia; one view is represented by the localizationist school and the other by the antilocalizationist philosophy. Even today the arguments are not entirely resolved. Aphasia disorders became associated with localized brain centers beginning with Broca's discovery of a center for the motor images of words and Wernicke's work on what he termed "sensory aphasia." By 1890, many forms of aphasia had been identified with each being associated with the destruction of a particular cortical center (Luria, 1972).

According to Head (1926), Hughlings Jackson offered the first serious challenge to this localizationist view of brain function. Jackson felt that the processes of speech were based on dynamic levels of sensorimotor integration and that when higher levels of propositional speech were disrupted as a result of an aphasia-producing lesion, lower nonpropositional or automatic levels of speech were released from control (Jackson, 1874/1913). Jackson's challenge questioned the propriety of ascribing specific behaviors to cortical "centers" while ignoring the contributions of the rest of the brain. These views polarized the thinking of investigators and had a profound effect on our understanding of brain function today.

Out of these two theories has arisen an intermediate position which attempts to harmonize the known evidence into a more unified concept of brain function. Schuell (1974) referred to this view as a "functional equivalence theory" and pointed out that, as such, it argues for a limited localization of brain function. Instead of considering that there are specific centers, as the localizationist view would hold, this more moderate view favors the concept of functional regions which may overlap. Although there is no clear-cut experimental evidence to confirm the functional equivalence theory, most aphasiologists probably hold this view today.

SUGGESTED READINGS

Brain, W. R. Speech Disorders: Aphasia, Apraxia and Agnosia (2nd Ed.). Washington, D.C.: Butterworths, 1965.

Schuell, H. Aphasia Theory and Therapy (edited by L. F. Sies). Baltimore: University Park Press, 1974.

REFERENCES

Annett, M. Hand preference and the laterality of cerebral speech. Cortex, 11, 305–328 (1975).

Benson, D. F. Fluency in aphasia: Correlation with radioactive scan localization. Cortex, 3, 373–394 (1967).

Benton, A. L. Contributions to aphasia before Broca. Cortex, 1, 314–327 (1964).

Benton, A. L., and Joynt, R. J. Early descriptions of aphasia. Archives of Neurology, 3, 205–222 (1960).

Bogen, J. E., and Bogen, G. M. Wernicke's region—Where is it? Annals of the New York Academy of Science, 280, 834–843 (1976).

Brain, W. R. Speech Disorders: Aphasia, Apraxia and Agnosia (2nd Ed.). Washington, D.C.: Butterworths, 1965.

Brown, J. R., and Simonson, J. A clinical study of 100 aphasic patients. Neurology, 7, 777–783 (1957).

Brust, J. C. M., Shafer, S. Q., Richter, R. W., and Bruun, B. Aphasia in acute stroke. Stroke, 7, 167–174 (1976).

Darley, F. L. A retrospective view: Aphasia. Journal of Speech and Hearing Disorders, 42, 161–169 (1977).

Duffy, R. J., and Ulrich, S. R. A comparison of impairments in verbal comprehension, speech, reading, and writing in adult aphasics. Journal of Speech and Hearing Disorders, 41, 110–119 (1976).

Gazzaniga, M. S. The split brain in man. Scientific American, 217, 24–29 (1967).

Geschwind, N. The paradoxical position of Kurt Goldstein in the history of aphasia. Cortex, 1, 214–224 (1964).

Geschwind, N. The organization of language and the brain. Science, 170, 940–944 (1970).

Geschwind, N. Current concepts: Aphasia. New England Journal of Medicine, 284, 654–656 (1971).

Geschwind, N. Language and the brain. Scientific American, 226, 76–83 (1972).

Gurdjian, E. S., Lindner, D. W., Hardy, W. G., and Webster, J. E. Cerebrovascular disease: An analysis of 600 cases. Neurology, 10, 372–380 (1960).

Head, H. Aphasia and Kindred Disorders of Speech (Vols. 1 and 2). London: Cambridge University Press, 1926.

Jackson, J. H. On the nature of the duality of the brain. Medical Press and Circular, Vol. 1 (1874). Reprinted in Brain, 38, 80–95 (1913).

Jackson, J. H. On affections of speech from disease of the brain. Brain, 1, 304–330 (1878).

Librach, G., Schadel, M., Seltzer, M., Hart, A., and Yellin, N. Stroke: Incidence and risk factors. Geriatrics, 32, 85–96 (1977).

Luria, A. R. Brain disorders and language analysis. Language and Speech, 1, 14–34 (1958).

Luria, A. R. The functional organization of the brain. Scientific American, 222, 66–78 (1970).

Luria, A. R. Aphasia reconsidered. Cortex, 8, 34–40 (1972).

Marks, M., Taylor, M., and Rusk, H. A. Rehabilitation of the aphasic patient: A survey of three years experience in a rehabilitation setting. Archives of Physical Medicine and Rehabilitation, 38, 219–226 (1957).

Matsumoto, N., Whisnant, J. P., Kurland, L. T., and Okazaki, H. Natural history of stroke in Rochester, Minnesota, 1955 through 1969: An extension of a previous study, 1945 through 1954. Stroke, 4, 20–29 (1973).

Meyer, A. The frontal lobe syndrome, the aphasias and related conditions. Brain, 97, 565–600 (1974).

Milner, B. Brain mechanisms suggested by studies of temporal lobes. In C. H. Millikan and F. L. Darley (eds.), Brain Mechanisms Underlying Speech and Language. New York: Grune & Stratton, 1967.

Penfield, W., and Roberts, L. Speech and Brain Mechanisms. Princeton, N.J.: Princeton University Press, 1959.

Schuell, H. Aphasia Theory and Therapy (edited by L. F. Seis). Baltimore: University Park Press, 1974.

Schuell, H., Jenkins, J. J., and Jimenez-Pabon, E. Aphasia in Adults. New York: Harper & Row, 1964.

Skelly, M. Aphasic patients talk back. American Journal of Nursing, 75, 1104–1142 (1975).

Smith, A. Diagnosis, Intelligence, and Rehabilitation of Chronic Aphasics: Final Report. Ann Arbor: University of Michigan, 1972.

Sperry, R. W. Hemisphere deconnection and unity in conscious awareness. American Psychology, 23, 723–733 (1968).

Weisenberg, T., and McBride, K. Aphasia—A Clinical and Psychological Study. New York: The Commonwealth Fund, 1935.

Whisnant, J. P., Fitzgibbons, J. P., Kurland, L. T., and Sayre, G. P. Natural history of stroke in Rochester, Minnesota, 1945 through 1954. Stroke, 2, 11–22 (1971).

Chapter 14
Intellectual and Memory Impairments

This chapter explores the problem of dementia and reviews the intellectual and memory impairments commonly associated with this condition. A brief explanation of several etiologies and the clinical signs of dementia is presented. Finally, there is a rather complete review of the literature regarding language disturbances among demented patients.

A cursory review of intellectual and memory capabilities of normal aging individuals was presented in Chapter 3. Briefly, it was noted that most older persons experience decrements in performance on standard intelligence tests. This seems to be relatively more true for tasks requiring acquisition of new ideas or adaptation to new situations. It was also observed previously that the elderly exhibit more difficulty in learning and retaining new information. Though some controversy exists, short-term memory appears more susceptible than long-term memory to the effects of senescence. In sum, nearly all aging persons exhibit mild impairment in intelligence and memory. However, some older people display marked deteriorations in mental functioning above and beyond the minimal decline observed in most cases of aging. In these more serious instances, the term "dementia" can be properly applied as a diagnostic label.

DESCRIPTION AND INCIDENCE OF DEMENTIA

Dementia refers to a disease or group of diseases in which there is cerebral atrophy and an associated deterioration in mental processes. There are multiple etiologies for dementia, as will be seen later, but all have in common a diffuse neuronal degeneration within the cerebral cortex. Inherent in the term "dementia" is the implication of a chronic, progressive deterioration in mental function that may have its onset in middle age or youth (Berry, 1975).

Miller (1977) has described some common clinical manifestations of dementia that include a prominent impairment of memory, particularly for recent events; impoverished, concrete thinking; emotional alterations, of which the most common is depression; and alterations in personality. It should be noted that not all demented patients will exhibit this profile of symptoms, and for some diseases this must not be considered a complete list of the clinical signs.

For several reasons, it is extremely difficult to estimate the incidence of dementia in the United States. As noted by Katzman and Karasu (1975), dementia or senile dementia is overdiagnosed, often confused with the general label "cerebral arteriosclerosis," and completely ignored in U.S. vital statistics tables. However, using several community surveys as a base, Katzman and Karasu were able to project certain percentage data to the total U.S. population over age 65. Their results are presented in Figure 14-1. In-

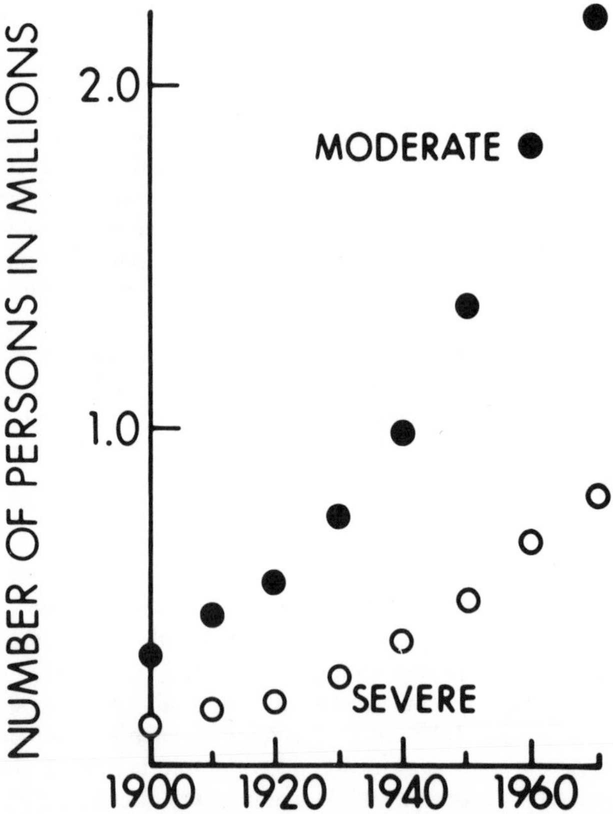

Figure 14-1. Estimated incidence of organic dementias in people age 65 or over in the United States. (Source: Katzman and Karasu, 1975.)

spection of this graph reveals that approximately 3 million people over age 65 were diagnosed as having dementia. Katzman and Karasu suggested that the term "severe" dementia would probably refer to the diagnosis of senile dementia or psychosis with cerebral brain disease, whereas "moderate" dementia would reflect the diagnosis of chronic brain syndrome without psychosis.

CAUSES OF DEMENTIA

Many of the pathological changes associated with dementia are seen to a much lesser degree in the normal aging brain. For example, a loss in brain weight, widening of sulci, shrinking of gyri, appearance of neurofibrillary tangles (condensing and coalescing of fibrils in the neuron), a depositing of starch-like material into senile plaques, and granulovacuolar changes may be seen in the normal aging brain but are particularly evident in varying degrees among the several forms of dementia (Berry, 1975).

It is beyond the scope of this chapter to present a detailed description of the several causes of dementia. However, a brief review of some of the more common etiologies is warranted. Specifically, four common etiologies of dementia are presented: 1) Alzheimer's disease/senile dementia, 2) Pick's disease, 3) Creutzfeldt-Jakob disease, and 4) arteriosclerotic brain disease. Malamud (1972) has presented a percentage distribution of these causes among 1225 autopsied cases of dementia and Table 14-1 reflects his observations.

Alzheimer's Disease/Senile Dementia

Perhaps the most common cause of dementia is the general category

Table 14-1. Distribution of types of degenerative disorders among 1225 cases

Type of disorder	Age range (years)	Number of cases (percent)	Male/Female ratio
Senile brain disease	65–98	416(34)	3:2
Alzheimer's disease	40–64	103(8.4)	2:3
Pick's disease	35–72	35(2.8)	1:1
Creutzfeldt-Jakob disease	43–86	32(2.7)	2:1
Arteriosclerotic brain disease	42–100	356(29)	2:1
Mixed senile-arteriosclerotic disease	62–94	283(23)	4:3

Source: Malamud (1972).

of Alzheimer's disease and senile dementia (senile brain disease). Traditionally, the clinical diagnosis of Alzheimer's disease and senile dementia has been based upon an arbitrary age level. If the symptoms occur before age 65, the diagnosis has usually been Alzheimer's disease; if after 65, the label "senile dementia" has been used. However, many authorities now call for abandonment of this age distinction and the use of a common diagnostic label, since the pathologic and clinical distinction of the two disorders is virtually impossible. The etiology of Alzheimer's disease is not known, though a hereditary predisposition has been reported (Busse, 1959). Whereas exact ratios differ from study to study, all agree that patients with this disease are more often females. Alzheimer's disease is characterized by diffuse brain atrophy with the presence of senile plaques, neurofibrillary tangles, and granulovacuolar changes. Focal atrophies are extremely uncommon.

The most serious clinical manifestation is loss of memory, beginning with a rather annoying forgetfulness and progressing to a more serious memory decay. This memory loss has been ascribed to deterioration in the hippocampal region, a noteworthy pathologic finding in Alzheimer's disease (Malamud, 1972). Typically, memories of recent events are lost first while past events may be well preserved. Often, the patient begins to neglect property and self, living almost entirely in the past. In addition, orientation and cognition may decline to such a degree that institutionalization is necessary. With this loss in mental capacity, many patients exhibit behavior and emotional changes such as restlessness, depression, paranoia, fantasy expression, stealing, and suicidal tendencies. Many of these alterations may be attributed to a loss of cortical inhibition over more primitive behaviors, a loss of memory for the social consequences of these actions, and patient insight regarding the pending deterioration of mental function.

Pick's Disease

As can be seen in Table 14-1, Pick's disease is a relatively rare disorder which does not reflect the female sex preponderance characteristic of Alzheimer's disease. Also, in contrast to Alzheimer's disease, Pick's disease is associated with focal atrophies usually involving bilateral degeneration of portions of the frontal, temporal, and parietal lobes (Malamud, 1972). Microscopically, there is an overall absence of neurofibrillary tangles and senile plaques but the presence of intracytoplasmic inclusions (Pick's bodies) is common (Berry, 1975).

Several clinical features distinguish Pick's disease from Alzheimer's disease. Most notable is the relatively well preserved memory function which characterizes Pick's disease. This is thought to reflect the relative sparing of the hippocampus (Malamud, 1972). In contrast, disturbances in memory and orientation are more common early features of Pick's disease (Katzman and Karasu, 1975). Usually, there is a lack of insight regarding the progressive dementia and depression is much less common than in Alzheimer's disease. It is important to note that because of the focal lobar atrophy associated with Pick's disease, symptoms of aphasia, apraxia, and agnosia may be observed (Malamud, 1972).

Creutzfeldt-Jakob Disease

Another rare cause of dementia is Creutzfeldt-Jakob disease, which has a rapid course and an unknown etiology. Pathologically, the gross changes are rather inconspicuous; however, microscopic alterations include a spongy degeneration of cortical tissues (Siedler and Malamud, 1963). Clinically, a variety of bizarre symptoms may be observed, including alterations in consciousness, myoclonus, cerebellar disturbances, sensory changes, and visual involvement.

Arteriosclerotic Brain Disease

Another very common, though perhaps overdiagnosed, cause of dementia is cerebral arteriosclerosis. With respect to the pathology of cerebral arteriosclerosis, Tomlinson et al. (1970) reported extensive softening of the brain in six patients. Usually patients are hypertensive and have a history of either a massive or multiple strokes. Depending upon the location of vascular insults, intellectual impairment and focal neurologic signs will be evident (Katzman and Karasu, 1975).

INTELLECTUAL AND MEMORY DEFICITS IN DEMENTIA

No attempt is made to present a complete review of the experimental effort related to intellectual and memory capabilities of the patient with dementia. However, a brief overview is warranted to provide a background for discussion of language disturbances typical of these patients.

With respect to intellectual functioning, perhaps the most common research strategy has been the administration of standardized intelligence tests. Miller (1977) has provided a rather extensive review of the literature in this area and has developed a table presenting the results of several studies involving the Wechsler-Bellevue and Wechsler Adult Intelligence Scales (see Table 14-2). This table reveals consistent depression in both verbal and performance scores across all studies. This is particularly evident for performance subtests where, according to Miller, response speed, manipulation of visual-spatial relationships, and adjustment to new situations are required.

Beyond these general observations of decrements in intelligence test scores, there have been few efforts to document the underlying nature or profile of changes characteristic of patients with dementia. One theoretical position regarding this problem has emerged with some strength and has been termed the "accelerated-aging" hypothesis. Very briefly, this theory holds that dementia is simply a more severe and rapid manifestation of the mental changes expected with normal aging. Miller (1974, 1977) has reviewed this position in some depth, but there are some serious reservations about the validity of such a concept.

In a rather extensive review of his work on memory loss among the aged, Kral (1966) proposed two forms of memory impairment commonly seen in this population. The first he termed a "benign" dysfunction characterized by an inability to recall certain relevant aspects of an experience (e.g., name, place, date, etc.). At a later time this information may be recalled and the subject is typically aware of the error. Most commonly, the memory loss is for events in

Table 14-2. Summary of studies applying the Wechsler intelligence scales to groups of demented patients expressed as mean IQs

	Number	Verbal	Performance	Full scale
Wechsler Bellevue				
Botwinnick and Birren (1951a)	31	—	—	84.1
Cleveland and Dysinger (1944)	17	89.5	52.8	—
Dorken and Greenbloom (1953)	67	—	—	77.6
Halstead (1943)	20	—	—	106
Lovett-Doust et al. (1953)	89	—	—	84.5
WAIS				
Bolton et al. (1966)	47	83.6	77.1	79.7
Kendrick et al. (1965)	20	93.1	79.2	—
Kendrick and Post (1967)	10	96.0	79.5	—
Miller (unpublished)	20	78.1	68.8	72.5
Sanderson and Inglis (1961)	15	89.0	—	—

Source: Miller (1977).

the remote rather than recent past. The second form of memory loss was called "malignant." In this case, complete events of the recent past may be totally forgotten and disorientation is apparent. Later, remote memories may also be lost.

Many psychometric studies have documented mild, benign memory impairments as a function of advancing age (Kral, 1958, 1966; Miller, 1977). However, the presence of the malignant form of memory loss is quite common among patients with dementia, particularly those having Alzheimer's/senile brain disease.

Miller (1971), in a series of experiments, provided some additional insight regarding the nature of malignant memory loss in subjects during early stages of dementia. His experimental strategy involved presenting subjects with a list of words, at the rate of one word per 1.5 seconds, and asking them to recall as many of the words as possible. For normal subjects the expected result of enhanced memory for first and last words in the list was confirmed. The increased recall of early words has been attributed to a passing of these items from short-term to long-term storage, whereas the easier recollection of later words reflects the strength of short-term storage (Glanger and Cunitz, 1966). With demented patients, however, Miller noted that, in addition to a generally poor performance on the task, there was an almost total lack of recall for the first words on the list. This was interpreted to mean that very little material was reaching the long-term store.

Miller was uncertain whether or not this latter finding was a reflection of an impaired short-term store or a problem in transferring information to the long-term store. He reasoned that a slower rate of word presentation should enhance recall of early words since there would be a greater opportunity for unhindered transfer to long-term storage. In a second experiment, he tested this hypothesis and discovered, in contrast to normal subjects, that demented subjects gained no advantage in early recall from a slower stimulus presentation rate. These data were collectively interpreted as evidence of a two-factor explanation for memory impairments in dementia. Specifically, there is impairment of both short-term memory capacity and establishment of new data in long-term storage.

LANGUAGE FUNCTIONING AMONG PATIENTS WITH DEMENTIA

Of particular concern to the central thesis of this book is the language functioning of patients with a diagnosed case of dementia.

To date, the research is fragmentary and incomplete, but several studies have been published and warrant brief review.

By far the greatest experimental effort has been devoted to word recall and object naming skills among these patients. Critchley (1964) described the language impairment of demented patients as a "... poverty of speech due to inaccessibility of those vocabularies which ordinarily we can utilize ..." (p. 354). Furthermore, he indicated that demented patients often use inappropriate labels for objects presented to them. Indeed, some experimental support for Critchley's notion was provided by Barker and Lawson (1968), who compared 100 patients with dementia to 40 normal gerontological subjects on several dimensions of an object-naming task. Briefly, they confirmed that demented subjects made significantly more errors in naming, and this effect was more dramatic for less common objects. These results are presented in Figure 14-2. It is also interesting to note that when the experimenter demonstrated the target object and/or the subject was allowed to handle it, the number of errors was significantly reduced for the patients with dementia but not for the normal subjects. These data were interpreted to mean that word-finding problems are a general feature of dementia, and in any clinical assessment of this feature the examiner should evaluate the factor of word frequency. In addition, Barker and Lawson argued that demonstration and handling of objects facilitates object identification more than the process of word finding.

Further insight regarding naming errors among demented patients was provided by Rochford (1971). He compared 43 aphasic subjects with 23 demented subjects on a simple object-naming task. In categorizing the pattern of errors, Rochford noted that the predominant error of aphasics was failure to name the object whereas that of the dements was misrecognition. Often, the demented subjects would offer a name of an object visually similar to the one being presented. Thus, there appeared to be more of an impairment of recognition without impairment of encoding ability. In a sense, this problem may be properly called agnosia. In examining this hypothesis more closely, Rochford also asked the two subject groups to identify the very familiar and highly overlearned names of body parts. Interestingly, the aphasics made no dramatic improvements but the patients with dementia did.

It should be noted that two experiments by Miller and Hague (1975) cast some doubt on the hypothesized word-finding difficulty suggested by Critchley and Barker and Lawson. In the experiments

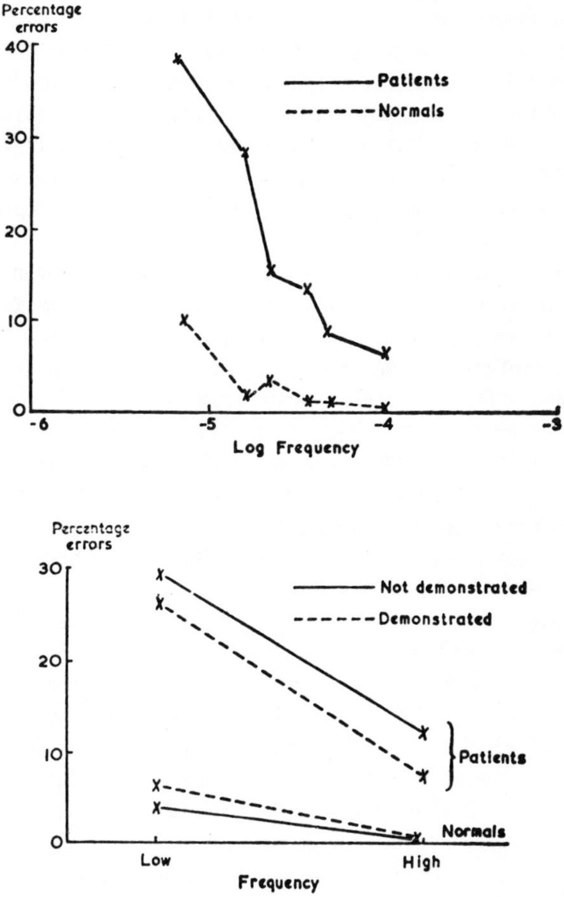

Figure 14.2. Naming errors for demented patients and normal gerontologic subjects as a function of frequency of stimulus (top) and frequency of stimulus with availability of object demonstration (bottom). (Source: Barker and Lawson, 1968.)

by Miller and Hague, subjects with dementia were compared with other institutionalized patients free of organic brain problems. In the first experiment, the subjects were asked to produce as many words beginning with "s" as possible in 5 minutes. As anticipated, the patients with dementia exhibited a much lower cumulative frequency of word output. Furthermore, the control group produced a much higher percentage of uncommon words. These findings would seem to support the idea that word-finding ability is depressed among demented subjects, particularly for rarer words. However, in the second experiment, the subjects' conversational speech samples were analyzed and no differences emerged between experimental groups with respect to frequency of rare and common word production. This later observation suggests that word retrieval among demented patients may be normal but the rate of expression is reduced.

Few other experiments are available regarding language functioning and dementia. One rather comprehensive study of language functioning by patients with aphasia, apraxia, general intellectual impairment, and confused language was reported by Halpern, Darley, and Brown (1973). The 10 subjects with intellectual impairments are of particular concern to this discussion. Basically, Halpern et al. discovered that these subjects exhibited "adequacy" disturbances with respect to their language output. Adequacy problems included erroneous responses to requests for definitions or in answering questions; reduced elaboration in answering; and substitution, deletion, or addition of substantive words. In addition, subjects with general intellectual impairments manifested problems with reading comprehension, arithmetic, and auditory comprehension.

In contrast to these rather consistent observations by Halpern et al., Ernst, Dalby, and Dalby (1970a) found no uniform pattern of aphasic disturbances for nine patients with pre-senile dementia except a "poverty of words" and "lack of language initiative" (p. 100). A similar lack of consistency for "gnostic-praxic" skills was observed in a second study by Ernst, Dalby, and Dalby, (1970b). This general lack of consistency was attributed to the variety of diffuse central lesions characteristic of the subject group examined.

A final study of interest in this discussion concerns perseverative (abnormal continuation of an act or idea) characteristics in the language production of demented patients. Freeman and Gathercole (1966) used 16 tests designed to elicit perseveration and compared a group of 20 schizophrenic and 20 demented subjects. The investigators found that demented subjects exhibit preservation errors of the "impaired switching type." Briefly, this error pattern occurs when the subject responds to an initial stimulus and then inappropriately reuses that response when a second stimulus is presented. Both Goldstein (1943) and Luria (1966) suggested that impaired switching is a manifestation of cortical involvement.

SUGGESTED READINGS

Halpern, H., Darley, F. L., and Brown, J. R. Differential language and neurologic characteristics in cerebral involvement. Journal of Speech and Hearing Disorders, 38, 162–173 (1973).

Miller, E. Abnormal Ageing. London: John Wiley & Sons, 1977.

REFERENCES

Barker, M. G., and Lawson, J. S. Nominal aphasia in dementia. British Journal of Psychiatry, 114, 1351–1356 (1968).

Berry, R. G. Pathology of dementia. In J. G. Howells (ed.), Modern Perspectives in the Psychiatry of Old Age. New York: Brunner/Mazel, 1975.

Busse, E. W. Psychopathology. In J. E. Birren (ed.), Handbook of Aging and the Individual. Chicago: University of Chicago Press, 1959.

Critchley, M. The neurology of psychotic speech. British Journal of Psychiatry, 110, 353–364 (1964).

Ernst, B., Dalby, M. A., and Dalby, A. Aphasic disturbances in presenile dementia. Acta Neurologica Scandinavia, 43, Supplement 99–100 (1970a).

Ernst, B., Dalby, A., and Dalby, M. A. Gnostic-praxic disturbances in presenile dementia. Acta Neurologica Scandinavia, 43, Supplement, 101–102 (1970b).

Freeman, T., and Gathercole, C. E. Perseveration—the clinical symptoms—in chronic schizophrenia and organic dementia. British Journal of Psychiatry, 112, 27–32 (1966).

Glauzer, M., and Cunitz, A. R. Two storage mechanisms in free recall. Journal of Verbal Learning and Verbal Behavior, 5, 351–360 (1966).

Goldstein, K. Concerning rigidity. Character and Personality, 11, 209–226 (1943).

Halpern, H., Darley, F. L., and Brown, J. R. Differential language and neurologic characteristics in cerebral involvement. Journal of Speech and Hearing Disorders, 38, 162–173 (1973).

Katzman, R., and Karasu, T. B. Differential diagnosis of dementia. In W. S. Fields (ed.), Neurological and Sensory Disorders in the Elderly. New York: Symposium Specialists, Inc., 1975.

Kral, V. A. Neuropsychiatric observations in an old peoples' home. Studies of memory function in senescence. Journal of Gerontology, 13, 169–176 (1958).

Kral, V. A. Memory loss in the aged. Diseases of the Nervous System, 27, Supplement, 51–54 (1966).

Luria, A. R. Higher Cortical Functions in Man. New York: Basic Books, 1966.

Malamud, N. Neuropathology of organic brain syndromes. In C. M. Gaitz (ed.), Aging and the Brain. New York: Plenum Press, 1972.

Miller, E. On the nature of the memory disorder in presenile dementia. Neuropsychologia, 9, 75–78 (1971).

Miller, E. Retrieval from long-term memory in presenile dementia. Paper presented at the Annual Conference of the British Psychological Society, Bangor, 1974.

Miller, E. Abnormal Ageing. London: John Wiley & Sons, 1977.
Miller, E., and Hague, F. Some statistical characteristics of speech in presenile dementia. Psychological Medicine, 5, 255–259 (1975).
Rochford, G. A study of naming errors in dysphasic and in demented patients. Neuropsychologia, 9, 437–443 (1971).
Siedler, H., and Malamud, N. Creutzfeldt-Jakob's disease. Journal of Neuropathological and Experimental Neurology, 22, 381 (1963).
Tomlinson, B. E., Blessed, G., and Roth, M. Observations on the brains of demented old people. Journal of Neurological Science, 7, 205–242 (1970).

Chapter 15
Cancer of the Larynx

The effects of laryngeal surgery because of cancer are presented in terms of anatomic change and speech production. Various management methods used to provide speech for the laryngectomee such as artificial larynges, surgical approaches, and esophageal speech are discussed.

Removal of the larynx because of cancer creates some special problems besides loss of speech. The challenge of meeting these problems constitutes a major hurdle for the aged patient. The elderly are often handicapped by pre-existing age-related complications which make learning how to speak again more difficult than for younger persons. Unfortunately, the evidence suggests that cancer of the larynx usually afflicts the elderly.

INCIDENCE OF LARYNGEAL CANCER

It has been recently estimated that during a given year approximately 8100 men and 1100 women in the United States will develop cancer of the larynx (Silverberg, 1977). In fact, a recent survey indicates that during the last 20 years the incidence of laryngeal cancer in males has increased, with the largest increase occurring in the United States (Barclay and Rao, 1975). These data suggest that the older male patient (75% were over age 55) is more likely to have cancer of the larynx that a woman of the same age. Furthermore, King, Everill, and Peirson (1968) reported that the mean age at surgery for patients who had their larynges removed was 62 years.

SURVIVAL FACTORS

According to Bryce (1975) only about 4% of the treated cases for laryngeal cancer back in the late 1800s lived more than 2 years postsurgery. Today the 5-year survival rate for all stages of treated laryngeal cancer is 62% and for treated local carcinoma of the larynx, 80% (Silverberg, 1977). These remarkable advances in the treatment of cancer can be largely attributed to medical advancements in the last 50 years.

In addition to the great strides which have been made in medicine, another important factor contributing to this remarkable improvement in survival has been early detection of laryngeal carcinomas. An important factor in early detection of laryngeal cancer is an awareness of the symptoms which signal the presence of a vocal disorder. Although "persistent hoarseness" is one of the more common symptoms among those elderly people who are subsequently diagnosed as having cancer of the larynx, other symptoms also deserve attention. Recently, Brewer (1975) compiled a list of terms used by patients to describe their voice problems which were subsequently shown to be related to laryngeal disease. Even though the symptoms Brewer reported (Table 15-1) are not specifically indicative of laryngeal cancer, they do have alerting value particularly in the elderly.

TREATMENT

When a patient is diagnosed as having a laryngeal cancer, the physician must decide which treatment procedure will produce the best chance of a cure, the least risk to life, and the best functional result (Cocke and Wang, 1976). The treatment modalities available for managing laryngeal cancer include radiation therapy and a variety of surgical procedures. These surgical procedures may involve either a total or one of several partial laryngectomy operations, depending on the site of lesion and other factors. When the laryngeal cancer is more extensive, additional neck tissue must be excised to remove any involved lymph nodes. A total laryngectomy operation typically includes removal of all laryngeal cartilages and associated intrinsic musculature, some extrinsic infrahyoid muscles, and the hyoid bone.

Removal of the larynx creates an anatomic and functional separation between the respiratory airway and the digestive tract. This separation completely deprives the laryngectomee of a pulmonary air supply for speech. As can be seen in Figure 15-1, the trachea in a laryngectomee ends at the base of the neck through an opening called a stoma. Hence, the laryngectomee has lost both the principal source of sound generation and the main source of air flow through the oral and nasal cavities.

LARYNGECTOMY COMPLICATIONS

Pre-existing Factors

Elderly patients who undergo surgical removal of their larynx usually have a number of pre-existing problems. These pre-existing factors

Table 15–1. Symptoms reported by patients with laryngeal disease

Phonatory	Sensory	Pain	Other
Loss of voice	Throat tickle	Pain: in side of neck in back of neck at base of tongue in ear (adults)	Nonproductive cough
Abrupt pitch breaks in adults	Frequent dry throat		Repetitive throat clearing
Reduced vocal range	Raw, scratchy, or burning throat		Blood tinged mucus
Tired voice	Tight throat	Frequent sore throat without fever	Audible respiration
Breathiness	Lump in throat	Sore or tender neck	Swollen neck glands and muscles
Huskiness			

Source: Brewer (1975).

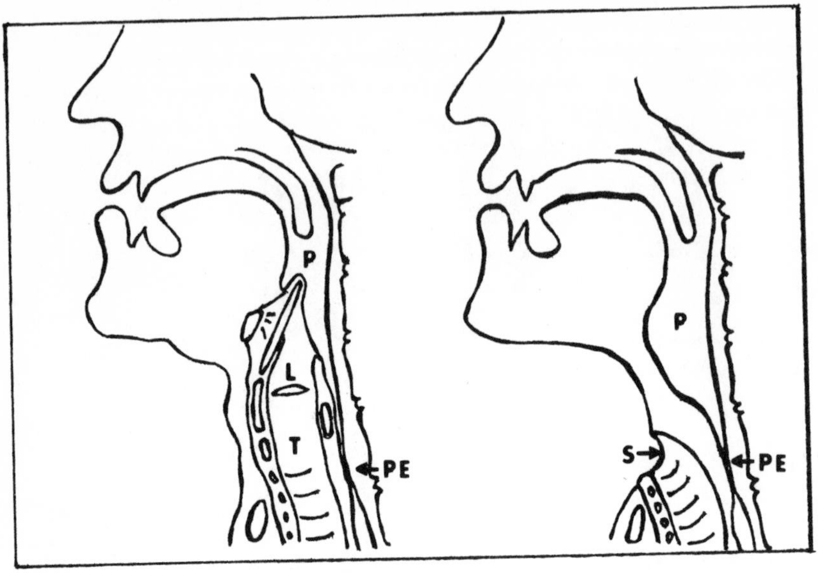

Figure 15.1. Vocal tract structures pre- and postlaryngectomy. P, pharynx; L, larynx; S, stoma; T, trachea; and PE, PE segment.

may include hearing loss (Berlin, 1964), frailty and general debility (Diedrich and Youngstrom, 1966), poor learning ability (Chen, Samberg, and Falsenstein, 1963), poor motivation (King et al., 1968), emotional problems (Stoll, 1958), and, in some instances, a previous stroke (Smith, Rise, and Gralnek, 1966). Hence, the elderly alaryngeal patient is frequently one who has a much broader problem of senescence associated with the specific difficulty of learning how to speak again. Of all these pre-existing factors the two which seem to have the largest impact on the elderly are loss of hearing acuity and psychological problems.

Berlin (1964) pointed out that elderly laryngectomees with a hearing loss cannot monitor stoma noise, are vulnerable to tissue-conducted masking noises if they use an artificial larynx, and generally have a difficult time acquiring esophageal speech. In the latter instance the problem is related to an inability to hear and monitor the sounds of speech in the higher frequencies (see Figure 6–8). The problem is further complicated if the spouse also has a hearing loss because the laryngectomee will not be heard very well and understood.

According to Stoll (1958), psychological factors really determine the success or failure of a laryngectomee in reacquiring speech. Many of the elderly have a reduced social need to talk, live alone, or just do not like the sound of alaryngeal speech. As one elderly woman wrote on her note pad, "I don't want to sound like an old frog." Emotional problems related to the grief of losing a body part and realizing that one is getting older may also contribute to a lack of motivation or aspiration. Berlin (1964) suggested that age at surgery and learning to speak again are more highly related to factors such as incentive, attitude, personality needs, anticipated social role, and how elderly patients view themselves. Hence, psychological factors appear to be more important than physiologic factors in acquiring a new voice (Snidecor, 1969).

Postlaryngectomy Factors

In addition to a loss of speech, total laryngectomy produces other directly related handicaps which impair normal everyday living. These difficulties may be grouped under two broad categories: loss of oral-nasal air flow and loss of laryngeal valving.

Loss of Oral-Nasal Air Flow Because normal respiration for a laryngectomee is accomplished through a neck stoma and not through the oral or nasal cavities, inhaled air is not properly warmed, filtered, or moistened. For these reasons the laryngectomee is more likely to have respiratory infections and be bothered to a greater extent by dust and other air pollutants. Nose blowing also becomes a problem and is usually reduced to nose wiping. Loss of nasal air flow also results in elevated thresholds for the sensations of taste and smell. That is, these sensations are reduced so that subtle odors and flavors are not easily detected.

Loss of Laryngeal Valving In normal individuals the larynx also serves to trap air in the lungs by closing the vocal folds. These laryngeal maneuvers are essential for activities such as physical exertion, coughing, bathing, and swimming. When the larynx is removed these kinds of activities present special problems for the laryngectomee (Snidecor, 1969). For example, lifting of heavy objects is difficult because air cannot be trapped in the lungs to help stabilize the thorax. Although lifting of heavy objects is not usually tried by the elderly, a similar situation is encountered when physical exertion is required during bowel elimination. Loss of laryngeal valving also makes tub bathing risky and even with showering special precautions must be taken to keep water out of the stoma.

ALARYNGEAL SPEECH

Probably the most profound handicap experienced by the elderly laryngectomee is the loss of speech. In fact, while most laryngectomees reacquire some form of speech, there are others who remain speechless and depend on writing for communication. A survey conducted by Watts (1975) indicated that 13% of 2730 responding laryngectomees did not speak at all, 11% spoke entirely with the aid of an artificial larynx, 70% spoke exculsively with an esophageal voice, and 6% used either an artificial larynx or esophageal speech depending on the situation. Unfortunately the elderly are too well represented in the nonspeaking group.

As suggested by Watts' report, there is more than one way to regain speech after laryngectomy. In fact, there are four general ways in which this particular feat may be accomplished: through the use of surgical-prosthetic approaches, surgical reconstruction of a new vibratory source, artificial noninvasive devices, and use of the remaining vocal tract structures to produce voice.

Surgical Approaches for Alaryngeal Speech

Most of the surgical-prosthetic approaches are experimental; consequently, they are not routinely used. Surgical reconstruction techniques have also been tried with a relatively few laryngectomees, but these cases also constitute a minority of the total laryngectomee population. Yet, in spite of these facts, most of the work in providing alaryngeal persons with a new voice has concentrated on surgical reconstruction and surgical-prosthetic approaches during the last 100 years. One major obstacle has prevented the wide acceptance of these particular procedures: how to prevent foods and fluids from entering the trachea and still use the respiratory tree as a power source for speech. Table 15-2 gives a summary of these surgically oriented procedures with references to further literature sources.

Artificial Larynx Speech

The first artificial larynx was devised by a physician named Czermak in 1859 (Kallen, 1934) for a young woman who had been tracheotomized. Czermak's device consisted of a tube with a reed inside that could be vibrated by directing the pulmonic air stream from the woman's lungs through one end of the tube. The other end of the tube was placed into the oral cavity and the channeled vibrations used for producing speech. Some of the artificial larynx devices now in use still use the same principle. Early in 1940, a more compact hand-held

Table 15-2. Surgical and surgical-prosthetic laryngeal rehabilitation approaches

Type of approach	Prosthesis required	Reference
Tracheo-esophageal shunt		
Internal shunt	No	Conley, De Amesti, and Pierce (1958)
	No	Calcaterria and Jafek (1971)
External shunt	Yes	Montgomery and Toohill (1968)
	Yes	Conley (1969)
	Yes	Taub and Bergner (1973)
Tracheo-pharyngeal shunt		
Internal shunt	Yes	McGrail and Oldfield (1971)
	No	Asai (1972)
External shunt	Yes/no	Montgomery (1972)
	Yes	Shedd et al. (1972, 1974)
	Yes	Sisson et al. (1975)
Implanted electronic prosthesis	Yes	Rodgers et al. (1975)
	Yes	Bailey et al. (1976)

electronic larynx was developed by Greene (1942). Since then a variety of small battery-powered, hand-held artificial larynges have appeared on the market. Table 15-3 gives the names of the more currently available artificial larynges, their approximate cost, power source, and where they can be obtained.

Esophageal Speech

The most widely used method of speech employed by alaryngeal persons is esophageal (Watts, 1975). This form of speech utilizes the remaining vocal tract structures to produce voice. To speak with an esophageal voice, the laryngectomee takes air into the esophagus and then uses this meager air supply (85 cc versus a former 700 cc) to vibrate the pharyngoesophageal (PE) spincter muscles located at the upper port of the esophagus (see Figure 15-1). The vocal excitations produced by this pseudoglottis are then resonated and articulated as the sound passes through the upper portions of the vocal tract (see Figure 2-14).

Esophageal Speech Problems Although esophageal speech has traditionally been advocated over other forms of alaryngeal speech, it also has problems. The two biggest difficulties with esophageal speech are: 1) not all laryngectomees are able to learn it, and 2) those who do typically have intelligibility problems (DiCarlo, Amster, and Herrer,

Table 15-3. Noninvasive artificial larynges

Brand name	Power source	Approximate cost ($)	Supplier
Aurex	Battery	190.00	Aurex Corp., 844 W. Adams Chicago, Ill. 60607
Barts Vibrator	Battery	195.00	Park Surgical Co., Inc. 5001 New Utrecht Ave. Brooklyn, N.Y. 11219
Cooper-Rand	Battery	175.00	Luminaud, P. O. Box 257 7670 Acacia Ave. Mentor, Ohio 44060
Neher #5000	Air	70.00	Neher Artificial Larynx Co. 1036th St., S. W. Kasson, Minn. 55944
Servox	Battery	395.00	Siemens Corp., 186 Wood Ave. Iselin, N. J. 08830
Tokyo Larynx	Air	25.00	Mr. Red Woodward, 3132 Waits Ave. Ft. Worth, Texas 76109
Western Electric-5	Battery	52.00	Bell Telephone Co. (Check the yellow pages under artificial larynx)

1955; Hyman, 1955). This lack of intelligibility has been traced in part to insufficient air support (Isshiki and Snidecor, 1964), altered vocal tract mechanics for voiceless consonant production (Christensen and Weinberg, 1976), and the phonatory properties of the PE segment (Weinberg and Bennett, 1972; Snidecor, 1975). These studies indicate that the esophageal speaker talks more quietly, usually utters three to four words per air charge, has a lower pitched voice, speaks at a slower rate, and has difficulty producing contrasts between voiced and voiceless sounds in speech (e.g., /p/ versus /b/).

Buccal and Pharyngeal Speech Other forms of speech that use existing structures of the vocal tract are pharyngeal and buccal speech. Pharyngeal speech sounds like the voice of Donald Duck. The laryngectomee has very little air available to produce these forms of speech since the vibratory source is formed by the tongue contacting either the pharyngeal wall or the cheek. This means that only the air between the PE segment and the point of vibration can be compressed and used for producing sound. A further problem with either of these forms of speech is that the tongue is restricted in its movements since it must also be used to form the vibratory source. The net result is a drastic loss in intelligibility. For these reasons both pharyngeal and buccal speech are not very desirable forms of alaryngeal speech even though there are a few laryngectomees who do resort to their use.

SUGGESTED READINGS

Gardner, W. H. Laryngectomee Speech and Rehabilitation. Springfield, Ill.: Charles C Thomas, 1971.

Snidecor, J. C. Speech Rehabilitation of the Laryngectomized. Springfield, Ill.: Charles C Thomas, Publisher, 1969.

REFERENCES

Asai, R. Laryngoplasty after total laryngectomy. Archives of Otolaryngology, 95, 114–119 (1972).

Bailey, B. J., Griffiths, C. M., and Everett, R. An implanted electronic laryngeal prosthesis. Annals of Otolaryngology, 85, 472–483 (1976).

Barclay, T. H. C., and Rao, N. N. The incidence and mortality rates for laryngeal cancer from total cancer registeries. Laryngoscope, 85, 254–258 (1975).

Berlin, C. I. Hearing loss, palatal function, and other factors in post-laryngectomy rehabilitation. Journal of Chronic Disorders, 17, 677–684 (1964).

Brewer, D. W. Early diagnostic signs and symptoms of laryngeal disease. Laryngoscope, 85, 499–515 (1975).

Bryce, D. P. The Conacher memorial lecture: 100 years of effort. Laryngoscope, 85, 241–253 (1975).

Calcaterra, T. C., and Jafek, B. W. Tracheo-esophageal shunt for speech rehabilitation after total laryngectomy. Archives of Otolaryngology, 94, 124–128 (1971).

Chen, L. Y., Samberg, H. H., and Falsenstein, B. Aspects of rehabilitation of the laryngectomized patient. Archives of Physical Medicine and Rehabilitation, 44, 267–272 (1963).

Christensen, J. M., and Weinberg, B. Vowel duration characteristics of esophageal speech. Journal of Speech and Hearing Research, 19, 678–689 (1976).

Cocke, E. W., Jr., and Wang, C. C. Cancer of the larynx: Selecting optimum treatment. Ca—A Cancer Journal for Clinicians, 26, 201–210 (1976).

Conley, J. J. Surgical techniques for the vocal rehabilitation of the laryngectomized patient. American Academy of Ophthalmology and Otolaryngology, 73, 288–299 (1969).

Conley, J. J., DeAmesti, F., and Pierce, M. K. A new surgical technique for the vocal rehabilitation of the laryngectomized patient. Annals of Otology, Rhinology and Laryngology, 67, 655–664 (1958).

DiCarlo, L. M., Amster, W., and Herrer, C. Speech After Laryngectomy. Syracuse, N.Y.: Syracuse University Press, 1955.

Diedrich, W. M., and Youngstrom, K. A. Alaryngeal Speech. Springfield, Ill.: Charles C Thomas, 1966.

Greene, J. S. Rehabilitating of the laryngectomized patient. Bulletin of the American Society for the Control of Cancer, 24, 5–8 (1942).

Hyman, M. An experimental study of artificial larynx and esophageal speech. Journal of Speech and Hearing Disorders, 20, 291–299 (1955).

Isshiki, N., and Snidecor, J. C. Air intake and usage in esophageal speech. Acta Otolaryngologica, 59, 559–574 (1964).

Kallen, L. A. Vicarious vocal mechanisms: The anatomy, physiology and development of speech in laryngectomized persons. Archives of Otolaryngology, 20, 460–503 (1934).

King, P. S., Everill, W. F., and Peirson, G. A. Rehabilitation and adaptation of laryngectomy patients. American Journal of Physical Medicine, 47, 192–203 (1968).

McGrail, J. S., and Oldfield, D. L. One-stage operation for vocal rehabilitation at laryngectomy. Transcripts of the American Academy of Ophthalomology and Otolaryngology, 75, 510–512 (1971).

Montgomery, W. W. Postlaryngectomy vocal rehabilitation. Archives of Otolaryngology, 95, 76–83 (1972).

Montgomery, W. W., and Toohill, R. J. Voice rehabilitation after laryngectomy. Archives of Otolaryngology, 88, 499–506 (1968).

Rodgers, J. H., Frederickson, J. M., and Bryce, D. P. New techniques for vocal rehabilitation. Canadian Journal of Otolaryngology, 4, 595–604 (1975).

Shedd, D. P., Bakamjian, V., Sako, K., Mann, M. B., Barba, S., and Schaaf, N. Reed-fistula method of speech rehabilitation. American Journal of Surgery, 124, 510–514 (1972).

Shedd, D. P., Bakamjian, V., Sako, K., Schaaf, N. G., and Mann, M. B. Postlaryngectomy speech rehabilitation by a simplified single-stage surgical method. American Journal of Surgery, 128, 505–511 (1974).
Silverberg, E. Cancer statistics, 1977. Ca—A Cancer Journal for Clinicians, 27, 26–41 (1977).
Sisson, G. A., McConnel, F. M. S., Logemann, J. A., and Yeh, S., Jr. Voice rehabilitation after laryngectomy: Results with the use of a hypopharyngeal prosthesis. Archives of Otolaryngology, 101, 178–181 (1975).
Smith, J. K., Rise, E. N., and Gralnek, D. E. Speech recovery in laryngectomized patients. Laryngoscope, 76, 1540–1546 (1966).
Snidecor, J. C. Speech Rehabilitation of the Laryngectomized (2nd Ed.). Springfield, Ill.: Charles C Thomas, 1969.
Snidecor, J. C. Some scientific foundations for voice restoration. Laryngoscope, 85, 640–648 (1975).
Stoll, B. Psychological factors determining the success or failure of the rehabilitation program of laryngectomized patients. Annals of Otolaryngology, 67, 550–557 (1958).
Taub, S., and Bergner, L. H. Air bypass voice prosthesis for vocal rehabilitation of laryngectomees. American Journal of Surgery, 125, 748–756 (1973).
Watts, R. F. Total rehabilitation of laryngectomees. Laryngoscope, 85, 671–673 (1975).
Weinberg, B., and Bennett, S. Selected acoustic characteristics of esophageal speech produced by female laryngectomees. Journal of Speech and Hearing Research, 15, 211–216 (1972).

Chapter 16
Speech and Language Assessment

This chapter presents an overview of most of the routine aspects of speech and language assessment with particular attention to geriatric patients. The topics covered include assessment of intellectual function, diagnosis of symbolization problems, determination of the presence of apraxia of speech, evaluation of peripheral execution problems, the case history, and special considerations with the laryngectomee.

The present chapter is designed to provide an overview of the assessment procedures used by the speech/language pathologist in determining the nature of various communication disorders. As such, the chapter is most helpful for those not in the profession of speech/language pathology. Organization of this discussion follows the model of language functioning depicted in Chapter 2. It must be recognized that examination procedures for intellectualization, symbolization, translation, and execution are extensive. Therefore, the techniques outlined in this chapter constitute typical assessment strategies, and no effort is made to review the many controversies that have developed with regard to some of these evaluation procedures.

ASSESSMENT OF INTELLECTUAL FUNCTION

As a general statement, most speech/language pathologists are not trained to administer traditional, standardized intelligence tests. Accordingly, in many instances the speech/language pathologist will refer patients to a psychometrist for such testing. However, some communication disorders specialists by virtue of unique training or professional setting are prepared to assess intelligence in a very thorough fashion.

As pointed out in Chapter 13, one of the common sequelae of aphasia is intellectual impairment. With the tremendous difficulty in partitioning intellectual functioning from symbolic performance, many tests of intelligence indirectly provide evidence of symbolization and vice versa. In the present section, however, attention is focused upon evaluative approaches specifically designed for the measurement of intellectual decline with particular attention to such deficits in the elderly.

An excellent discussion of intellectual assessment may be found in Miller (1977), who divided the evaluation process into two components: measurement of the amount of deterioration and differential diagnosis. A brief review of his observations in both areas is warranted.

Intellectual Deterioration

Perhaps the major difficulty in assessing intellectual deterioration in elderly patients, particularly those with dementia or traumatic brain damage, is the absence of premorbid intelligence data. Therefore, determination of the amount of decline is usually a very general or cursory approximation based upon previous education level, profession, etc. Clearly, such a strategy is very hazardous and often grossly inaccurate.

There has been, according to Miller, a historical effort to evaluate subtests of various intelligence batteries to identify a "deterioration index." For example, it has been argued that vocabulary performance is a good predictor of intelligence (Yates, 1956) and is more resistant to the impact of aging and brain damage (Yates, 1956; Gonen and Brown, 1968). Accordingly, administration of a vocabulary test to patients should give a close approximation of premorbid intellectual status with which other test data may be compared to determine the degree of deterioration. However, this strategy has been seriously challenged for many reasons, including poor test-retest reliability for many vocabulary instruments, strong evidence that vocabulary is susceptible to deterioration with progressive dementia and brain damage, large overlap of normal subjects and demented subjects on such tests, and validity problems in fracturing a full IQ test and examining only individual subtests. Miller summarized these points by stating:

> For a few psychologists, the search for right Wechsler subtest combination goes on, rather like the mediaeval alchemists (*sic*) search for the philosopher's stone, and with as little likelihood of ultimate success. (p. 109)

Differential Diagnostic Assessment

The second problem in intellectual assessment confronting most psychometrists, according to Miller, is the differential diagnosis of dementia and functional psychiatric disorders, namely, depression.

Conventionally, two forms of testing have been employed to permit this differentiation.

The first form involves learning and memory tests on which demented patients generally perform much worse than depressed patients. Two such tests have been developed specifically for use with geriatric patients and both have excellent validity. The first is referred to as the Synonym Learning Test (Kendrick, Parboosingh, and Post, 1965) and the second, the Inglis Paired Associate Learning Test (Inglis, 1957). The details of these tests may be studied in the listed references provided.

The second form of testing involves reproduction of geometric designs, where again the demented patients usually exhibit markedly reduced scores when compared with depressed subjects. Miller has attributed this reduced performance to memory problems and disturbed spatial perception among dements. Several tests have design-copying subtests including the Memory-for-Designs Test (Graham and Kendall, 1960), Visual Motor Gestalt Test (Bender, 1946), and the Revised Visual Retention Test (Benton, 1963). These tests appear to have reasonably good discriminatory power but are of lesser value than learning and memory tests in differential diagnosis (Brilliant and Gynther, 1963).

By way of summary, Miller described a typical test battery for investigation of intellectual decline in the elderly, and his suggestions are provided in Table 16-1.

Special Concerns When Testing Intelligence in the Elderly

Obviously, the assessment of elderly patients requires some variations in clinical procedure from that used with young adults. This is particularly true with cases of dementia and brain damage. Table 16-2 describes several variables often encountered when testing the elderly and suggestions for minimizing these problems are offered.

ASSESSMENT OF SYMBOLIZATION FUNCTION

A variety of standardized tests have been developed for evaluating a broad range of central language problems. It is beyond the scope of this chapter to present a detailed discussion of these procedures. Therefore, only a brief description of the more common tests is offered. A trained speech/language pathologist will select one or more of these tests during a language assessment depending upon training, personal preference, and type of data sought. Information obtained from such

Table 16–1. Suggested battery of intelligence tests for use with geriatric patients suspected of having intellectual and memory impairments

Stage	Information gained
Intelligence test (preferably Wechsler)	Possible indication of intellectual deterioration Base against which further changes can be measured
Diagnostic tests	
Learning tests (as appropriate for age)	Poor performance excludes functional disorder but is consistent with all other neurologic conditions that produce severe amnesia
Memory-for-designs test	May exclude functional disorder but results often equivocal
Neuropsychological examination for aphasia, apraxia, etc.	Positive findings indicate organic pathology
Retest on any cognitive test for which previous test results are available	Rarely possible but good indication of intellectual decline
Repeat all or part of stages 1 to 3 after several weeks	Evidence of progressive deterioration

Source: Miller (1977).

tests can be of considerable value in developing and predicting the course of a therapy program. Furthermore, such information can be of inestimable value to health professionals and family members in appreciating the patient's communicative strengths and limitations. Following is a cursory overview of several common tests for assessment of adult language problems.

Examining for Aphasia

The test developed by Eisenson (1954) is perhaps less frequently used than some to be described later. It is arranged to permit testing for the following deficits: 1) receptive-evaluative problems (visual, auditory, and tactile agnosia; auditory-verbal aphasia; alexia), and 2) productive-expressive problems (apraxia of speech and nonverbal apraxia; automatic speech; writing numbers, letters, and from dictation; spelling; naming; word finding; arithmetic; clock setting; and oral reading). The clinician has an opportunity to estimate degree of severity and thereby develop a profile of deficits.

Language Modalities Test for Aphasia (LMTA)

Wepman and Jones (1961) developed a language test based upon their

Table 16-2. Some problems and suggested solutions when testing the elderly

Problem	Possible solutions
Confusion	Repeat instructions, give examples or demonstrations where possible Present information slowly Allow adequate response time
Anxiety	Familiarization with the examiner and testing situation A brief period of conversation before examination Positive reinforcement and encouragement during the testing
Memory loss	Repeat instructions and test items where possible Complete only short segments of the test each session if possible
Fatigue	Same as above for memory loss
Failure on test items	Positive reinforcement and encouragement during testing Understanding and comforting attitude
Bizarre response	Lack of reaction or reinforcement for unusual and disturbed behaviors Patient but firm reiteration of required task and response
Lack of cooperation	Often very difficult to overcome May require several contacts or encouragement by trusted friend or family member to participate in testing
Language difficulties	Choice of an alternate test upon which patient can perform or adaptation of required response form to meet patient's need (may sacrifice standardization requirements in so doing)
Severe confusion or intellectual deterioration	If patient has not lost contact, very simple informal testing involving common actions or selection from two-item multiple choice questions.
Hearing loss	Face examinee, articulate precisely, repeat and rephrase questions or instructions. (Note: Simply talking louder may not always help greatly)

five-item classification system, which includes: 1) pragmatic aphasia, an inability to conceptualize or obtain meaning from a given stimulus; 2) semantic aphasia, present when the patient cannot readily recall names and substantive words; 3) syntactic aphasia, wherein the patient's grammatical structure is disrupted, resulting in telegraphic speech; 4) jargon aphasia, defined as the absence of intelligible utterances though proper intonation may be observed; and 5) global aphasia, a disorder where production and probably comprehension are severly reduced, thereby limiting the patient to short, automatized utterances. Both verbal and graphic responses to picture, word, number, and sentence stimuli are scored in accordance with the above classification scheme, permitting the examiner ultimately to designate the type of aphasia.

Minnesota Test for Differential Diagnosis of Aphasia (MTDDA)

One of the more popular examination tools is the MTDDA (Schuell, 1965), which was developed after extensive observation of aphasic patients. Schuell's basic contention was that aphasia is a disorder "... that crosses all language modalities and ... is characterized by a reduction of available vocabulary, impaired verbal retention span, and impaired perception and production of messages" (Schuell, Jenkins, and Jiminez-Pabon, 1964, p. 113). The MTDDA is an extensive test comprised of 62 subtests designed to assess auditory disturbances, visual and reading disturbances, speech and language production disturbances, visual-motor and writing disturbances, and numerical relation problems. Based on a variety of response patterns, the examiner may classify the patient with respect to type and severity. The five types developed by Schuell are: 1) simple aphasia; 2) aphasia with involvement of central visual processing; 3) aphasia with sensorimotor involvement; 4) aphasia with some residual language, visual problems, and dysarthria; and 5) aphasia with irreversible and almost complete loss of language skills.

Porch Index of Communicative Ability (PICA)

Porch (1967) identified two critical dimensions or criteria of a good aphasia test, namely, multidimensional scoring of the patient's response (accuracy, promptness, completeness, responsiveness, efficiency) and reliability of scoring. The PICA was developed to meet these criteria and involves 18 subtests that assess verbal, gestural, and graphic responses to 10 common objects placed before the examinee. Profiles of responses across the 18 subtests are plotted; they have diagnostic, prognostic, and therapeutic significance (Porch, 1971). Recently, the PICA was administered to 130 normal, predominantly elderly, adult subjects, thereby providing substantive normative data (Duffy, Keith, Shane, and Podraza, 1976).

The Boston Diagnostic Aphasia Test

One of the major motivations for the Boston Test (Goodglass and Kaplan, 1972) was the need for an instrument which would permit localization of the cerebral insult or nature of the neuropathologic substrate. The Boston Test evaluates input and output by modality and also permits a rating of severity of aphasia as well as a profile of speech characteristics. By examining results of the subtests and rating scales, the examiner can approximate localizable aphasic syndromes by comparison to several presented in the manual. In addition, provision is made for separate assessment of apraxia, arithmetic problems, and visual-spatial disturbances.

The Token Test

The Token Test was developed by De Renzi and Vignolo (1962) to provide a sensitive tool for evaluation of receptive language disturbances that would not be contaminated by intelligence problems. Basically, the Token Test involves presentation of a series of increasingly more difficult commands. The patient responds by manipulating or arranging plastic tokens of different shapes, sizes, and colors. Several variations of the Token Test have been used (for example, Berry, 1976), but the test is now available in standardized, published form (McNeil and Prescott, 1978).

Other Tests

As mentioned earlier, there are many other tests of aphasia that are not discussed here, and the reader is referred to sources such as Bay (1962), Sklar (1966), Luria (1964), and Benton (1967) for additional information. It should also be mentioned that many of the full diagnostic tests, such as the LMTDA and MTDDA, have provisions or forms for screening. It should be emphasized that most of the tests have comprehensive assessment items sensitive to the problem of agnosia described in Chapter 10. However, frequently the disorder of motor speech programming is evaluated independently of tests for aphasia. Therefore, special procedures for assessment of apraxia are discussed in the next section.

ASSESSMENT OF TRANSLATION FUNCTION

Many nonstandardized techniques for diagnosis of apraxia of speech have been suggested. A partial list of these techniques includes the following. First, the patient may be asked to utter a series of words of increasing difficulty and complexity such as "door-doorknob-doorkeeper-dormitory" (Darley, Aronson, and Brown, 1975, p. 97). The apraxic subject will exhibit increasing difficulty. Second, the examiner can require the subject to repeat words with difficult phonetic combinations such as "tincture of merthiolate," "Methodist Episcopal," "statistician," etc. This will usually precipitate considerable difficulty for apraxic patients and should elicit much of the articulatory variability noted earlier in Chapter 11. Third, if the examiner compares intelligibility and accuracy of production for oral reading during normal and accelerated rate, the apraxic may be expected to perform better in the second condition. Fourth, oral-motor examination will usually reveal no weakness or paralysis if the apraxia is isolated. Fifth, the examiner may try to elicit automatic or more non-propositional forms of speech such as counting, naming the days of the week, reciting the Lord's Prayer, etc. In these cases, the apraxic will be apt to exhibit normal or near normal performance. Sixth, tests of auditory perception, reading, and writing may be depressed but, if the apraxia of speech is isolated, only mildly so. Aphasics, on the other hand, will probably present notably lower performance in at least one or more of such tests.

In some cases of apraxia of speech, particularly those that are more severe, a concomitant oral apraxia may be present (see Chapter 11). It is important that the speech language pathologist ascertain the presence of oral apraxia, and this may be achieved by determining the client's ability to perform nonspeech oral movements such as tongue protrusion and smiling. Poeck and Kerschensteiner (1973) and Moore, Rosenbek, and LaPointe (1976) have developed more formalized assessment techniques for oral apraxia.

ASSESSMENT OF EXECUTION FUNCTION

Evaluation of peripheral speech production capability involves several aspects. Integrity of respiratory support for speech, laryngeal control, valving, and articulatory function must be assessed. From a composite view of all of these functions, the speech/language pathologist can determine isolated peripheral deficits and can make logical inferences regarding probable deficits further up the neurologic stream (see Chapter 12).

Respiration

Since speech is usually accomplished within midrange lung volumes, a person must sustain rather extensive neuromuscular damage or reduction in ventilatory function to seriously impair speech. However, in many disorders this does occur and the pulmonary support for speech is reduced.

The speech/language pathologist will usually use one or more of three strategies to assess pulmonary function for speech. First, evaluation of respiratory performance during tidal volume exchange will be completed. Here, rate of breathing may be calculated. Darley et al. (1975) have suggested that rates exceeding .5 Hz may result in speech problems though this has not received broad, data-based support. In addition, the clinician may observe the breathing pattern. It has been documented that some normal talkers employ primarily thoracic enlargement and some abdominal excursions (Hixon, Mead, and Goldman, 1976) and hence, the old idea of "right way" to breathe is no longer widely held. However, a trained speech/language pathologist can, by palpation and observation, usually discern respiratory fixations (probably caused by antagonistic movements of diaphragm-external intercostal and internal intercostal-abdominal musculature), emergency breathing, respiratory control problems, reduced chest wall expansion-contraction, and possible associated rib cage deformities.

The second strategy used to assess respiratory function for speech involves careful listening to utterance characteristics. As noted in Chapter 12, reduced respiratory support for speech, diminished chest wall control, and irregular respiratory patterns may result in distinctive speech disturbances. To a large extent, these speech problems may reflect interactive deviations of the phonatory or respiratory systems, but the competent speech/language pathologist can usually determine the locus of difficulty. Usually, perceptual evaluation of contextual speech is the most revealing, but several special tasks may be required of the client including sustaining the vowel "ah" and rapid repetition of a syllable such as "puh" (diadochokinesis). More on these assessments is provided in the next section, but in the case of sustaining "ah," if it is too brief, or in the case of repeating "puh" if it is too slow, the respiratory system may be implicated.

The final approach to evaluation of respiratory function for speech involves instrumental evaluation. This is still largely experimental, but use of electromyography, body plethysmography, spirometry, chest wall kinematics, etc., have been used in the evaluation of speech respiration. Most of the research has focused upon normative data collection, and only a limited number of studies have been designed to relate respiratory function to speech disorders. (For additional information, see Chapters 5 and 12.)

Phonation

As with respiration, three general clinical approaches have been proposed for evaluating phonatory adequacy. The first involves perceptual assessment of voice characteristics during contextual speech. Typically, the speech/language pathologist will make judgments with respect to pitch, loudness, rate, integrity of laryngeal valving, pitch variability, loudness variability, phrasing, and consistency or pervasiveness of any potential disorder. Certain formal scaling procedures are available to the speech/language pathologist to assist in making these judgments (Wilson, 1971; Thurman, 1977; Wilson and Rice, 1977). Though final determination of a voice disorder should rest with a trained speech/language pathologist, other health professionals may assist in identifying potential voice patients by reference to the following set of questions adapted from Darley et al. (1975, p. 85):

1. Does the pitch of the voice sound consistently too low or too high for the individual's age and sex?
2. Does the pitch of the voice show sudden and uncontrolled variations, possibly extending into the falsetto range?
3. Is the voice a monotone or monopitch, lacking normal pitch and inflectional changes?
4. Does the voice sound tremulous or tremorous?
5. Is the voice insufficiently or excessively loud?
6. Does the voice show monotony of loudness or absence of loudness variations?
7. Does the voice show sudden, uncontrolled alterations in loudness, sometimes becoming excessively loud and at other times excessively weak?
8. Is there a progressive diminution or decay of loudness as speech continues?
9. Are there alternating changes in loudness?
10. Does the voice sound harsh, rough, or raspy?
11. Does the voice sound "gurgly" or "wet," as associated with hoarse voice quality?
12. Is the voice continuously breathy, weak, and thin?
13. Is the breathiness constant, or is it transient, periodic, or intermittent?
14. Does the voice sound strained or strangled, as if the patient is exerting effort in squeezing the voice through the glottis?

15. Are there sudden stoppages or arrests of the voiced air stream, suggesting momentary impedance of the air flow?
16. Is the speech interrupted by sudden forced inspirations or expirations?
17. Are phrases excessively short, possibly associated with the need to inhale more frequently than normal? Does the speaker sound as though he has run out of air or does he produce a gasp at the end of a phrase?
18. Is the voice audibly breathy on inhalation?
19. Are there grunts at the end of exhalations?
20. Does the speech show a reduction in normal stress of emphasis patterns?
21. Is excess stress placed on usually unstressed parts of speech, as on monosyllabic words or unstressed syllables of polysyllabic words?

The speech/language pathologist may also wish to evaluate the capabilities of the vocal mechanism by determining the influence of various tasks upon voice function. For example, as mentioned previously, duration of a sustained vowel is frequently determined. Though no absolute minimum has been determined for intelligible speech, McDonald and Chance (1964) claimed that the duration should exceed 1 second. In addition, pitch and loudness ranges may be determined on a subjective basis by having the patient sing the scale and amplify the voice from inaudibility to a shout. Rapidity and regularity of diadochokinesis may also be indicative of laryngeal adequacy.

Finally, several instruments have been developed in recent years to permit careful quantification of various parameters of voice. Perhaps the most versatile of these is the TONAR II (Fletcher, 1976), which allows acoustic analysis of average fundamental frequency, fundamental frequency contours, vocal intensity, and intensity contours. The FLORIDA I (Holbrook, 1977) apparatus, though largely a therapeutic aid, may be used to determine fundamental frequency characteristics. Other less common instruments, often engineered locally, are used in many settings.

Articulation

Several formal tests are available for measuring the number, type, and position of various articulation errors. Though most of these tests are used with children, several, such as the Fischer-Logemann Test of Articulation Competence, the Templin-Darley Tests of Articulation, and the McDonald Deep Test of Articulation have procedures applicable to adults as well and could easily be used with gerontologic subjects. In addition, the speech/language pathologist usually assesses intelligibility and the nature of articulation deviations in contextual speech (see Chapters 11 and 12 for examples of such disturbances). The health professional can be of considerable value in identifying elderly people with clinically significant articulation by considering the following list of questions (adapted from Darley et al., 1975, p. 96):

Palatopharyngeal system:

1. Does the voice sound hypernasal?
2. Does the voice sound hyponasal (denasal)?
3. Is there nasal emission of the air stream?

Articulatory system:

1. Do consonants lack precision? Do they show slurring, inadequate sharpness, distortions, or lack of crispness? Is there clumsiness in transition from one consonant to another?
2. Do vowel sounds seem distorted throughout their total duration?
3. Are there prolongations of phonemes?
4. Are there repetitions of phonemes?
5. Is the rate of speech abnormally slow or rapid (not including silent periods between words)?
6. Does the rate increase progressively within given segments of connected speech?
7. Does the rate increase progressively from the beginning to the end of the sample?
8. Does the rate change alternately from slow to fast?
9. Are there prolongations of interword or intersyllable intervals?
10. Are there inappropriate silent intervals?
11. Are there short rushes of speech separated by pauses?
12. Are there intermittent nonsystematic breakdowns in accuracy of articulation?

With particular reference to velopharyngeal adequacy, several special approaches may be used. One formal articulation test that is sensitive to hypernasality is available to the speech/language pathologist, namely the Iowa Pressure Articulation Test (Morris, Spriestersbach, and Darley, 1961). In addition, various instrumental measures are available, including the TONAR II and FLORIDA II (Holbrook, 1977), aerodynamic assessment of nasal pressures or flows, and cineradiographic, videofluoroscopic, and ultrasonic evaluation of palatal and pharyngeal wall movement patterns. One neurologic disorder, myasthenia gravis, primarily manifested in progressive hypernasality (Wolski, 1967), can be evaluated by stressing the speech system. Typically, the speech/language clinician will apply such stress by having the patient count or read continuously. If after several minutes the client exhibits considerable fatigue and deterioration of articulation, particularly with respect to velopharyngeal adequacy, myasthenia gravis may be suspected and neurologic referral should be made.

Examination of the Peripheral Speech Mechanism

One very important component of any speech examination is evaluation of oral sensorimotor function. The reader is referred to the appendix of this chapter for an examination form used at Idaho State University that summarizes several dimensions commonly assessed. This form is a variation of the one employed for many years by Ewanowski and his colleagues at the University of Wisconsin Health Sciences Center in Madison. The authors are indebted to this fine service for original development of the form.

As can be seen from inspection of this form, anatomic structures and physiologic function are evaluated including the head and face, lips, mandible, teeth, tongue, palate, oropharynx, and fauces. In addition, provision is made for determination of oral sensory capabilities through two-point discrimination and/or oral stereognosis.

THE CASE HISTORY

Routinely, regardless of the nature of the problem, the speech/language pathologist will obtain a comprehensive case history. Such information provides considerable insight regarding causes, predisposing factors, and maintenance of many disorders. Furthermore, information regarding perceived severity of the disorder, family and social interaction difficulties, variability of the problem, and intellectual, emotional, and occupational status may be ascertained. Often, history information will signpost the need for referral to other health care professionals. With the elderly, particularly those with intellectual, memory, or language impairments, it may be necessary to obtain case history information from a family member, cooperating professional, or close friend. This information may be particularly critical for assessment of postmorbid changes by comparison to reported premorbid capabilities.

SPECIAL CONSIDERATIONS WITH THE LARYNGECTOMEE

As mentioned in Chapter 15, not all laryngectomees, particularly the older laryngectomee, will develop adequate alaryngeal speech. Therefore, assessment of the laryngectomized patient pre- and postoperatively is very important. Diedrich and Youngstrom (1966) have advised assessment of three factors: physical characteristics of the oral, pharyngeal, esophageal, and related structures; general physical status; and psychological adjustment. Table 16-3 outlines several conditions likely to hinder the development of esophageal speech. Careful evaluation of

Table 16–3. Potential reasons for failure to acquire esophageal speech

Physical (concerned with the surgery or original disease)
- Cicatrix
- Recurring fistulas
- Innervation disorder
- Postradiation fibrosis
- Stenosis of the esophagus
- Recurrence of the carcinoma
- Strictures of the hypopharyngeal space
- Extensive surgery, especially excision of the pharynx, base of the tongue, and floor of the mouth

Other physical reasons
- Hernia
- Senility
- Arthritis
- Colostomy
- Aerophagia
- Hearing loss
- Abdominal surgery
- Cleft or paralysis of palate
- Edema and secretions in hypopharynx
- Pulmonary disease (tuberculosis, asthma, emphysema, etc.)
- Either too much tonicity (spasm) or inadequate approximation of the PE segment tissues

Psychological
- Living alone
- Emotional problems
- Inability to accept the new voice
- Inability to learn a new motor function
- Lack of speech instruction
- Lack of practice
- Poor motivation

Source: Diedrich and Youngstrom (1966).

these factors may aid substantially in prognosis. Inspection of this table shows that the speech/language pathologist is obviously heavily dependent upon the surgeon, otolaryngologist, and psychologist or social worker for information regarding the physical and psycho-emotional variables. The table also indicates that many of the negative signs will be more common among the elderly including innervation disorders, senility, arthritis, hearing loss, edema and secretions in the hypopharynx, pulmonary disease, living alone, inability to learn a new motor function, and poor motivation.

Despite these potential hinderances to development of esophageal speech, the speech/language pathologist will usually attempt to teach air intake and expulsion. Unfortunately, it must be recognized that many older patients may not be able to master esophageal speech even if the air intake-expulsion problems are overcome. This can result from other coordination problems or psychological variables. If esophageal speech fails, an artificial larynx may be recommended but again, not all older laryngectomees may be expected to become proficient with such devices.

SUGGESTED READINGS

Darley, F. L., Aronson, A. E., and Brown, J. R. Motor Speech Disorders. Philadelphia: W. B. Saunders, 1975.

Miller, E. Abnormal Ageing. London: John Wiley & Sons, 1977.

Nation, J. E., and Aram, D. M. Diagnosis of Speech and Language Disorders. St. Louis: C. V. Mosby, 1977.

REFERENCES

Bay, E. Aphasia and non-verbal disorders of language. Brain, 85, 411–426 (1962).

Bender, L. Instructions for the Use of the Visual Motor Gestalt Test. New York: American Orthopsychiatric Association, 1946.

Benton, A. Revised Visual Retention Test. Iowa City: State University of Iowa, 1963.

Benton, A. Problems in test construction in the field of aphasia. Cortex, 3, 32–58 (1967).

Berry, W. R. Testing auditory comprehension in aphasia: A clinical alternate to the Token Test. In R. H. Brookshire (ed.), Clinical Aphasiology: Proceedings of the Conference. Minneapolis: BRK Publishers, 1976.

Brilliant, P. J., and Gynther, M. D. Relationship between performance on three tests for organicity and selected patient variables. Journal of Consulting Psychology, 27, 474–479 (1963).

Darley, F. L., Aronson, A. E., and Brown, J. R. Motor Speech Disorders. Philadelphia: W. B. Saunders, 1975.

De Renzi, E., and Vignolo, L. A. The Token Test: A sensitive test to detect receptive disturbances in aphasics. Brain, 85, 665–678 (1962).

Diedrich, W. M., and Youngstrom, K. A. Alaryngeal Speech. Springfield, Ill.: Charles C Thomas, 1966.

Duffy, J. R., Keith, R. L., Shane, H., and Podraza, B. L. Performance of normal (non-brain-injured) adults on the Porch Index of Communicative Ability. In R. H. Brookshire (ed.), Clinical Aphasiology: Proceedings of the Conference. Minneapolis: BRK Publishers, 1976.

Eisenson, J. Examining for Aphasia. New York: Psychological Corp., 1954.

Fletcher, S. G. Theory and use of TONAR II: A status report. Unpublished report, University of Alabama in Birmingham, 1976.

Gonen, J. Y., and Brown, L. Role of vocabulary in deterioration and restitution of mental functioning. Proceedings of the Annual Congress of the American Psychological Association, 1968.

Goodglass, H., and Kaplan, E. The Boston Diagnostic Aphasia Test. Washington, D.C.: Lea & Febiger, 1972.

Graham, F. K., and Kendall, B. S. Memory for designs test: Revised general manual. Perceptual and Motor Skills, Monograph Supplement 11, 1960.

Hixon, T. J., Mead, J., and Goldman, M. D. Dynamics of the chest wall during speech production: Function of the thorax, rib cage, diaphragm, and abdomen. Journal of Speech and Hearing Research, 19, 297–356 (1976).

Holbrook, A. Instrumental analysis and control of vocal behavior. In M. Cooper and M. H. Cooper (eds.), Approaches to Vocal Rehabilitation. Springfield, Ill.: Charles C Thomas, 1977.

Inglis, J. A paired associate learning test for use with elderly psychiatric patients. Journal of Mental Science, 103, 796–803 (1957).

Kendrick, D. C., Parboosingh, R.-C., and Post, F. A synonym learning test for use with elderly psychiatric subjects: A validation study. British Journal of Social and Clinical Psychology, 4, 63–71 (1965).

Luria, A. R. Factors and forms of aphasia. In A. De Reuk and M. O'Connor (eds.), Disorders of Language. London: J. A. Churchill, 1964.

McDonald, E. T., and Chance, B. Cerebral Palsy. Englewood Cliffs, N.J.: Prentice-Hall, 1964.

McNeil, M. R., and Prescott, T. Revised Token Test. University Park Press, Baltimore, 1978.

Miller, E. Abnormal Ageing. London: John Wiley & Sons, 1977.

Moore, W. M., Rosenbek, J. C., and LaPointe, L. L. Assessment of oral apraxia in brain-injured adults. In R. H. Brookshire (ed.), Clinical Aphasiology: Proceedings of the Conference. Minneapolis: BRK Publishers, 1976.

Morris, H. L., Spriestersbach, D. C., and Darley, F. L. An articulation test for assessing competency of velopharyngeal closure. Journal of Speech and Hearing Research, 4, 48–55 (1961).

Poeck, K., and Kerschensteiner, M. Analysis of sequential motor events in oral apraxia. Paper presented at the Academy of Aphasia, Albuquerque, 1973.

Porch, B. E. Porch Index of Communicative Ability: Theory and Development (Vol. I). Palo Alto: Consulting Psychologists Press, 1967.

Porch, B. E. Porch Index of Communicative Ability: Administration, Scoring, and Interpretation (Vol. II). Palo Alto: Consulting Psychologists Press, 1971.

Schuell H. Differential Diagnosis of Aphasia with the Minnesota Test. Minneapolis: University of Minnesota Press, 1965.

Schuell, H., Jenkins, J., and Jiminez-Pabon, E., Aphasia in Adults. New York: Harper & Row, 1964.

Sklar, M. Sklar Aphasia Scale. Beverly Hills: Western Psychological Services, 1966.

Thurman, W. L. Restructuring voice concepts and production. In M. Cooper and M. H. Cooper (eds.), Approaches to Vocal Rehabilitation. Springfield, Ill.: Charles C Thomas, 1977.

Wepman, J., and Jones, L. Studies in Aphasia: An Approach to Testing. Chicago: University of Chicago Education-Industry Service, 1961.

Wilson, D. K. Voice Problems of Children. Baltimore: Williams & Wilkins, 1971.

Wilson, F. B., and Rice, M. A Programmed Approach to Voice Therapy. Austin, Tex.: Learning Concepts, 1977.

Wolski, W. Hypernasality as the presenting symptom of myasthenia gravis. Journal of Speech and Hearing Disorders, 32, 36–38 (1967).

Yates, A. J. The use of vocabulary in the measurement of intellectual deterioration—A review. Journal of Mental Science, 102, 409–440 (1956).

APPENDIX:
Examination of the Speech Mechanism

Clinic number______

Name: ____________________ Father's name: ______________

Address: ____________________ Date of birth: ________ Age: ____

____________________ Sex: ______________

Phone: ____________________ Date of examination: ________

I. Head and face:
  A. Size of head: Normal ________ Too large ________
     Too small ______________________
  B. Symmetry of head: Normal________ Deviation ______
  C. Size of face: Normal __ Too large______ Too small____
  D. Symmetry of face: Normal________ Deviation________
  E. Scars: ______________________
  F. Other: ______________________
  G. Comments: ______________________
  ____

II. Lips: (facial nerve: C VII)
  A. Shape: ______________________
  B. Upper length: Normal____Too long____Too short___
  C. Lower length: Normal____Too long____Too short___
  D. Position at rest:______________________
  E. Other: ______________________
  F. Function:
    1. Protrusion: Normal ______ Diminished ______
       Absent ______________________
    2. Retraction (R): Normal ______ Diminished _____
       Absent ______________________
    3. Retraction (L): Normal ______ Diminished _____
       Absent ______________________
    4. Retraction (bilateral): Normal _____ Deviated __
    5. Pucker: Normal ______ Diminished ______
       Absent ______________________
    6. Press and tense: Normal_____ Diminished_____
       Absent ______________________

Source: Idaho State University Speech and Hearing Center.

7. Diadochokinesis (Repetition of the syllable /p∧/):
   a. Trial 1: . . . . /5 seconds
   b. Trial 2: . . . . /5 seconds
   c. Trial 3: . . . . /5 seconds
   d. Average: . . . . /5 seconds

G. Comments: ____
____

III. Mandible: (trigeminal nerve: C V)

A. Maxillary-mandibular relationship:
   1. Maxilla in relation to mandible (anterio-posterior dimensions):
      Normal ________ Anterior ________ Posterior ______
   2. Maxilla in relation to mandible (lateral dimension):
      Normal ________ Wider ________ Narrower ______

B. Mandible size: ____

C. Mandible shape: ____

D. Mandibular function:
   1. A-P movement: Normal ________ Deviated ________
      Absent ____
   2. Lateral movement against resistance: Normal ______
      Diminished (R): ______ Diminished (L): ______
      Absent ____
   3. Diadochokinesis (chatter of the teeth):
      a. Trial 1: . . . . /5 seconds
      b. Trial 2: . . . . /5 seconds
      c. Trial 3: . . . . /5 seconds
      d. Average: . . . . /5 seconds

E. Comments: ____
____

IV. Teeth:

A. Condition: ____

B. Missing teeth: ____

C. Occlusion: ____

D. Comments: ____
____

V. Tongue: (hypoglossal nerve: C XII)
  A. Size in relation to dental arch: Normal ____________
     Too large ________________ Too small ______________
  B. Position during rest: ________________________________
  C. Frenulum: Normal ____________ Short ____________
  D. Function:
     1. Shorten: Normal __________ Diminished ________
        Absent ________________________________
     2. Curl: Normal ____________ Diminished ________
        Absent ________________________________
     3. Protrusion: Normal ________ Diminished ________
        Absent ________________________________
        Deviation (R): ________ Deviation (L): ________
     4. Elevation (tip): Normal ________ Diminished ______
        Absent ________________________________
     5. Elevation (Dorsum): Normal ______ Diminished ____
        Absent ________________________________
     6. Lateralization (R): Normal ______ Diminished ______
        Absent ________________________________
     7. Lateralization (L): Normal ______ Diminished ______
        Absent ________________________________
     8. Diadochokinesis (tip) (repetition of the syllable /t∧/):
        a. Trial 1: ..../5 seconds
        b. Trial 2: ..../5 seconds
        c. Trial 3: ..../5 seconds
        d. Average: ..../5 seconds
     9. Diadochokinesis (dorsum) (repetition of the syllable (/k∧/):
        a. Trial 1: ..../5 seconds
        b. Trial 2: ..../5 seconds
        c. Trial 3: ..../5 seconds
        d. Average: ..../5 seconds
  E. Comments: ________________________________
     ____

VI. Alveolus:
  A. Cleft (describe): ________________________________
  B. Repaired or fused: ________________________________
  C. Other: ________________________________

VII. Premaxilla:
- A. Cleft (describe): ____________________
- B. Floating: ____________________
- C. Repaired or fused: ____________________
- D. Other: ____________________

VIII. Hard Palate:
- A. Cleft (describe): ____________________
- B. Height: Normal ________ High vault ________
  Low vault ____________________
- C. Width: Normal ________ Too high ________
  Too narrow ____________________
- D. Comments: ____________________
  ____

IX. Soft palate: (facial nerve: C VII; glossopharyngeal nerve: C IX; vagus nerve: C X)
- A. Length: Normal ________ Too short ________
  Too long ____________________
- B. Symmetry at rest: Normal ________ Deviated ________
- C. Function:
  1. Elevation: Normal ________ Deviated ________
  2. Dimple (% of distance along A-P length of velum where dimple occurs during elevation) ________
  3. Velopharyngeal closure: Definite ________
     Probable ______ Improbable ______ Absent ______
  4. Gag reflex: Normal ________ Diminished ________
     Absent ____________________
- D. Comments ____________________
  ____

X. Oropharynx: (vagus nerve: C X)
   A. Size: Normal ______ Capacious ______ Too small ______
   B. Condition: ______________________________
   C. Function:
      1. LPW Movement (R): Normal ______________
         Diminished ______________ Absent ______________
      2. LPW Movement (L): Normal ______________
         Diminished ______________ Absent ______________
      3. PPW Movement: Normal ______ Diminished ______
         Absent ______________________________
   D. Comments: ______________________________
      ____

XI. Fauces:
   A. Size of isthmus: ______________________________
   B. Condition of faucial tonsils: Normal ______________
      Hypertrophied ______________ Absent ______________
   C. Condition of faucial pillars: ______________________________

XII. Oral sensory function:
   A. Two-point discrimination: (Identify test sites and d.1.'s)____
      ____
      ____
      ____
   B. Oral stereognosis: (Identify form types and results) ____
      ____
      ____
      ____

General comments: ______________________________
____
____
____
____
____

Section IV
REHABILITATIVE CONSIDERATIONS

Chapter 17
Role of the Audiologist

This chapter contains a short history of audiology and a listing of the services which the audiologist can be expected to perform. A general review of the training and certification requirements of the audiologist is also presented. To aid the health professional seeking audiologic services, a list of work settings is given to indicate where this specialist may be located. Finally, there are descriptions of three different active roles that the alert, interested audiologist may take in serving the elderly when health professionals and community officials fully recognize the potential contribution of this hearing specialist.

AUDIOLOGIC BEGINNINGS

Audiology is a relatively new profession. The name "audiology" and this unique area of expertise emerged as a recognizable profession during World War II. This happened as otologists, speech pathologists, and other professionals began to deal with the needs of servicemen who had become hearing impaired in service-related injuries. Raymond Carhart, a speech pathologist, and Norton Canfield, an otologist, both worked in the Veterans Administration hospitals during this period and were principal figures both in the use of the term "audiology," which they each suggested in about 1945, and in the subsequent development of the profession (Berger, 1976). Carhart helped establish a program for the training of audiologists at Northwestern University, where he was the first university professor of audiology (NHAJ, 1948). Canfield authored one of the first texts in the field entitled, *Audiology: The Science of Hearing* (*1949*). In December 1947, the American Speech Correction Association council voted to include hearing rehabilitation in the name of the association. Since that time this organization has been known as the American Speech and Hearing Association. Further details about this association and its activities are contained in Chapter 20.

AUDIOLOGIC SERVICES

The needs which prompted the emergence of this new specialty caused the development of many audiologic procedures which are listed in this chapter and described in more detail in Chapters 6 and 18. The audiologist's major clinical responsibilities include: 1) hearing measurement, 2) diagnostic assistance for the physician, 3) medical rehabilitation assistance, and 4) aural rehabilitation. Many audiologists are also engaged in teaching and/or research.

Hearing Measurement

The accurate assessment of hearing loss is a necessary preliminary to handling any hearing disability. The procedures evolved to do this include pure tone air and bone conduction testing and speech audiometric tests such as speech reception threshold (SRT) and speech discrimination. (See Chapter 6 for additional detail on these tests). Hearing measurement involves basic testing to determine the hearing sensitivity by pure tones and SRT's and the clarity of hearing by speech discrimination so that an intelligent course of therapy may be prescribed.

Diagnostic Assistance for the Physician

The physician is able to perform an examination of the ear canal and eardrum, but to diagnose and properly treat many forms of hearing loss he needs other information. The results of basic hearing measurement (pure tone and speech tests) are invaluable in diagnosis. Even those physicians who use tuning forks and informal conversation to make a gross assessment of hearing generally turn to the complete audiogram with pure tone and speech results when a diagnosis is to be made. In addition to routine assessment, the audiologist has developed a large battery of sophisticated tests to assist the physician in diagnosing the many different forms of auditory pathology and the exact site of the lesion. Tests to detect conductive losses like otosclerosis, cochlear pathologies like Ménière's disease, neural lesions such as VIIIth nerve tumor, and central auditory disorders are available. These include impedance tests like tympanometry, acoustic reflex, and Eustachian tube function. Other procedures include SISI, tone decay, Bekesy, loudness balance, electroencephalic response audiometry, and electronystagmography. Functional hearing losses can also be detected through auditory tests, including Stenger, delayed auditory feedback, and galvanic skin response audiometry. See Chapter 6 for more detail.

Medical Rehabilitation Assistance

If medical rehabilitation is indicated after preliminary diagnosis, it may take the form of surgical intervention or the use of medication. In either case, the measurement of hearing is an important monitoring device to determine the effectiveness of these procedures. In the case of otologic surgery like a stapedectomy, the physician will generally have a pre- and postsurgical audiogram derived. Pre- and post-audiograms are also needed to determine the effectiveness of medication, as in treating otitis media. When ototoxic drugs like streptomycin are used, as, for example, in treating tuberculosis, physicians generally want to monitor hearing on a regular basis to determine if the medication is having an adverse effect on hearing.

Aural Rehabilitation

In addition to medical intervention, hearing loss often requires nonmedical rehabilitation. The purpose of such therapy is to help the person adjust to his loss, to help him learn alternative methods to communicate, and to help him properly select and use a hearing aid if indicated. The methods employed here include the use of hearing aid evaluation, hearing aid orientation and counseling, and communication rehabilitation, including auditory training and speechreading. Chapter 18 describes these approaches in some detail. When properly applied, aural rehabilitation is based upon a consideration of the individual communication, social, and emotional needs of the patient. Therapy is aimed at helping the client cope with his immediate needs whether they relate to interaction in the family setting, the institutional setting, or elsewhere.

It should be noted that physicians recently have been thrust into the position of providing medical clearance for all persons who obtain hearing aids in this country (Federal Register, 1977). See additional details on this regulation in Chapter 19.

This approach appears excellent in that physicians will now be able to manage medical treatment for persons who have serious or correctable losses. It may, however, put many doctors in an awkward position in needing to advise persons about buying a hearing aid. In this regard, a referral to an audiologist who will provide complete hearing measurement and rehabilitative services is the procedure of choice for the physician. In fact, the federal regulations require such referrals for those under 18. It is most important that the physician recognize that hearing aids are appropriate for "nerve type" or sensorineural deafness, assuming medical care is not indicated. Most users of hearing aids these days do, in fact, have sensorineural losses. Further discussion of these factors is contained in Chapters 6 and 18.

AUDIOLOGIC TRAINING

To provide these services, it is apparent that the audiologist must have rather comprehensive training. The American Speech and Hearing Association (ASHA) has established training requirements and a certification procedure for the audiologist. This organization is to the audiologist what the American Medical Association is to the physician or what the American Psychological Association is to the psychologist.

To meet the ASHA certification requirement, audiologists must obtain a master's degree or its equivalent, and their coursework includes training in speech pathology, psychology, and the biologic sciences. Additionally, the audiologist generally takes coursework in education, physics, and electronics.

To conduct good basic *hearing measurement,* the audiologist needs to be familiar with the electronic equipment he must utilize, and he must understand, as the psychologist does, how to measure behavior of the human organism.

To *assist in the diagnostic work of the physician,* it is important for the audiologist to understand the anatomy, physiology, and neurology of the hearing mechanism and to be familiar with psychophysics, the study of man's perceptual responses to various physical parameters of sound.

To work effectively with the physician and the surgeon in *medical rehabilitation,* audiologists must be familiar with all of the various hearing disorders, their causes, their symptoms, typical audiologic findings, and possible surgical or medical procedures. In functional or non-organic losses, it is important for the audiologist to understand the psychology of abnormal behavior.

In the case of *aural rehabilitation,* the audiologist must use therapeutic methods drawn from his exposure to training in speech pathology and education of the deaf. Many of his clients will have substantial speech and language problems. In addition, psychological training in counseling will be needed here, not that the audiologist assumes a heavy counseling role, but in all dealings with the patient he must use sound principles to establish rapport and provide motivation. Equally important is exposure to other health professions and to special clinical populations such as pediatric and geriatric groups. In an increasing number of training programs, audiologists are receiving coursework in gerontology and related health care professions (Leutenegger and Stovall, 1971; Hull and Traynor, 1975; Colton, 1977; Erickson, 1977). Exposure to electronics is also urgently needed when the rehabilitation audiologist is assisting the patient in selecting or adjusting to a hearing aid.

Besides the specific coursework required by ASHA, the student in audiology must complete 300 clock hours of supervised clinical practicum, some in diagnostic work and some in therapeutics. After graduation a Clinical Fellowship Year (CFY) is required during which the new professional must have his work monitored by a certified member. Finally, it is required that a national examination be passed before the Certificate of Clinical Competence in Audiology (CCC-A) is awarded. This entire training process, though not the exact coursework, is similar to that required of speech pathologists, as explained in Chapter 20.

AUDIOLOGIC WORK SETTINGS

With this type of broad training focused on the specific problems of hearing impairment, the audiologist is well qualified to serve a key role in a variety of work settings. When audiologic services are needed, this trained professional may be found in a number of settings or may provide consultant services in such locations as the following:

1. Hospital or mental hospital
2. Rehabilitation center
3. Nursing home or senior citizen center
4. Public health clinic
5. Office of ear, nose, and throat specialists
6. Community speech and hearing center
7. College- or university-sponsored hearing center
8. Armed services medical corps
9. Veterans administration facility
10. Medical schools
11. Public schools
12. Schools for the deaf or the retarded
13. Safety divisions of various industries
14. Private practice

Responsibilities in these settings thrust the audiologist into a role as a key professional or advocate for the hearing-impaired person. Whether dealing with the newborn infant, a child in the schools, young adults, or the elderly, audiologists have provided leadership and expertise in helping to identify hearing impairment and to obtain proper remediation. Audiologists provide screening programs for newborns and at preschool and school levels. They provide hearing measurement and rehabilitation in public schools, schools for the deaf, hospitals, physicians' offices, rehabilitation centers, senior citizen centers, and nursing homes. As advocates for the hard of hearing they take responsibility in referring the person to other appropriate professionals once identification of the loss occurs. It can be said that audiologists have a broader understanding of the problems of hearing impairment than any other specialist, even though they are definitely not experts in areas of medicine or education of the deaf. This broad training and advocacy role are needed, especially, in dealing with the complex rehabilitation problems of the elderly hard-of-hearing person.

APPROACHES TO SERVING THE ELDERLY

Traditional Clinical Approach

In most of the settings listed above, the audiologist serves as a member of a clinical staff. He most likely will have an array of complex equipment located in a sound-proof booth to facilitate testing without the interference of environmental noise. In these settings the audiologist's role is to provide services to those who are referred or who come by self-referral to such a facility. Many of those who apply for services will be elderly because of the high incidence of hearing loss in those 65 years and older. It is currently estimated that 23–40% of all persons over 65 years possess some degree of impaired hearing (see Chapter 4). In addition, many elderly will be referred because of medical conditions like stroke that often have an effect upon hearing or because of the need to diagnose symptoms like dizziness that are associated with hearing disorders.

Once the audiologist has administered the appropriate battery of audiologic diagnostic tests, his attention will turn to the rehabilitation of the patient. If medical rehabilitation is not indicated he may be chiefly responsible for aural rehabilitation, which could include hearing aid evaluation and orientation, counseling, and communication rehabilitation through speechreading and auditory training. There are a number of traditional and not so traditional approaches which may be used in these clinical situations to provide aural rehabilitation. These are described in detail elsewhere (Sanders, 1971; Northern, 1972; O'Neill and Oyer, 1973) and in the next chapter (Chapter 18).

There are many of the elderly, however, who will not be served in the traditional clinical setting. Often, cost is a factor which prevents the elderly person from seeking professional assistance, but there are other factors, including a natural reluctance on the part of some to admit to the debilitating processes of growing older. Campanelli (1968) suggested that part of this reluctance is related to the belief that hearing deficiencies must be accepted as an inevitable part of growing older and that nothing positive can be done to compensate for the resulting handicap. To increase service to the elderly, the active, interested audiologist has used some other approaches besides the traditional clinical one.

Community Outreach Programs

Community outreach programs take a variety of forms, but they generally involve an abbreviated form of testing at various locations away from the clinic. Often, creativity must be used to find a reasonably quiet test area since sound-proof booths are not usually available. Portable equipment is used for test purposes.

One example of such a program was recently reported by Adair and Keiser (1976). In their community in Iowa, the county public health department conducts regular monthly well-elderly clinics at various locations throughout the county. The goal of these clinics is to detect and prevent chronic disease and to provide a point of contact between the elderly and the physicians in the community. Audiologists were invited to participate in these clinics, since many of the patients were noted to have hearing problems. Some of the elderly had expressed concern about whether they should buy a hearing aid, seek medical treatment, or just learn to live with their problem. Basic pure tone testing is performed by the audiologists and a case history is taken, after which the patient is counseled about the findings. Recommendations are made in conjunction with the geriatric nurse working with the clinic. Those with middle ear conditions are referred to their physicians. Others are advised to go to an audiology clinic for a hearing aid evaluation and/or for other forms of aural rehabilitation. Some patients are given simple help with and instruction about their hearing aids. In this way audiologic services have been provided to a group not previously served.

In Illinois a similar program was initiated throughout the state under auspices of the Chicago Hearing Society (Schow and Brunt, 1974; Colton and O'Neill, 1976). Under this program free hearing screening was provided at a variety of locations including retirement apartment houses, senior citizen centers, and churches. As a part of the program, hearing aid evaluations were provided to some clients at hearing clinics. Also, when indicated, aural rehabilitation sessions were provided on a weekly basis for neighborhood groups and were located at the same setting where the screening was conducted.

Alpiner (1963) ran a similar program at a golden age center in Cleveland. Schallenkamp, Condon, and Willis (1975) staffed satellite hearing clinics in a rural 10-county area in South Dakota. Kaplan and Rickerson (1976) have served a variety of centers in the Washington, D.C., area with such an outreach program. Rupp, McLauchlin, Harless, and Mikulas (1971) have reported on efforts of this type developed in Michigan. In a slightly different approach, McCartney, Maurer, and Sorenson (1974) have described a mobile audiology service for the elderly which is functioning out of Portland, Oregon, and serving a three-county area. This program utilizes a well equipped mobile van in which screening as well as follow-up services may be performed in a variety of locations.

Several of these programs were federally or privately funded. Some were sponsored by university training programs, and still others were provided as voluntary service by hearing clinic personnel to the communities in which they live. Whatever the source of support, it is obvious that audiologists may play a community role outside of the traditional clinical setting.

Consultant Services to Nursing Homes

In still another variation, the audiologist may serve the elderly as a consultant in nursing homes or other long-term care facilities. It has been shown that the percentage of hearing loss among nursing home residents may be as high as 97% (Miller and Ort, 1965). Approximately 50% may be expected to have losses which are substantial, i.e., 40 dB or greater (Rupp, 1970; Schow and Nerbonne, 1976). It is evident, therefore, that the audiologist has a potential role to play in these settings, and in recent years a number of programs have been developed to meet this need. Hull and Traynor (1975) have recently reported a community-wide program to serve nursing home residents, and Schow (1977) has described a statewide effort to improve hearing services to this population. A number of pioneering efforts have been important in the development of these programs (Heffler, 1960; Alpiner, 1963; Walle, 1971; Harless and Rupp, 1972).

In these programs the audiologist typically performs an abbreviated pure tone test on all new residents and then follows through with appropriate rehabilitative techniques. Hearing aid evaluations and other therapy procedures are often, by necessity, done within the nursing home setting, so that traditional techniques have had to be modified accordingly. Even so, forms of tympanometry and speech discrimination testing, as well as hearing aid evaluations, can be conducted in these settings. In the nursing home it is important that the audiologist maintain a program over an extended period of time, since this is required to develop rapport and familiarity with the residents and staff found in the long-term care facility. Additional detail on these programs is contained in Chapter 18.

Some audiologists have taken little interst in the elderly, assuming, along with many other professionals, that hearing loss in the very aged is virtually nonremedial because of phonemic regression and other vicissitudes of age (Busse, 1960). This, however, is not a common attitude, and most audiologists take an active role with the elderly in a clinical setting at least. It is obvious that many more elderly will be served as audiologists and health professionals in many communities develop programs similar to those described above.

SUGGESTED READINGS

Garwood, V., Bergman, M., Dixon, J., and Haspiel, G. Roles played by audiologists. Journal of the Academy of Rehabilitative Audiology, 6:1, 20–21 (1973).

Hodgson, W. R. Role of audiology. In W. R. Hodgson and P. H. Skinner (eds.), Hearing Aid Assessment and Use in Audiologic Habilitation. Baltimore: Williams & Wilkins, 1977.

Newby, H. A. The profession of audiology. In H. A. Newby (eds), Audiology (3rd Ed.). New York: Appleton-Century-Crofts, 1972.

Rupp, R. R. The roles of the audiologist. Journal of the Academy of Rehabilitative Audiology, 10:1, 10–17 (1977).

REFERENCES

Adair, J. R., and Keiser, J. H. Well elderly clinics: New horizons for the audiologist. Paper presented at the Annual Convention of the American Speech and Hearing Association, Houston, 1976.

Alpiner, J. G. Audiologic problems of the aged. Geriatrics, 18, 29–26 (1963).

Berger, K. W. Genealogy of the words "audiology" and "audiologist." Journal of the American Audiology Society, 2, 38–44 (1976).

Busse, E. Aging and personal relations. In N. W. Shock (ed.), Aging: Some Social and Biological Aspects. Washington, D. C.: American Association for the Advancement of Science, 1960.

Campanelli, P. A. Audiological perspectives on presbycusis. Eye, Ear, Nose, and Throat Monthly, 47, 3 (1968).

Canfield, N. Audiology: The Science of Hearing. Springfield, Ill.: Charles C Thomas, 1949.

Colton, J. C. Student participation in aural rehabilitational programs. Journal of the Academy of Rehabilitative Audiology, 10:1, 31–35 (1977).

Colton, J. C., and O'Neill, J. J. A cooperative outreach program for the elderly. Journal of the Academy of Rehabilitative Audiology, 9, 38–41 (1976).

Erickson, J. G. Pragmatics of the development of community resources or why university programs should provide training in public relations. Journal of the Academy of Rehabilitative Audiology, 10:1, 23–30 (1977).

Federal Register. Department of Health, Education, and Welfare, Food and Drug Administration, Hearing Aid Devices, Professional and Patient Labeling and Conditions for Sale, Part IV. Tuesday, February 15, pp. 9286–9296 (1977).

Harless, E. L., and Rupp, R. R. Aural rehabilitation of the elderly. Journal of Speech and Hearing Disorders, 37, 267–273 (1972).

Heffler, A. J. The Montefiore Home hearing conservation program. Geriatrics, 15, 180–186 (1960).

Hull, R. H., and Traynor, R. M. A communitywide program in geriatric aural rehabilitation. Asha, 17, 33 (1975).

Kaplan, H., and Rickerson, C. University based aural rehabilitation programs: Geriatric programs. Paper presented at the Annual Convention of the American Speech and Hearing Association, Houston, 1976.

Leutenegger, R. R., and Stovall, J. D. A pilot graduate seminar concerning speech and hearing problems of the chronically ill and the aged. Asha, 13, 61–66 (1971).

McCartney, J. H., Maurer, J. F., and Sorenson, F. D. A mobile audiology service for the elderly: A preliminary report. Journal of the Academy of Rehabilitative Audiology, 7, 25–36 (1974).

Miller, M. H., and Ort, R. G. Hearing problems in a home for the aged. Acta Otolaryngologica, 59, 33–44 (1965).

NHAJ (National Hearing Aid Journal), February, 1948. As cited in K. W. Berger, Genealogy of the words "audiology" and "audiologist." Journal of the American Audiology Society, 2, 38–44 (1976).

Northern, J. L. Visual and auditory rehabilitation for adults. In J. Katz (ed.), Handbook of Clinical Audiology. Baltimore: Williams & Wilkins, 1972.

O'Neill, J. J., and Oyer, H. J. Aural rehabilitation. In J. Jerger (ed.), Modern Developments in Audiology (2nd Ed.). New York: Academic Press, 1973.

Rupp, R. R. Understanding the problems of presbycusis. Geriatrics, 25, 100–107 (1970).

Rupp, R. R., McLauchlin, R. M., Harless, E., and Mikulas, M., The specter of aging—Golden years or tarnished? Hearing and Speech News, 39:6, 10–13 (1971).

Sanders, D. Aural Rehabilitation. Englewood Cliffs, N. J.: Prentice-Hall, 1971.

Schallenkamp, K., Condon, M., and Willis, V. The use of satellite clinics and computerization to facilitate hearing testing and remedial services to rural dwelling senior citizens. Paper presented at the Annual Convention of the American Speech and Hearing Association, Washington, D.C., 1975.

Schow, R. L. How to promote and provide speech and hearing help in nursing homes: Experiences in a state-wide program. Paper presented at the Annual Convention of the California Speech and Hearing Association, San Francisco, 1977.

Schow, R., and Brunt, M. Identification of hearing loss in senior citizens with remediation by amplification and lipreading. Final Report. State of Illinois Department of Aging, June, 1974.

Schow, R. L., and Nerbonne, M. A. Hearing levels in nursing home residents. Research Laboratory Report, 1, pp. 1–10. Department of Speech Pathology and Audiology, Idaho State University, Pocatello, 1976.

Walle, E. L. Communication problems of the chronically ill and aged in the institutional setting. Hearing and Speech News, 39:6, 16–17 (1971).

Chapter 18
Aural Rehabilitation

Aural rehabilitation is defined in this chapter in its traditional form along with more recent approaches. The various procedures of aural rehabilitation are described, including speechreading, auditory training, hearing aid evaluation, hearing aid orientation, and counseling. These methods of therapy are also discussed in the context of their use with the elderly person and also with the institutionalized elderly. The general characteristics and living conditions of elderly patients are listed with a discussion of how these affect aural rehabilitation.

DEFINITIONS AND NEEDS

Traditionally, aural rehabilitation has been considered to consist of hearing aid evaluation and orientation, counseling for client and family, auditory training, speechreading, and speech conservation (Newby, 1972). More broadly defined, it is any effort made to rehabilitate the hearing impaired through nonmedical procedures.

Generally, traditional aural rehabilitation has not been popularly received by the adult hearing impaired (Rassi and Harford, 1968; Northern and Sanders, 1972; Oyer, Freeman, Hardick, Dixon, Donnelly, Goldstein, Lloyd, and Mussen, 1976). It is reported, for example, that some clinics have tried everything but "dancing girls" to lure clients in for therapy, but without success (Alpiner, 1973a). Nevertheless, there is some evidence to indicate that aural rehabilitation can be successful. For instance, at the Army's Walter Reed General Hospital, at National Technical Institute for the Deaf, in clinics throughout the San Francisco Bay area, and in Denmark there have been ongoing programs that have proved to be of great value (Northern, Ciliax, Roth, and Johnson, 1969; Binnie, 1976; Ewertsen, 1974).

The importance of aural rehabilitation is underscored by the fact that there are so many hearing-impaired persons needing rehabilitation. It is estimated that 6 million Americans over 65 have sufficient bilateral hearing loss to warrant consideration of hearing aids, and yet only 21% of them use an aid (U.S. Senate Hearings, 1973). When compared to persons with other disabilities, the hard-of-hearing person is grossly neglected. Yarington (1976) observed:

> Modern society has been trained to rush to the assistance of the blind, identifying them with white canes and dark glasses and even the seeing eye dog ... On the other hand, the attitude toward individuals with hearing loss is decidedly different. They are generally ignored, hearing aids are designed to be invisible, (and) hearing conservation programs are difficult to establish ... In general, the individual with slowly deteriorating hearing is faced with the prospect of gradual estrangement from his associates and family, will gradually be looked on as a social outcast, may develop symptoms of paranoia, and faces a significant handicap. Perhaps this explains the tranquil expression on the face of the blind as compared to the frustrated appearance and introverted attitude exhibited by those with significant hearing problems. (p. 178)

Failure to recognize and rehabilitate people with hearing impairment may have serious consequences besides the demoralizing effects pointed out by Yarington. Gardner (1975), for example, has studied interpersonal relationships and communication in the elderly and is convinced that serious hearing impairment is one of the most important factors triggering what is commonly called senility. It is fairly obvious that persons who cannot effectively communicate will often make inappropriate comments and appear confused. Somewhat more surprising is the finding that a substantial proportion of elderly psychiatric patients diagnosed as schizophrenics of late onset (paranoid type) had a severe auditory deficit (Kay, Beamison, and Roth, 1964). Another study has revealed that the older family member with a hearing and speech deficit that makes communication difficult is more likely to be placed in a nursing home by his family than is the incontinent or bedridden elderly person who requires a great deal of physical care (Elconin, Egeberg, and Dunn, 1964).

It is apparent, then, that hearing loss may have devastating effects, especially when it is present in the elderly. If medical management is not indicated for correcting the disability, and only infrequently does it help the presbycusic, then aural rehabilitation is needed. Of course, such rehabilitation is used with children and adults, as well as with the gerontologic population. Several forms of a total adult aural rehabilitation program have been suggested in recent publications, including those by Sanders (1971), Northern (1972), Ross (1972), ARA (1973), O'Neill and Oyer (1973), ASHA

(1974), Oyer and Frankmann (1975), Binnie (1976), and Oyer and Hodgson (1977). All of these programs suggest a broadly based approach to aural rehabilitation, and most include the following areas after preliminary hearing assessment aspects are completed:

1. Hearing aid evaluation
2. Hearing aid orientation
3. Counseling of client and family
4. Communication rehabilitation including auditory training and speechreading
5. Comprehensive planning for emotional, social, and vocational adjustment

What follows in this chapter is a general description of various rehabilitative procedures and, in connection with each, a discussion of how these methods are used with the elderly.

HEARING AID EVALUATION

Usually the first effort in aural rehabilitation is to determine if a hearing aid can be used by the patient. If amplication is indicated, then the most appropriate aid needs to be selected. The hearing aid evaluation is an audiologic procedure designed to deal with these two matters. It would generally follow a thorough audiologic assessment as explained in Chapter 6. With audiometric and nonaudiometric results from that assessment, the need for a hearing aid evaluation can be determined.

Federal regulations now require that all individuals consult with a physician before purchase of a hearing aid (Federal Register, 1977). Individuals over 18 may, however, sign a waiver form and skip medical examination under certain conditions. The new program puts the physician in a position to frequently make decisions about the need for hearing aids and aural rehabilitation. After physical examination and medical treatment, the ideal situation will be one in which the physician can refer these patients to the audiologist for assessment and for decisions about amplification.

Hodgson (1977) has suggested a cursory guideline which outlines when individuals should be referred for hearing aid evaluation. It is based on the pure tone average or speech reception threshold (SRT) in the better ear (see Table 18-1). There are exceptions to this guide, as in the case of persons with unilateral loss or for those with unusual audiograms, who may need hearing aids.

Table 18-1. General guide to relationship between hearing loss and need for amplification, based on pure tone average or speech reception threshold in better ear (see text for important qualifications)

Hearing loss in dB (re: ANSI 1969)	Need for amplification
0–25	No need
25–40	Part time need for special occasions
40–55	Frequent need
55–80	Area of greatest satisfaction
80+	Great need—partial help

Source: Hodgson 1977

Nevertheless, the information in Table 18-1 provides a useful set of general rules.

The nonaudiometric self-evaluation of hearing through a scale such as the Hearing Handicap Scale (HHS) also provides a helpful guideline regarding the need for rehabilitative help (High, Fairbanks, and Glorig, 1964; see Chapter 6). When a person's scores are greater than 30% on the HHS, full audiologic assessment is advisable, and when scores are in excess of 40%, as shown in Table 6-1, there is an indication that the handicap is sufficient to warrant amplification.

When a hearing aid evaluation is undertaken, a number of approaches may be used. A study by Burney (1972) showed that the most popular method is still the one originally proposed by Carhart (1946). In this procedure, the subject is clinically tested in several conditions, both with and without amplification. Nevertheless, other approaches are being applied, including the use of a master hearing aid (Wasson, 1963), a prescription procedure (Berger, 1976), and referral to a hearing aid dealer for selection after audiometric assessment and counseling by an audiologist (Resnick and Becker, 1963).

The role of audiologists and hearing aid dealers in the selection and dispensing of hearing aids has recently stimulated controversy (RPAG, 1973; HEW, 1975; ASHA,1977a). Some audiologists now select and dispense hearing aids, whereas dealers have generally been responsible for the dispensing in the past. Regardless of the extent to which audiologists may distribute aids in the future, hearing aid dealers will probably continue to take some part in the hearing aid delivery system. In the past the dealers have sold between 70 and 80% of all hearing aids in this country without the involvement of medical or audiologic consultants (Stutz, 1969; HEW, 1975). The Retired Professional Action Group and other organizations have expressed great concern about the sale of hearing aids when the professionals from medicine and audiology are not involved (RPAG, 1973; HEW, 1975; ASHA, 1977b). It would appear from the evidence cited and from personal experience in working with the hearing impaired that hearing aids are sometimes dispensed to persons who do not benefit from using these devices. This is particularly serious in the case of elderly persons where numerous problems may emerge in obtaining a good fit and in achieving an adequate adjustment to the aid. Far too many elderly are unable to use aids, which eventually end up in dresser drawers.

Audiologists who are taking an active role in clinical rehabilitation programs can provide very helpful services before and after an aid is sold, especially in the case of elderly persons. Through aural rehabilitation programs much can be done in helping the new user in the adjustment process. In addition to the potential problems of misfitting and adjustment, however, there are many who have not yet obtained an aid who should. The hearing aid industry estimates that there are 7.5 million potentially successful hearing aid users who do not have an aid, and at least one-half are thought to be over 65 (HEW, 1975). This industry and their associated dealers are working vigorously to reach these nonusers. In short, there is a potent need to involve physicians, audiologists, and dealers in the process of hearing aid selection. Hopefully, through the united efforts of all these groups more persons who need hearing aids will receive them, and rehabilitation assistance will be available so that all who have aids will receive maximum benefit from them.

One advantage of having an audiologist perform a hearing aid evaluation is that if a hearing aid is not indicated, then the person having hearing troubles may obtain help through other forms of aural rehabilitation. These rehabilitation services are seldom provided by hearing aid dealers (Libby, 1974) and then only when an aid is sold. It may be noted that hearing aids are not recommended for approximately 10–20% of those persons who go to speech and hearing centers for hearing aid advice (Hoople, 1960; Hardick, 1977).

Through audiologic procedures decisions can be made as to whether or not a person can benefit from an aid, what type of aid (ear level or body) should be used, the ear(s) for which aid(s) should be used, and specific characteristics (such as frequency response, gain, maximum power, ear mold coupling) which the aid should have. Once a person obtains an aid, periodic hearing aid re-evaluations are recommended to ascertain that optimal help is being achieved from the amplification. The exact procedures used in a hearing aid evaluation are described in detail in other sources (Berger and Millin, 1971; Ross, 1972; Alpiner, 1975; Hodgson, 1977).

For the Elderly in General

While hearing aid evaluations are conducted with all age groups, in most clinics a substantial proportion, if not a majority, are performed for the elderly (Alpiner, 1973b; Blood and Danhauer, 1976). Bowman (1974) reported that of the 1163 clients seen the preceding year at the Philadelphia Hearing Society, the average age was 72 years. Thus, regular hearing aid evaluation procedures are generally appropriate for the elderly.

The elderly require special considerations that are not as important with younger subjects (Canfield, 1973). For example, Rupp, Higgins, and Maurer (1977) have developed a scale for predicting the feasibility of hearing aid use with older individuals. This scale incorporates the following factors: magnitude of the hearing loss, self-assessment scores, motivation to hear better, adaptability, attitude toward hearing aids, age, manual dexterity, visual ability, financial resources, and family support (see Appendix A). All of these things play some part in predicting the prospects for success. However, it is interesting that the first four factors are given the greatest weight and account for 55% of the potential score.

Another procedure designed, in part, for use with the elderly calls for the utilization of the sentence portion of the Utley Lipreading Test. Dodds and Harford (1968) use this test to allow for visual input along with auditory input which is heard under two conditions, both with and without amplification. In this way, some elderly clients who do very poorly on both aided and unaided auditory discrimination tests can be shown to benefit from an aid. This can serve as encouragement to patients who might otherwise reject amplification. Sometimes with the elderly, the opposite problem is encountered. Namely, patients show such good speech discrimination without an aid that amplification is not indicated even though the person is experiencing some hearing handicap in daily life. In these cases, it should be remembered that most experts agree that the person with presbycusis should get a hearing aid before the time of intense need is upon him (Rupp, McLauchlin, Harless, and Mikulas, 1971). The elderly person will probably be able to make the adjustment to amplification better before he has an extreme loss and before he reaches an advanced age. Thus, careful monitoring of the loss from year to year is indicated, and in some cases an aid will be recommended for an elderly person sooner than when it would be for a younger client.

One problem with the traditional hearing aid evaluation is that the procedure is too lengthy for some elderly subjects. Oyer et al. (1976) have suggested that one reason rehabilitation has not been successful with the elderly is that they have become discouraged after enduring the tedium of the usual hearing aid evaluation. Instead of one extensive procedure, Hardick (1977) uses a procedure in which a hearing aid is selected in a series of shorter sessions over an extended period of time. Various aids are tried with different earmold arrangements over a 6–12 week therapy period until the best hearing adjustment is made or until amplification is ruled out as a form of remediation.

For the Institutionalized Elderly

According to Buch, Basavaraju, Charatan, and Kamen (1976) there are over 1 million institutionalized elderly in this country. When the hearing-impaired person is located in an institutional setting, such as a nursing home, a radically different approach may be needed for hearing aid evaluation. As a group, the hearing-impaired institutionalized elderly have been sadly neglected. There have been a number of reports for over 30 years emphasizing the hearing problems of residents in nursing homes (Grossman, 1955; Kleemeier and Justiss, 1955; Bloomer, 1960; Heffler, 1960; Mitchell, 1962; Alpiner, 1963; Gaitz and Warshaw, 1964; Miller and Ort, 1965; Chafee, 1967; Walle and Newman, 1967; Walle, 1971; Hull and Traynor, 1975b; Leutenegger, 1975; Schow and Nerbonne, 1976; McCartney and Alexander, 1976; Smith and Fay, 1977).

Among other things, these reports have emphasized a high incidence of hearing impairment that varies from 20% to 97% depending on the nursing home involved and the definition of loss. According to Schow and Nerbonne (1976) a good overall figure is that 80% have slight hearing loss of 26 dB HTL (ANSI) or greater, and about 50% have a more serious loss of at least 40 dB HTL. Despite this high prevalence of loss, very few residents seem to have careful monitoring of their hearing problems. Buch et al. (1976) found, for example, that many residents at the Jewish Institute for geriatric care in New York had never consulted a physician for advice about their deafness or hearing loss. Consistent with this is the report of McCartney and Alexander (1976). One-third of the 616 ears they examined among nursing home residents had excessive cerumen plugging the ear canal.

In the use of hearing aids, Grossman (1955) reported that in one nursing home only 29% of the possible candidates for hearing aids were using them. In two other homes, Alpiner (1963) similarly found only 33% (19 out of 58) of the potential users wearing aids. Beginning in 1975, in a state-wide program of hearing screening, in Idaho, the authors discovered that only about 11% of potential candidates were using aids. Another 20% of the potential group had aids but were not using them.

It would appear, then, that despite three decades of discussion, there are still many unresolved hearing problems among elderly nursing home residents. Part of the problem lies with the reluctance of residents to seek care, to use aids, or to admit they have a loss. Even when given the opportunity to have hearing aid evaluations and to receive hearing aids, nursing home residents often refuse. Gaitz and Warshaw (1964) found that when aids were recommended for and freely offered to eight persons in one nursing home of 40 residents, five of the eight refused. Alpiner (1973a) had even worse luck in recommending hearing aid evaluations to the residents of two facilities, since only six of 48 residents referred for evaluation were willing to follow this advice.

In general, audiometric screening and nonaudiometric assessment can be done in the nursing home without difficulty (Schow and Nerbonne, 1977), but when the residents have been asked to journey to a speech and hearing clinic for a hearing aid evaluation, many refuse. This is not surprising when one considers the medical and psychological problems of these residents, as well as their frequent nonambulatory status. Recognizing this, Traynor and Hull (1975) have suggested a modified evaluation procedure. They persuasively argue that testing in the nursing home is defensible since it is possible to predict quite precisely where the clients will be using the aid. Evaluation in the nursing home allows a meaningful interaction with a typical environment, whereas this would not be true of any one testing site for the active elderly. They suggested the following steps:

1. Pure tone and impedance screening results are utilized, and speech discrimination is estimated by informal conversation
2. No more than three trial aids are selected based on frequency response, gain, maximum power output and manual dexterity of the patient
3. The aids are successively placed on the patient and speech discrimination is assessed by presenting the PB-50 word lists live voice at about a 6-foot distance; scores are derived with or without visual clues.
4. The resident is counseled about use and care of the aid and then allowed to use the aid for a 1-week period

The present authors have likewise used a modified hearing aid evaluation procedure within nursing homes. In the Idaho State University Speech and Hearing program, which is offered to nearby nursing homes, an attempt has been made to obtain a preliminary assessment of hearing aid candidacy for all hearing-impaired residents as part of the initial screening in these facilities. All residents were given a pure tone air conduction screening test, a simple otoscopic examination, impedance testing, and both self and staff hearing handicap scales (see discussion of special assessment procedures and Nursing Home Hearing Handicap Index in Chapter 6). These procedures comprised an overall approach to specify hearing status. From this evaluation the need for cerumen removal, middle ear treatment, and further hearing rehabilitation was determined. For those residents with hearing loss, an initial assessment of hearing aid benefit was attempted. However, recognizing the problems of evaluating several aids with a 50- or even a 25-word PB list, a 10-item list was employed. The 10-word lists were developed by Rose, Schreurs, Keating, and Miller (1974) (see Appendix B). For one group of 28 patients, these lists were presented via a tape recorded signal which was broadcast through a speaker at a normal conversation level of 45 dB HTL. Residents were tested individually both with and without a master hearing aid. The aid was fit to the best ear or when the ears were equal it was fit to the right ear because of cerebral dominance considerations (see Chapter 9). This testing showed good improvement through amplification in some cases, but for the majority no improvement was noted. Mean data are shown in Table 18-2.

This aided and unaided performance in preliminary tests must be evaluated along with all the other assessment information, and it

Table 18–2. Data obtained on a sample (N = 28) of residents from one nursing home who were seen as part of the Idaho State University nursing home aural rehabilitation program

	Number	Mean PTA[a] (dB)	Unaided Discrimination (%)	Aided Discrimination (%)	Self handicap (%)	Staff handicap (%)
Mean	28	43	33	37	26	26
SD		15	37	34	34	38

Subjects with improved discrimination: 6

Pearson (r) correlations;

Self handicap with PTA	.62
Staff handicap with PTA	.76
Self handicap with Discrimination	−.45
Staff handicap with Discrimination	−.64
Staff and self handicap	.53

[a] PTA, Pure tone average (500,1000,2000 Hz).

certainly does not preclude further, more extensive hearing aid evaluation procedures (on both ears) as described by Traynor and Hull (1975). It became obvious, however, that even 10-item, single-word discrimination tests were too difficult for some residents in the evaluation process. Several other 10-item tests were therefore selected, utilizing simple unrelated phrases from the Utley Lip-reading Test and a series of related sentences devised especially for the nursing home situation (see Appendix B). These various discrimination tasks have allowed a semiformal evaluation of hearing aid performance as compared to unaided scores for residents who could not cope with the usual discrimination test. Use of visual clues can also be allowed or denied, depending on the difficulty of the task. In working with the resident to select a trial aid, it is important that the discrimination task be of appropriate difficulty so that all scores are not extremely poor or extremely good. Under these conditions it is most feasible to learn the effect of amplification and also to demonstrate benefit to the resident. After hearing aid selection, the trial period in the ISU program may go on for several weeks or months. This is possible when a small "bank" of hearing aids is available for use in the nursing home. The aids are new and used instruments gathered through donation by philanthropic groups or individuals. All aids are electroacoustically analyzed to assure good performance.

Smith and Fay (1977) have reported an extended hearing aid selection process which they operate in a 1600-bed, long-term-care facility in New York. They found, as did Schow and Nerbonne (1977), that in the institutionalized setting the loss generally needs to reach 40 dB HTL before it becomes a handicap. They use some preliminary listening training with desk auditory trainers before fitting a hearing aid. The aid is then worn for up to several weeks before more formal testing is attempted. Several aids are generally tested in this relaxed manner before a selection is made. They have spent as long as 5 months in selecting aids which were ultimately purchased and successfully used. Even longer time periods have been required for other residents who never were able to find a successful fit. This program also has access to a bank of hearing aids that were used for trial purposes.

In a report of their program, Smith and Fay (1977) claimed the most successful fitting was found with the conventional body aid, and 35 of the 49 successful users employed such aids. Only 14 used eyeglass or other ear level aids, even though 18 others could have used aids with less power than the body aid had it not been for the oldsters' difficulty in handling the smaller aids. Hull and Traynor (1975a) also reported that most selections were of body aids in their nursing home work. Smith and Fay further reported that virtually none of the users objected to any type of aid by reason of personal vanity. In the ISU program, however, there have been cases where residents would not wear a body aid because of its cosmetic appearance even though they needed more volume that a larger aid could have provided.

HEARING AID ORIENTATION AND COUNSELING

After selection of an appropriate hearing aid, it should be obtained for use in a trial period. The new user is sometimes able to adjust quickly to amplification, but quite often there is a somewhat more difficult and longer coping process. Occasionally this adjustment is extremely problematic, and these users are the ones whose aids will either be returned at the conclusion of the trial period or eventually end up in the dresser drawer. A dilemma posed by this variability in adjustment is that it is very difficult to predict which clients will have the greater adjustment problems. Hardick (1977) estimated that of all new hearing aid users about 75% need only a brief introduction to the benefits, limitations, and care of hearing aids. He claimed that among the elderly, a smaller percentage make such a quick adjustment and many need extensive orientation. However, he said it is difficult to predict the ones who will need this in-depth service.

In Denmark the attitude is taken that all new users should be given some extended training, and four weekly 2-hour sessions are held for groups of new users (Ewertsen, 1974). The classes are taught by a hearing and speech therapist who has over 6 years of education as preparation for this job. Even more extensive rehabilitation is provided for those who desire it. The benefits of this program are indicated by the fact that only about 6% do not use their hearing aids after these training sessions.

By contrast, in this country, while surveys give an incomplete picture because of only partial returns, the same degree of success is notably lacking. Blood and Danhauer (1976), for example, reported getting only a 48% return on a survey of persons for whom aids were evaluated or recommended. It appeared that 11% of this group were not regularly using their hearing aids, and the percentage is probably greater for those who did not return the questionnaire. In fact, some probably did not even get an aid, much less use it, if the experience of Rassi and Harford (1968) may be taken as an example. They found that only 70% purchased a hearing aid when advised to do so. In one survey, Alpiner (1973b) received responses from 119 persons following 1 year of hearing aid use. Only 67% said they received the benefits they expected from their aids. There were 17% who felt they had not been adequately counseled on hearing aid use, and 75% of these dissatisfied persons were 65 years or older.

One American survey (Northern et al., 1969) showed that 97% were using the recommended aid, but this was in an Army program where hearing aid orientation is required. In this and other VA and service-related programs in the United States, extended hearing aid orientation of about 20 hours is routinely provided by audiologists (Altshuler, 1974). Otherwise, there is a great deal of variation in the orientation offered to new users in America. It is claimed that hearing aid dealers spend an average of 11 hours with persons to whom they sell an aid (Payne, 1975). This time estimate may include interaction extending over several years and probably includes a substantial amount of time in sales-related activities. Also, the dealers' training is generally limited when compared to the instructors used in the hearing aid orientation program offered in Denmark or in the U.S. VA facilities. Of course, many dealers do provide valuable orientation to those who return to them for follow-up service. It must be recognized, however, that it is difficult for the dealer to get some clients to return (Altshuler, 1974). Furthermore, Libby (1974) pointed out that there are only a few hearing aid dealers who provide or arrange for their customers to return for a series of structured orientation sessions. Therefore, he claims that intensive counseling and orientation are not given "the same priority and attention" (p. 29) by the dealer when compared to the time spent in hearing evaluation and fitting.

In audiologic facilities, hearing aid rechecks, orientation, and follow-up may or may not be stressed. Fleming, Birkle, Kolman, Miltenberger, and Israel (1973) reported that in the Washington, D.C., area, with a population of about 3 million, and more than a dozen speech and hearing clinics, no clinics (except for service-related personnel) offered comprehensive follow-up services. Hardick (1977) also reported that in the Detroit area, among a half dozen major audiologic facilities and a dozen or so audiologists in private practice with otologists, only two facilities offer extensive rehabilitative follow-up. By comparison, Fleming et al. (1973) found good continuing services in 10 of 21 non-VA facilities in the San Francisco Bay area. In short, while brief hearing aid orientation is provided for most clients by the audiologist or the dealer, extensive orientation is only occasionally provided in this country despite the fact that some persons have a substantive need for such services.

The important components of hearing aid orientation and counseling sessions have been described by Sanders (1975) and Kasten and Warren (1977). In these sessions, they suggest inclusion of the following hearing aid orientation information:

1. Introducing the hearing aid, including its components and controls
2. Putting the aid on and listening to amplification
3. Caring for earmolds and batteries
4. Using the telephone, TV, alarm clocks, and other communication devices
5. Checking the aid and getting it repaired

In counseling they suggest:

1. Describing the levels of hearing such as primitive, warning, and symbolic (Ramsdell, 1970)
2. Explaining the audiologic findings
3. Discussing the handicapping aspects of hearing loss
4. Describing the benefits and limitations of aids
5. Analyzing total communication needs
6. Finding solutions for communication problems

Tannahill (1973) developed a hearing aid adjustment program with six consecutive weekly meetings which included most of the above components. He incorporated with this program a public charting procedure to monitor the progress of clients in: 1) gradually increasing their wearing time, 2) using appropriate volume settings, and 3) increasing their speech discrimination performance. A spirit of comradery developed in the groups as individuals tried to achieve their goals in this program. Through such a process, clients were helped to make the initial adjustment to amplification while learning and sharing experiences in a group setting. This program has also been applied with as few as four sessions through a combination of group and individual therapy or individual therapy alone. It has been used now for about 6 years with clients at Illinois State University and Idaho State University, and there are over 150 graduates of these adjustment sessions. Data in Table 18-3 show the mean improvement of SRT and discrimination that occurred with a sample group of 21 clients over a four-session period.

Table 18-3. Mean data on a sample ($N = 21$) of clients seen in a hearing aid adjustment program used at Idaho State University and Illinois State University

		Aided			
	Unaided	Session 1	Session 2	Session 3	Session 4
Pure tone average (dB) (500, 1000, 2000 Hz)	40.7	30.7	31.2	25.5	23.3
Speech discrimination (%)			72.2	75.0	76.3

For the Elderly in General

As with hearing aid evaluations, the usual procedures with hearing aid orientation are generally appropriate for the elderly, and, in fact, a large portion of regular clients in these programs are 65 years or older. It has been previously mentioned that the need for orientation is often greater in the elderly. In Canada the efforts of senior citizen groups were instrumental in arranging for long-term instruction in the care and use of aids (Gough, 1977). Canadians over 65 are eligible to receive hearing aids free of charge through a governmental program, but extensive follow-up orientation sessions are not included as part of the service. Only a brief introduction to hearing aids is provided along with an instructional booklet from the manufacturer. It is interesting that a majority of the elderly people interviewed who had gone through this brief program reported that they "could not recall much of the information and did not fully comprehend the instructions and suggestions contained in the manufacturers' brochures" (Gough, 1977, p. 40). In response, a program has been instituted in Alberta to provide more extensive orientation services.

Such experiences demonstrate the value of hearing aid adjustment programs in meeting the special needs of the elderly. Miller (1967) has stated:

> No presbycusic patient who has not used a hearing aid should purchase one without the opportunity to use the aid first under supervision and with at least a short program of training in the essentials of auditory training and speechreading. (p. 4)

Without this he feels the successful elderly hearing aid user will seldom be found. Happily, a number of programs for the aged have incorporated hearing aid orientation as a part of an overall, total rehabilitation effort for new hearing aid users (Alpiner, 1965; Miller, 1967; Barr, 1970; Harless and Rupp, 1972). These programs are similar to those already described and also include emphasis on auditory training and speechreading, as described later in this chapter. Greater detail on hearing aids, their care, and other communication devices is contained in Chapter 19.

For the Institutionalized Elderly

Smith and Fay (1977) have an excellent approach to this challenge, which actually blends with their hearing aid evaluation procedures previously described. During the extended process of hearing aid selection, lasting up to 5 months or longer, Smith and Fay provided regular individual listening training. This was combined with in-service training for staff members. Demonstrations, instructions and assistance were offered to the staff on a continuing basis since in some cases, the ward personnel had to take the responsibility for management of the hearing aids.

After a trial hearing aid was selected, the audiologist continued to work with the patient on a regular basis (usually two times per week) for up to 15 months. The average time was 9–10 months. Apparently this time was spent primarily in solving adjustment problems, interacting with the client to provide listening practice, and evaluating the patient's progress. In some cases a number of aids were tried, and finally it was concluded that there was no reasonable hope for success. Of the 62 patients who went through the program, 12 (19%) adjusted to their aids through these orientation activities within 1 month. Another 37 (60%) required up to 5 months for auditory rehabilitation. There were also 13 (21%) who were on the program for as long as 15 months but without success. The following points were used as indicators of success:

1. Consistent use of the hearing aid
2. All possible independence in care of the aid
3. Improvement in daily communication
4. Enhancement of interaction with staff members
5. Increased participation in recreational and other activities
6. Positive personality changes

The most important factors in predicting success were health, mental status, and language function. Age, visual impairment, motor disturbance, and personality were of limited influence. According to Smith and Fay (1977) the extent of auditory impairment was also a secondary factor in predicting success. They stated, "Poor speech discrimination predicted nothing, except the need for much training" (p. 419). Hull and Traynor (1975a) have developed a rather detailed handout which they give to nursing home residents to help in hearing aid adjustment. The instructions, however, seem better suited for use with the noninstitutionalized elderly.

COMMUNICATIVE REHABILITATION INCLUDING AUDITORY TRAINING AND SPEECHREADING

Auditory training and speechreading are usually the procedures that first come to mind when aural rehabilitation is mentioned. Actually, both terms are used to refer to a wide variety of techniques. To some professionals, auditory training includes the various activities discussed in the section on hearing aid orientation and counseling. To others it means a series of listening activities, and to still others it simply means learning about the dynamics of conversational situations and how to better control them. Auditory training may, in fact, include any or all of these elements.

Speechreading, or lipreading as it is frequently called by the lay person, is thought by some to be a skill which, when mastered, would prepare a person for "private eye" work. Others consider it to be a skill worthy of months and years of analytic or synthetic training through methods developed by Mueller-Walle, Nitchie, and others (Sanders, 1971). Even so, it is recognized that speechreading rarely provides total understanding by itself. Still others, including many audiologists, emphasize that speechreading is simply a process of being visually alert to all lip, facial, gestural, and environmental clues. According to this view, speechreading is a skill which nearly all people have to some degree, and the focus is not so much on teaching speechreading as on encouraging the hearing impaired to utilize the skills they already possess.

These two procedures, then may be used in many ways. Fleming et al. (1973) reported a variety of activities of an auditory training or speechreading nature that would be included in communication rehabilitation. These consisted of teaching and encouraging the patient to:

1. Physically position himself to maximize lighting, reverberation, and signal-to-noise factors.
2. Develop expertise in interacting with conversational partners.
3. Maximize acoustic and lighting conditions in his usual conversational locations.
4. Become a better listener by being more interested and attentive.
5. Deal with the impatient normal hearing conversational partner.

Lundborg, Linzander, Rosenhamer, Lindstrom, Svard, and Fransson (1973) recommended a selective use of such communication training. They examined the need for and success of various auditory rehabilitation procedures in a group of 3850 Swedish patients. For subjects with 40–60 dB loss, they routinely recommend hearing aid orientation, but they advise auditory training and speechreading only when there is a steeply falling audiogram. For patients with 60–80 dB loss, they found that 10% benefited from speechreading and auditory training. If there was 80 dB or greater loss, they stated that 40% received help from a full rehabilitation program. However, they inferred that age and other factors reduced what would otherwise have been a higher success rate. This would suggest that more extensive therapy is required in cases with more extreme loss, and that these procedures become more difficult to apply to the elderly.

While communication aspects may thus be applied on a selective basis, they can also be merged in a total therapy program. The bias of the authors of this book is that they fit best as part of a total hearing rehabilitation process which should be generally applied to the elderly client.

For the Elderly in General

Several total rehabilitation programs have been described for the elderly in which auditory training and speechreading aspects may be noted. Hardick (1977) described an aural rehabilitation program for the aged. He feels that the following are important characterisitics of a program for the elderly:

1. It is client-centered to meet individual needs. This is done through a combination of individual and group therapy.
2. The program revolves around amplification and/or modifying the communication environment. Hardick works "mightily" to find suitable amplification, and formal speechreading work is not emphasized. He states: "I have no evidence that people can lipread any better after any form of therapy so I do not wish to infer to my patients or their families that they get better if they practice a lot" (p. 63). He feels the maximum benefit will come from visual clues if a person is attentive to them, but relaxed, and speechreading as a part of total listening.
3. He requires the attendance of a relative or friend to gain admittance to the group.
4. His programs are all short-term, involving a weekly meeting for 6–12 weeks, depending on how quickly the goals of the group are accomplished.
5. As much consumer information as possible is disseminated to the group.

The goals Hardick describes for the program include the major aspects of aural rehabilitation. Clients are told about their hearing loss and their hearing aid. There is extensive experimentation with hearing aid use until the right aid is selected. The electroacoustic aspects of the aid are then measured and recorded. Listening practice is given to awaken the person's interest in hearing again. Hardick feels that the elderly, in particular, enjoy the peace and quiet of hearing loss and need to be sold on the benefits of hearing. They are informed about speechreading, with its difficulties, and encouraged to use their native skill. Attitudes and behaviors are discussed, and some are discouraged, such as bluffing, self depreciation, and guilt. Finally, helpful suggestions are given about alarm clocks, TVs, telephones, and personal safety. Hardick admittedly takes a conservative view of the benefits of speechreading and auditory training. He promises no dramatic improvement, but he says:

> I submit that whether or not we can materially improve a person's ability to read lips or significantly improve their auditory discrimination, that we can provide answers to many perplexing problems faced daily by the hearing impaired, those who live with them, and those who interact with them in the employment setting and socially. (p. 60)

The philosophy promoted by Hardick is very consistent with the aural rehabilitation program at Idaho State University. The therapy is set up on a short-term basis with weekly 1.5-hour sessions for 5–6 weeks. Family members or friends are encouraged to come and are given a chance to wear a hearing aid and participate in discussions. The sessions incorporate both group and individual therapy and may be extended on an individual basis for those who still need additional help. When the client is a new hearing aid user, these sessions are incorporated with the hearing aid adjustment class previously described. When the person is not deemed a candidate for hearing aid use but has hearing problems, the program is tailored to focus on specific communication difficulties and solutions. For example, the class may spend time analyzing the situation of the weekly bridge game, with suggestions on lighting, seating position, anticipating the conversation, and so forth.

The basic approach is to present to the client a variety of ways by which he may improve his overall communication. Thus, by pooling all information available to him (as discussed by Sanders, 1975), it is possible to compensate for the loss of audition. Alternative sources of information include amplification, knowledge of language, awareness of situational constraints, and visual attentiveness to lip movements, facial expressions, and gestures. In addition, attentive listening is discussed with suggestions for improving one's listening skills (see Appendix C). In this therapy program speechreading is discussed in terms of those factors which make it easier or more difficult. However, no extensive drillwork is undertaken, and the emphasis is on visual attentiveness rather than visual phonemic (viseme) reception.

The audiologist monitors progress and attainment of goals in these sessions with auditory, visual, and handicap measures. Auditory testing includes SRT, discrimination, and electroacoustic aid performance. Molds can be made or adjusted with instamold equipment and by arrangement with the hearing aid dealer. Basic vision and pre- and postspeechreading scores are measured with an eye chart and with the Utley word and sentence portions. Scoring is based not only on response accuracy but also on the attempts made, so that the client's listening strategy can be assessed. Some clients lack confidence and others are overconfident, making many mistakes. These factors may have an important influence, and adjustment in listening strategy may be indicated (Kelly and Tobin, 1974). Pre- and postscores from scales like the HHS and the Communicative Performance Questionnaire (Sanders, 1975) allow measurement of the reduction in hearing handicap.

The programs employed by Hardick and at Idaho State University emphasize the general listening and visual attentiveness aspects of auditory training and speechreading as important communicative skills in total aural rehabilitation. Several other programs for the elderly do the same (Alpiner, 1965; Fleming, 1972; Bowman, 1974). Others working with the elderly continue to emphasize these two procedures in a more traditional approach which would employ drillwork and extensive practice in mastering these skills (Pang and Fujikawa, 1969; Barr, 1970; Harless and Rupp, 1972; McCartney, Maurer and Sorenson, 1974; Kaplan and Rickerson, 1976).

Drillwork in speechreading has been emphasized to some extent as an isolated therapy approach. Hearing societies in Chicago, Detroit, and other large cities traditionally have offered such lipreading classes (Hardick, 1977). These courses were popularized by Nitchie, Bruhn, and others in the early 1900s and have been given "lip service" ever since. Because of public awareness of these classes, lipreading may be the first remedy which an elderly hearing-impaired person considers as a solution for his problem. Even after training in speechreading, many clients maintain a high interest in further therapy (Northern et al., 1969; Hardick, 1977). It is possible that they continue to feel the need for more training because it is so hard to master. However, from their experience, Colton and O'Neill (1976) felt that, while the social interaction aspects are beneficial, an isolated speechreading program is considerably weakened as therapy unless residual hearing and auditory training procedures are stressed also. Alpiner (1973a) was more adamant when he referred to the "...invalid procedures of Nitchie, Kinzie, Jena, and Mueller-Walle" (p. 55). Earlier Alpiner (1965) had stated:

> Studies on aged persons with regard to speechreading and auditory training are most limited. The general feeling is that these procedures are not too successful but this remains either to be proved or disproved. (p. 458)

Colton and O'Neill (1975) have recently produced some evidence which seems to support traditional drillwork. They applied two different auditory training procedures on 22 geriatric subjects (60–85 years of age) who had mild to moderate sensorineural losses. Two subgroups of 11 were selected and matched prior to therapy for age, schooling, SRT, and speech discrimination. The experimental group then received 10 hours of therapy which focused on the three most common phoneme confusions (/p/, /t/, /s/) found in these subjects. The drillwork was divided into 4 hours on isolated phonemes, 3 hours on syllable drill of these phonemes, and 3 hours on word drill. The experimental subjects were given feedback when they made errors, and reasons for misperception were discussed. The control group also received 10 hours of training, but they simply listened to stories without feedback or discussion. Both experimental and control subjects used the same amplification, an auditory training unit with a setting that produced a frequency response closely resembling a typical hearing aid.

After training, the experimental subjects showed a statistically significant average improvement of about 10% on an NU-6 speech discrimination test (pre, 73.45%; post, 83.63%). The control group showed no improvement in mean scores (pre, 74.72%; post, 74.90%). No improvement was noted for either group on pre- and post-SRTs, HHS scores, or individual phoneme errors of /p/, /t/, /s/. Colton and O'Neill concluded that drillwork is more beneficial than simple listening with amplification. However, they suggested that the experimental group therapy seemed primarily to increase listening and attending skills, since no improvement was noted in specific phoneme perception. They observed that a word, sentence, and paragraph approach to such listening drill may be beneficial. A question raised by this research is whether listening and attending skills increased because of the feedback or because of the auditory trainer drillwork. Perhaps the same result could be obtained through group listening and individual therapy which provide feedback and emphasize the development of better listening skills.

For the Institutionalized Elderly

As previously noted, the prevalence of extreme loss is greater in the nursing home population. Accordingly, the need for extensive auditory rehabilitation is even greater in the institutionalized patient than in other elderly subjects, but it is also more fraught with difficulty. Traynor and Hull (1975) have described a speechreading and auditory training program for use in nursing homes, senior citizen centers, or retirement communities. However, the group procedures they describe, including synthetic speechreading and listening activities, seem better suited for senior citizen centers than nursing homes, and the benefits they state seem to be primarily social. They did report some success with an interesting type of communication rehabilitation, namely, the use of manual signs to help patients with extreme impairments to communicate their basic needs. Such a program may have merit in certain cases.

Miller (1976) undertook an extensive aural rehabilitation program in the nursing home setting. Through 12 hours of individual help, residents were given auditory training and speechreading instruction which could be either analytic or synthetic depending on the resident's personality, needs, and vision. Miller was able to locate 22 residents for this therapy approach from a population of over 300 residents. Many were unwilling to undergo pretherapy testing. Even use of the word "test" frequently had a traumatic effect. Standardized test procedures, though designed for use in the homes, were often too difficult for the residents. Despite this fact, a significant improvement was noted in pre- and posttest mean scores of the 11 experimental subjects. Speech discrimination improved an average of 8% (55.6–63.6%), and speechreading of the Utley sentence test went from 23.7% to 38.5%, a 15% increase. In contrast, the control group had received no therapy, and they showed only about 1% improvement on each test. While this report demonstrates the potential for traditional rehabilitation procedures even in a nursing home setting, Miller concluded that relatively small numbers of residents have adequate motivation and ability to profit from training.

After working with a nursing home rehabilitation program for about 2 years, the authors of this book feel that the primary emphasis of such programs should be in assessment, hearing aid evaluation, orientation, and individual counseling and inservice training. While some social benefits may derive from communication therapy, it is felt that the greatest yields will come from these other efforts.

COMPREHENSIVE PLANNING OF REHABILITATION

A complete aural rehabilitation program will include consideration of emotional, social, and vocational matters. In addition, speech or psychiatric therapy may be indicated. The needs and methods for speech therapy for the elderly are discussed in Chapter 21, and psychological treatment would be handled by referral. But the emotional and social needs of the elderly deserve some special consideration. Lack of motivation has frequently been mentioned as a deterrent to effective aural rehabilitation, and other general characteristics of the elderly can present challenges to the aural rehabilitationist.

If aural rehabilitation is to be effective it must focus on the total individual, not just the hearing loss. As previously discussed in Chapter 3, there are a number of physiologic and psychological changes and circumstantial factors which affect the elderly. To call attention to these and their effect in the case of hearing impairment and rehabilitation, a brief summary is included here.

Physiologic Changes

The biologic changes in aging are associated with the deterioration of bodily functions and produce greater susceptibility to disease. Indeed, when aged persons contract acute disease, they suffer longer than the average younger person (Cottrell, 1974), and they are twice as likely as younger persons to have chronic disability (Muskie, 1971). The most common illnesses are arthritis, various forms of cardiovascular diseases, and cancer, according to Cottrell (1974). Cottrell also reported that when sensory types of chronic disability such as hearing loss are added to the list, almost everybody over 60 has at least one chronic condition. It is understandable that elderly persons tend to be more concerned about life-threatening forms of illness than they are about sensory handicaps, and this explains in part the failure of many to seek rehabilitative help for hearing loss. Nevertheless, more attention would probably be given to hearing disorders if hearing were carefully screened in the physical examination as often as vision.

The decline in fluid intelligence and long-term memory storage along with increased time requirements for learning (see Chapters 3 and 14) have implications for therapy also. These changes produce a reduced ability to adapt to new situations, solve problems, and think creatively. This will be noted in some clinical cases more than others, of course, but a good rule for the clinician is to be willing to go over information repeatedly, and great patience may occasionally be required. The reader will recall that Smith and Fay (1977) exhibited such patience in working with elderly patients for as long as 15 months to obtain an appropriate hearing aid fitting and adjustment. Kleemeier and Justiss (1955) have pointed out that physiologic conditions may hinder the elderly client in learning to care for and maintain an aid. They may forget to turn the aid off at night, to change batteries, or they may get old and new batteries mixed up. Other problems such as poor vision or manual dexterity may make it difficult to change batteries, to get the mold in the ear, or to feel when the aid controls "click" into new positions. These factors may make it necessary for another person to help in caring for the hearing aid.

Psychological Changes

A number of personality changes associated with aging may be related to hearing loss. It will be recalled that disengagement (i.e., withdrawal or isolation), cautiousness, rigidity, and depression may often be found in the elderly (see Chapter 3). When consideration is given to the effect of hearing loss, it is apparent that remediation of the loss should prevent the occurrence of these symptoms, or, if they are present, should help alleviate them. Patients with loss sometimes deny having a hearing impairment. This may signify an inability to accept still another disability in addition to those already acknowledged. One may wonder whether the hearing impaired deny loss deliberately as part of the disengagement process and because of the peace and quiet the loss provides (Hardick, 1977) or whether the isolation is actually brought on by the hearing impairment. In the latter case, the person may subconsciously compensate for poor communication abilities by socializing less frequently and, as a consequence, may not be aware of the loss. This person is perhaps a better candidate for rehabilitation, while the person seeking disengagement should probably be allowed to follow his desires (Kübler-Ross, 1969).

Circumstantial Factors

Family Relations and Social Interaction According to Oyer (1976), more older people (40% of men and 15% of women) live with a spouse than in any other of five common arrangements. About one-third of older individuals live alone and less than 25% live with adult children. Thus, on a routine basis, there are important communications involving other family members in many elderly persons' homes. Family relations can be very much strained in these communications when there is hearing disability, particularly since there are a number of other potentially explosive issues, like changing roles of retired spouses or disagreements in child-rearing practices between different generations. It is therefore important that the hearing-impaired person have members of his family or friends participate with him in the rehabilitative process. In fact, Hardick (1977) refuses entry into his rehabilitative groups unless the client is accompanied by such a partner.

Financial Security It is estimated that one in every four persons over 65 lives beneath the poverty level (Muskie, 1971). A study by Harris (1976) showed the median income for older people to be $4800. When rehabilitation is offered to older persons, there must be a recognition that finance is a concern for many. Indeed, it would appear that if rehabilitative needs are to be fully met, sources of funding must be located and legislation must be enacted. Fortunately, interest in the elderly at the federal government level is high as evidenced by increased spending for aging research and medicare expansion proposals, which would include audiologic rehabilitative services (Hull, 1977). Other local and state agencies and service organizations, such as Lions Clubs, have also been helpful in financial support. Mussen (1977) believes, however, that when elderly persons are able to pay for services that they should do so, since the chances for successful completion of therapy will be better when a personal financial investment is involved.

Relocation The average American moves 14 times in his lifetime. However, according to Oyer (1976), there is less movement among older persons, although a large number move immediately after retirement. Moving may be welcomed, according to Oyer, or it may be a traumatic adjustment, particularly in cases where the move is into a nursing home. Rosenwasser (1964) pointed out that in nursing homes, often the resistence or outright refusal to wear a hearing aid may in fact represent an unwillingness to adjust to a new strange environment. At the same time, patients may use their hearing losses as an excuse for their unwillingness to participate in the social activities of their new surroundings. A move into a nursing home signifies a loss of freedom and independence as well as impending death. For some, patience and understanding may help the client to make this adjustment.

Death Coping with death is one of the major concerns of the elderly. When death appears to be near at hand, it can be a strong deterrent to motivation in auditory rehabilitation. Alpiner (1965) has noted this hopelessness in some individuals who, when approached about rehabilitative help, would say, "I am going to die soon, so what is the use of any kind of help? Spend your time on young people" (p. 3). Imminent death does not always produce such responses, however. When one elderly gentleman was approached in a nursing home served by the Idaho State University rehabilitation program, he responded, "Sonny, this home is Grand Central Station, you know. This is the last stop. But I want to make the most of it while I'm here." He was a motivated participant despite his age and condition.

Summary In rehabilitation, much depends upon the patient's health, attitudes, and circumstances, and these will influence the acceptance of the disability and the response to therapy. Understanding and awareness of these factors should therefore be evident in auditory rehabilitation efforts for the elderly. The words of Beckinridge previously quoted by Alpiner (1963) provide a fitting conclusion for this chapter. She advised (p. 26) that in working with the elderly one should remember that they are:

1. Not as old as they used to be, physically or mentally
2. Not like children; they must be approached on a mature level
3. As individual and varied as any age group
4. Subject to basic human needs; they need to love and be loved, to feel useful, to belong somewhere, to laugh, to believe in something.
5. Generally much more flexible and capable of learning new things than we give them credit for

SUGGESTED READINGS

Alpiner, J. G. Diagnostic and rehabilitative aspects of geriatric audiology. Asha, 7, 455–459 (1965).

Binnie, C. A. Relevant aural rehabilitation. In J. L. Northern (ed.), Hearing Disorders. Boston: Little, Brown, 1976.

Hardick, E. J. Aural rehabilitation programs for the aged can be successful. Journal of the Academy of Rehabilitative Audiology, 10, 51–66 (1977).

Harless, E. L., and Rupp, R. R. Aural rehabilitation of the elderly. Journal of Speech and Hearing Disorders, 37, 267–273 (1972).

Hearing Aid Journal. Topic-of-the-month: Geriatrics. October (1977).

Hull, R. H. Hearing impairment among aging persons. Lincoln, Neb.: Cliffs Notes, 1977.

Kasten, R. N., and Warren, M. P. Learning to use the hearing aid. In W. R. Hodgson and P. H. Skinner (eds.), Hearing Aid Assessment and Use in Audiologic Habilitation. Baltimore: Williams & Wilkins, 1977.

Kodman, F., Jr. Techniques for counseling the hearing aid client. Audecibel, 22, 214–217 (1973).

Leutenegger, P. R. Patient Care and Rehabilitation of Communication-Impaired Adults. Springfield, Ill.: Charles C Thomas, 1975.

Liden, G. (ed.). Geriatric Audiology. Stockholm: Almquist and Wiksell, 1968.

Mussen, E. F. Problems of rehabilitative audiology in the retirement community setting. Journal of the Academy of Rehabilitative Audiology, 10, 68–70 (1977).

Northern, J. L. Visual and auditory rehabilitation for adults, In J. Katz (ed.), Handbook of Clinical Audiology. Baltimore: Williams & Wilkins, 1972.

Oyer, H. J., and Hodgson, W. R. Aural rehabilitation through amplification. In W. R. Hodgson and P. H. Skinner (eds.), Hearing Aid Assessment and Use in Audiologic Habilitation. Baltimore: Williams & Wilkins, 1977.

Ross, M. Principles of Aural Rehabilitation. Indianapolis: Bobbs-Merrill, 1972.

Sanders, D. A. Hearing aid orientation and counseling. In M. C. Pollack (ed.), Amplification for the Hearing-Impaired. New York: Grune & Stratton, 1975.

Tannahill, J. C. Hearing aids: Trial and adjustment by new users. Audecibel, 22, 90–97 (1973).

REFERENCES

Alpiner, J. G. Audiologic problems of the aged. Geriatrics, 18, 19–26 (1963).

Alpiner, J. G. Diagnostic and rehabilitative aspects of geriatric audiology. Asha, 7, 455–459 (1965).

Alpiner, J. G. The hearing aid in rehabilitation planning for adults. Journal of the Academy of Rehabilitative Audiology, 6:1, 55–57 (1973a).

Alpiner, J. G. Client opinions of clinical hearing aid evaluations. Journal of the Academy of Rehabilita·ive Audiology, 6:1, 58–60 (1973b).
Alpiner, J. G. Hearing aid selection for adults. In M. C. Pollack (ed.), Amplification for the Hearing-Impaired. New York: Grune & Stratton, 1975.
Altshuler, M. As I see it .... Hearing Instruments, 25:9, 16–25 (1974).
ARA Task Force on Aural Rehabilitation for Adults. Journal of the Academy of Rehabilitative Audiology, 6:1, 50–53 (1973).
ASHA. ASHA challenges new FDA hearing aid regulation. Asha, 19, 261, 264–265 (1977a).
ASHA. FTC's presiding officer report cites hearing aid sales abuse, need for control. Asha, 19, 779, 782 (1977b).
ASHA Committee on Rehabilitative Audiology. The audiologist: Responsibilities in the habilitation of the auditorily handicapped. Asha, 16, 68–70 (1974).
Barr, D. F. Aural rehabilitation and the geriatric patient. Geriatrics, 25, 111–113 (1970).
Berger, K. W. Prescription of hearing aids: A rationale. Journal of the American Audiology Society, 2:3, 71–78 (1976).
Berger, K. W., and Millin, J. P. Hearing aids. In D. E. Rose (ed.), Audiological Assessment. Englewood Cliffs, N.J.: Prentice-Hall, 1971.
Binnie, C. A. Relevant aural rehabilitation. In J. L. Northern (ed.), Hearing Disorders. Boston: Little, Brown, 1976.
Blood, I., and Danhauer, J. L. Are we meeting the needs of our hearing air users? Asha, 343-347 (1976).
Bloomer, H. H. Communication problems among aged county hospital patients. Geriatrics, 15, 291–295 (1960).
Bowman, Z. M. Aural rehabilitation for the elderly. Hearing Instruments, 25:9, 15 (1974).
Buch, J., Basavaraju, N. G., Charatan, F. B., and Kamen, S. Preventive medicine in a long-term care institution. Geriatrics, 31, 99–108 (1976).
Burney, P. A survey of hearing aid evaluation procedures. Asha, 14, 439–444 (1972).
Canfield, C. H. The geriatric population—Are they good candidates for hearing aids. Hearing Instruments, 24, 13 (1973).
Carhart, R. Selection of hearing aids. Archives of Otolaryngology, 44, 1–18 (1946).
Chafee, C. E. Rehabilitation needs of nursing home patients: A report of a survey. Rehabilitation Literature, 28, 337–382 (1967).
Colton, J. C., and O'Neill, J. J. The effects of auditory training on audiologic measures obtained with geriatric subjects. Paper presented at the Annual Convention of the American Speech and Hearing Association, Washington, D.C., 1975.
Colton, J. C., and O'Neill, J. J. A cooperative outreach program for the elderly. Journal of the Academy of Rehabilitative Audiology, 9, 38–41 (1976).
Cottrell, F. Aging and the Aged. Dubuque, Iowa: William C. Brown, 1974.
Dodds, E., and Harford, E. Application of a lipreading test in a hearing aid

evaluation. Journal of Speech and Hearing Disorders, 33, 167–173 (1968).

Elconin, A. F., Egeberg, R. O., and Dunn, O. J. An organized hospital based home care program. American Journal of Public Health, 54, 1106–1117 (1964).

Ewertsen, H. W. Hearing rehabilitation in Denmark. Hearing Instruments, 25:9, 20–21 (1974).

Federal Register. Rules of the Food and Drug Administration for the hearing aid industry. Federal Register, February 15, 9286–9296 (1977).

Fleming, M. A total approach to communication therapy. Journal of the Academy of Rehabilitative Audiology, 5:1, 2, 28–31 (1972).

Fleming, M., Birkle, L., Kolman, I., Miltenberger, G., and Israel, R. Development of workable aural rehabilitation programs. Journal of the Academy of Rehabilitative Audiology, 6, 35–36 (1973).

Gaitz, C. M., and Warshaw, H. E. Obstacles encountered in correcting hearing loss in the elderly. Geriatrics, 19, 83–86 (1964).

Gardner, W. G. Hearing loss the route to senility? Audecibel, 24, 74–76 (1975).

Gough, K. H. Hearing rehabilitation for the elderly: A report on a project for the training of hearing aides. Hearing Aid Journal, 30, 9 (1977).

Grossman, B. Hard of hearing persons in a home for the aged. Hearing News, September, 11–20 (1955).

Hardick, E. J. Aural rehabilitational programs for the aged can be successful. Journal of the Academy of Rehabilitative Audiology, 10, 51–66 (1977).

Harless, E. L., and Rupp, R. R. Aural rehabilitation of the elderly. Journal of Speech and Hearing Disorders, 37, 267–273 (1972).

Harris, L., and Associates, Inc. The Myth and Reality of Aging in America. National Council on the Aging, 1975, as cited in H. J. Oyer and E. J. Oyer (eds.), Aging and Communication. Baltimore: University Park Press, 1976.

Heffler, A. J. The Montefiore home hearing conservation program. Geriatrics, 15, 180–186 (1960).

HEW. Final Report to the Secretary on Hearing Aid Health Care. Springfield, Virginia: U.S. Department of Commerce, 1975.

High, W. S., Fairbanks, G., and Glorig, A. Scale of self assessment of hearing handicap. Journal of Speech and Hearing Disorders, 29, 215–230 (1964).

Hodgson, W. R. Clinical measures of hearing aid performance. In W. R. Hodgson and P. H. Skinner (eds.), Hearing Aid Assessment and Use in Audiologic Habilitation. Baltimore: Williams & Wilkins, 1977.

Hoople, G. D. Care of hearing in the elderly. Geriatrics, 15, 106–109 (1960).

Hull, R. H. Aural rehabilitation for the aging hearing impaired person. Journal of the Academy of Rehabilitative Audiology, 10, 46–50 (1977).

Hull, R. H., and Traynor, R. M. The pathologic and audiologic manifestations of presbycusis. Short course presented at the Annual Convention of the American Speech and Hearing Convention, Washington, D.C., 1975a.

Hull, R. H., and Traynor, R. M. A communitywide program in geriatric aural rehabilitation. Asha, 17, 33 (1975b).

Kaplan, H., and Rickerson, C. University based aural rehabilitation programs: Geriatric programs. Paper presented at the Annual Convention of the American Speech and Hearing Convention, Houston, 1976.

Kasten, R. N., and Warren, M. P. Learning to use the hearing aid. In W. R. Hodgson and P. H. Skinner (eds.), Hearing Air Assessment and Use in Audiologic Habilitation. Baltimore: Williams & Wilkins, 1977.

Kay, D. W. K., Beamison, P., and Roth, M. Old age mental disorders in Newcastle-Upon-Tyne. Part 1: A study of prevalence. British Journal of Psychiatry, 116, 146–158 (1964).

Kelly, B. R., and Tobin, H. Quantification of psychological variables pertinent to aural rehabilitation. Journal of the Academy of Rehabilitative Audiology, 7:2, 55–64 (1974).

Kleemeier, R., and Justiss, W. Adjustment to hearing loss and hearing aids in old age. In I. Webber (ed.), Aging and Retirement. Gainesville: University of Florida Press, 1955.

Kübler-Ross, E. On Death and Dying. New York: MacMillan, 1969.

Leutenegger, R. R. Patient Care and Rehabilitation of Communication-Impaired Adults. Springfield, Ill.: Charles C Thomas, 1975.

Libby, E. R. Aural rehabilitation 1974. Hearing Instruments, 25:9, 11 (1974).

Lundborg, T., Linzander, S., Rosenhamer, H., Lindstrom, B., Svard, I., and Fransson, A. Experiences with hearing aids in adults. Scandinavian Audiology, Supplement 3, 9–46 (1973).

McCartney, J. H., and Alexander, D. Geriatric audiology in nursing homes. Paper presented at the Annual Convention of the American Speech and Hearing Association, Houston, 1976.

McCartney, J. H., Maurer, J. F., and Sorenson, F. D. A mobile audiology service for the elderly: A preliminary report. Journal of the Academy of Rehabilitative Audiology, 7:2, 25–35 (1974).

Miller, M. Audiologic management of presbycusis patients. Fenestra, 4:4, special insert article (1967).

Miller, M. H., and Ort, R. G. Hearing problems in a home for the aged. Acta Otolaryngologica, 59, 33–44 (1965).

Miller, W. E. An investigation of the effectiveness of aural rehabilitation for nursing home residents. Paper presented at the Annual Convention of the American Speech and Hearing Association, Houston, 1976.

Mitchell, J. A program for the geriatric patient. ASHA, 4, 167–171 (1962).

Muskie, E. S. Some perspectives on the problems of the elderly. Hearing and Speech News, 39:6, 3–5 (1971).

Mussen, E. F. Problems of rehabilitative audiology in the retirement community setting. Journal of the Academy of Rehabilitative Audiology, 10, 68–70 (1977).

Newby, H. A. Audiology. New York: Appleton-Century-Crofts, 1972.

Northern, J. L. Visual and auditory rehabilitation for adults. In J. Katz (ed.), Handbook of Clinical Audiology. Baltimore: Williams & Wilkins, 1972.

Northern, J., Ciliax, D., Roth, R., and Johnson, R., Jr. Military patient attitudes toward aural rehabilitation. Asha, 11, 391–395 (1969).

Northern, J. L., and Sanders, D. A. Philosophical considerations in aural rehabilitation. In J. Katz (ed.), Handbook of Clinical Audiology. Baltimore: Williams & Wilkins, 1972.

O'Neill, J. J., and Oyer, H. J. Aural rehabilitation. In J. Jerger (ed.), Modern Developments in Audiology (2nd Ed.). New York: Academic Press, 1973.

Oyer, E. J. Exchanging information within the older family. In H. J. Oyer and E. J. Oyer (eds.), Aging and Communication. Baltimore: University Park Press, 1976.

Oyer, H. J., and Frankmann, J. P. The Aural Rehabilitation Process: A Conceptual Framework Analysis. New York: Holt, Rinehart and Winston, 1975.

Oyer, H. J., Freeman, B., Hardick, E., Dixon, J., Donnelly, K., Goldstein, D., Lloyd, L., and Mussen, E. Unheeded recommendations for aural rehabilitation: Analysis of a survey. Journal of the Academy of Rehabilitative Audiology, 9, 20–30 (1976).

Oyer, H. J., and Hodgson, W. R. Aural rehabilitation through amplification. In W. R. Hodgson and P. H. Skinner (eds.), Hearing Aid Assessment and Use in Audiologic Habilitation. Baltimore: Williams & Wilkins, 1977.

Pang, L. Q., and Fujikawa, S. Hearing impairment in the aged: Incidence and management. Hawaii Medical Journal, 29, 109–113 (1969).

Payne, J. Statement of James Payne, Public Hearing of HEW. In Final Report to the Secretary on Hearing Aid Health Care. Springfield, Virginia: U.S. Department of Commerce, 1975.

Ramsdell, D. A. The psychology of the hard-of-hearing and deafened adult. In H. Davis and S. R. Silverman (eds.), Hearing and Deafness (3rd Ed.). New York: Holt, Rinehart and Winston, 1970.

Rassi, J., and Harford, E. An analysis of patient attitudes and reactions to a clinical hearing aid selection program. Asha, 10, 283–290 (1968).

Resnick, D., and Becker, M. Hearing aid evaluation—A new approach. Asha, 5, 695–699 (1963).

Rose, D. E., Schreurs, K. K., Keating, L. W., and Miller, K. E. A 10-word speech-discrimination screening test. Paper presented at the Annual Convention of the American Speech and Hearing Association, Las Vegas, 1974.

Rosenwasser, H. Otitic problems in the aged. Geriatrics, 19, 11–17 (1964).

Ross, M. Principles of Aural Rehabilitation. Indianapolis: Bobbs-Merrill, 1972.

RPAG (Retired Professional Action Group). Paying Through the Ear: A Report on Hearing Health Care Problems. Philadelphia: Public Citizen, Inc., 1973.

Rupp, R. R., Higgins, J., and Maurer, J. F. A feasibility scale for predicting hearing aid use (FSPHAU) with older individuals. Journal of the Academy of Rehabilitative Audiology, 10, 81–104 (1977).

Rupp, R. R., McLauchlin, R. M., Harless, E., and Mikulas, M. The specter of aging—Golden years or tarnished? Hearing and Speech News 39:6, 10–13 (1971).

Sanders, D. A. Hearing aid orientation and counseling. In M. C. Pollack (ed.), Amplification for the Hearing-Impaired. New York: Grune & Stratton, 1975.

Schow, R. L. How to promote and provide speech and hearing help in nursing homes: Experiences in a state-wide program. Paper presented at the Annual Convention of the California Speech and Hearing Association, San Francisco, 1977.

Schow, R. L., and Nerbonne, M. A. Hearing levels in nursing home residents. Research Laboratory Report, 1, pp. 1–10. Department of Speech Pathology and Audiology, Idaho State University, Pocatello, 1976.

Schow, R. L., and Nerbonne, M. A. Assessment of hearing handicap by nursing home residents and staff. Journal of the Academy of Rehabilitative Audiology, 10, 2–12 (1977).

Smith, C. R., and Fay, T. H. A program of auditory rehabilitation for aged persons in a chronic disease hospital. Asha, 19, 417–420 (1977).

Stutz, R. The American hearing aid user. Asha, 11, 459–461 (1969).

Tannahill, J. C. Hearing aids: Trial and adjustment by new users. Audecibel, 22, 90–97 (1973).

Traynor, R. M., and Hull, R. H. University of Northern Colorado geriatric aural rehabilitation program. Short course presented at the Annual Convention of the American Speech and Hearing Association, Washington, D.C., 1975.

U.S. Senate Hearings. Subcommittee on Consumer Interests of the Elderly of the Special Committee on Aging, Hearing Aids and the Older American. September 10, 1973.

Utley, J. A test of lipreading ability. Journal of Speech Disorders, 11, 109–116 (1946).

Walle, E. L. Communication problems of the chronically ill and aged in the institutional setting. Hearing and Speech News, 39:6, 16–17 (1971).

Walle, E. L., and Newman, P. W. Rehabilitation services for speech, hearing, and language disorders in an extended care facility. Asha, 9, 216–218 (1967).

Wasson, H. W. A multifilter circuit simulating representative hearing aids suggested for hearing aid selections. Journal of Auditory Research, 3, 185–188 (1963).

Weaver, C. H. Human Listening: Processes and Behavior. Indianapolis: Bobbs-Merrill Co., Inc., 1972.

Yarington, C. T., Jr. Presbycusis. In J. L. Northern (ed.), Hearing Disorders. Boston: Little, Brown, 1976.

APPENDIX A: FEASIBILITY SCALE FOR PREDICTING HEARING AID USE (FSPHAU)

An Analytic Approach to Predicting the Probable Success of a Provisional Hearing Aid Wearer

(Ralph R. Rupp, Ph.D., Audiology Area, Section of Speech and Hearing Sciences
The University of Michigan Medical School, Ann Arbor, Michigan)

Prognostic factors/descriptions (continuum, high to low)	Assessment (5-high: 0-low)	Weight	Weighted score (Possible) Actual	
1. Motivation and referral (self....family)	5 4 3 2 1 0	×4	(20)____	1.
2. Self-assessment of listening difficulties (realistic... denial)	5 4 3 2 1 0	×2	(10)____	2.
3. Verbalization as to "fault" of communication difficulties (self-caused... projection)	5 4 3 2 1 0	×1	(5)____	3.
4. Magnitude of loss: amplification results.				4.
A. Shift in spondaic threshold:____________	5 4 3 2 1 0	×1	(5)____	
B. Discrimination in quiet:____________ at____dB HTL	5 4 3 2 1 0	×1	(5)____	
C. Discrimination in noise:____________ at____dB HTL	5 4 3 2 1 0	×1	(5)____	
5. Informal verbalizations during hearing aid evaluation re: quality of sound, mold, size (acceptable...awful)	5 4 3 2 1 0	×1	(5)____	5.

Source: Rupp et al., 1977.

Prognostic factors/descriptions (continuum, high to low)	Assessment (5-high: 0-low)	Weight	Weighted score (Possible) Actual	
6. Flexibility and adaptability versus senility (relates outwardly...self)	5 4 3 2 1 0	×2	(10)____	6.
7. Age: 95 90 85 80 75 70 65 ≤ (0 0 1 2 3 4 5)	5 4 3 2 1 0	×1.5	(7.5)____	7.
8. Manual hand, finger dexterity, and general mobility (good... limited)	5 4 3 2 1 0	×1.5	(7.5)____	8.
9. Visual ability (adequate with glasses...limited)	5 4 3 2 1 0	×1	(5)____	9.
10. Financial resources (adequate...very limited)	5 4 3 2 1 0	×1.5	(7.5)____	10.
11. Significant other person to assist individual (available...none)	5 4 3 2 1 0	×1.5	(7.5)____	11.
12. Other factors, please cite	?	?	?	12.

Client________ FSPHAU:[a]	Very limited	0 to 40%	
Age__________	Limited	41 to 60%	
Date__________	Equivocal	61 to 75%	%
Audiologist____	Positive	76 to 100%	Total Score

[a] Four prognostic predictions are possible from the employment of the FSPHAU: positive (scores of 76-100%); equivocal (scores of 61-75%); limited (scores of 41-60%; and very limited (scores less than 41%).

Source: Rupp et al. (1977).

Scoring the FSPHAU Factors

1. Motivation/referral

5. Completely on own behalf
4. Mostly on own behalf
3. Generally on own behalf
2. Half self; half others
1. Little self; mostly others
0. Totally at urging of others

2. Self-assessment	5. Complete agreement 4. Strong agreement 3. General agreement 2. Some agreement 1. Little agreement 0. No agreement
3. Verbalization as to "fault" of communicative difficulties	5. Clearly created by hearing loss 4. Usually by loss 3. Loss and others 2. Environments and others 1. Mostly of others 0. Others totally at fault

4. Magnitude of loss; and results of amplification[a]	ST shift	Understanding in quiet at _dB HTL	Understanding in noise at _dB HTL
	5. 30 + db	90%	70%
	4. 25	80–88	60–68
	3. 20	70–78	50–58
	2. 15	60–68	40–48
	1. 10	50–58	30–38
	0. 5	48	28

5. Informal verbalizations during hearing aid evaluation re: quality of sound, mold, size, weight, look	5. Completely positive 4. Generally positive 3. Somewhat positive 2. Guarded 1. Generally negative 0. Completely negative
6. Flexibility and adaptability A. Questionnaire and observation B. Raven's Progressive Matrices C. Face/Hand Sensory Test	5. 90th percentile 4. 70 3. 50 2. 25 1. 10 0. 5

7. Age	5. 65 years 4. 70 3. 75 2. 80 1. 85 0. 90+
8. Manual/hand dexterity via Purdue Peg Board and Symbol Digit Modalities Test	5. Superior 4. Adequate 3. Slow but steady 2. Slow and shaky 1. Slow and awkward 0. "Arthritic"
9. Visual ability (with glasses)	5. Very good—no problems 4. Corrected, adequate 3. Adequate but safeguarded 2. Limited visibility 1. Very limited 0. Blind
10. Financial resources	5. Unlimited resources 4. Generally unrestricted 3. Adequate 2. Adequate but close 1. Dipping into savings 0. Poverty level, on assistance
11. Significant other person	5. Always available 4. Often 3. Sometimes 2. Occasionally 1. Seldom 0. Never

[b] Alternate scoring scheme for factor 4 in cases where the ST shift was minimal due to loss in high frequencies only.

(Average threshold shift at 2000 and 3000 Hz)	5. 25 × dB 4. 21–25 dB 3. 16–20 dB 2. 11–15 dB 1. 6–10 dB 0. 0–5 dB

APPENDIX B: SELECTED SAMPLES OF 10-ITEM LISTS FOR INFORMAL SPEECH DISCRIMINATION TESTING

Rose et al. (1974)

List A	List B
1. Knees	1. Knee
2. Else	2. Bathe
3. Owl	3. Ace
4. Rooms	4. Wool
5. Thin	5. Chew
6. Owes	6. Deaf
7. Bells	7. Dolls
8. Ache	8. Ease
9. Dull	9. Been
10. Felt	10. Few

Adapted from Utley (1946)

List A	List B
1. All right	1. How old are you?
2. Where have you been?	2. What did you say?
3. That's right	3. OK
4. Look out	4. No
5. How have you been?	5. That's pretty
6. How tall are you?	6. Pardon me
7. Good night	7. Good afternoon
8. Excuse me	8. You're welcome
9. What do you want?	9. I know
10. Of course	10. Come again

Schow (1977)

1. Do you have any children?
2. How many children do you have?
3. Where does (nearest relative) live?
4. How long ago did you see him/her?
5. Did he/she come to visit you here?
6. Who is your roommate?
7. Is he/she older or younger than you are?

8. How long have you been rooming together?
9. Do you like to do things together?
10. Does he/she have family close by?

APPENDIX C: LISTENING IMPROVEMENT

1. Develop a desire to listen.
   Suppress the desire to talk. Develop a strong desire to listen and to learn by listening.
2. Reflect the message to the talker.
   Use provocative (probing) questions and follow-up questions. This helps in clarifying instructions and directions from employers.
3. Try to guess the talker's intent or purpose.
   We always do this to some extent; if you do this badly, your listening will be poor.
4. Try to bring the quality of your "usual" listening up to your maximum potential. Don't expect to do this overnight. Work on it a few minutes each day. If you gradually increase this, the habit will eventually become more automatic.
5. Try to find out if important words mean the same thing to you as they do to the talker. This is a common source for misunderstandings or communication problems. To clarify this, ask for meanings or explain your own.
6. You should try to determine your purpose in every listening situation. This is especially true in a lecture or formal situation. As you listen in more informal situations, sometimes the details are most important, at other times the central theme is crucial, and at other times you need to focus on the intent rather than specific words.
7. Become aware of your own biases and attitudes. Discussion on certain topics may bring a strong emotional reaction. If you are aware of these biases, it may help you to resist the emotional reaction and thus listen better.
8. Learn to use your spare time as you listen. Sometimes there is no spare time if the message comes very fast; if there is, use it. Review what has been said, put things in perspective, judge relationships, relevance, etc.
9. Analyze your listening errors. Introspection may help you to avoid similar errors in the future.

Source: Adapted from Weaver (1972).

10. Be aware of how long the listening process takes you. Listening is an active not a passive process, and if you are slow at it maybe you need to work at it harder. Concentrate on exactly what you want to listen to, sort the information as it comes in, try to figure out its meaning. If you are slow at these processes try to speed them up.

Don't expect your listening ability to improve drastically in a short time. If you work at it though, improvement will come over a period of years.

Chapter 19
Hearing Aids

This chapter explores the nature of hearing aids, with emphasis on function, components, styles, earmolds, and controls. Sections on hearing aid use and on care and maintenance of the aid are also included. Other types of amplification devices are described.

A hearing aid is a special amplifying device that makes sounds louder or more intense. These aids are important in common rehabilitation procedures and are frequently used by elderly hearing-impaired persons. Such amplifying devices cannot entirely compensate for a loss, especially when there is very poor hearing clarity. However, even for the older patient with a high frequency hearing loss, an aid can often provide a great deal of help by simply making faint sounds louder. Hearing aids are actually quite complex electronic instruments, as evidenced by the fact that complete volumes have been devoted to discussions about them (Berger, 1970; Miller, 1972; Donnelly, 1974; Pollack, 1975a; Rubin, 1976; Hodgson and Skinner, 1977).

Despite their complexity, hearing aids are relatively simple to operate. Nevertheless, some special problems occasionally develop because users do not comprehend how the aid generally functions or what various controls are designed for. This is especially true in the case of elderly persons who have hearing aids. When the hearing aid does not work, it is not only perplexing but it may have serious consequences to the elderly hearing aid user or to those who may assist him. Accordingly, this chapter is intended to serve as a primer to acquaint persons with hearing aids and some other amplifying devices, as well as to provide a ready reference in cases of difficulty. Special attention is given to matters that may be relevant in hearing aid use by the elderly.

COMPONENTS

A hearing aid is made like many other amplifying devices. It has a *microphone* to pick up the sound and change it to an electrical signal. An *amplifier* then magnifies this signal, and a *receiver* or speaker changes the signal back to sound which is louder than the original (see Figure 19-1).

STYLES

Body and Ear Level Styles

Hearing aids come in several styles, as shown in Figure 19-2. The *body aid* is quite bulky, and it fits in a pocket, clips to a shirt, or is worn in a harness underneath the clothing. There are three

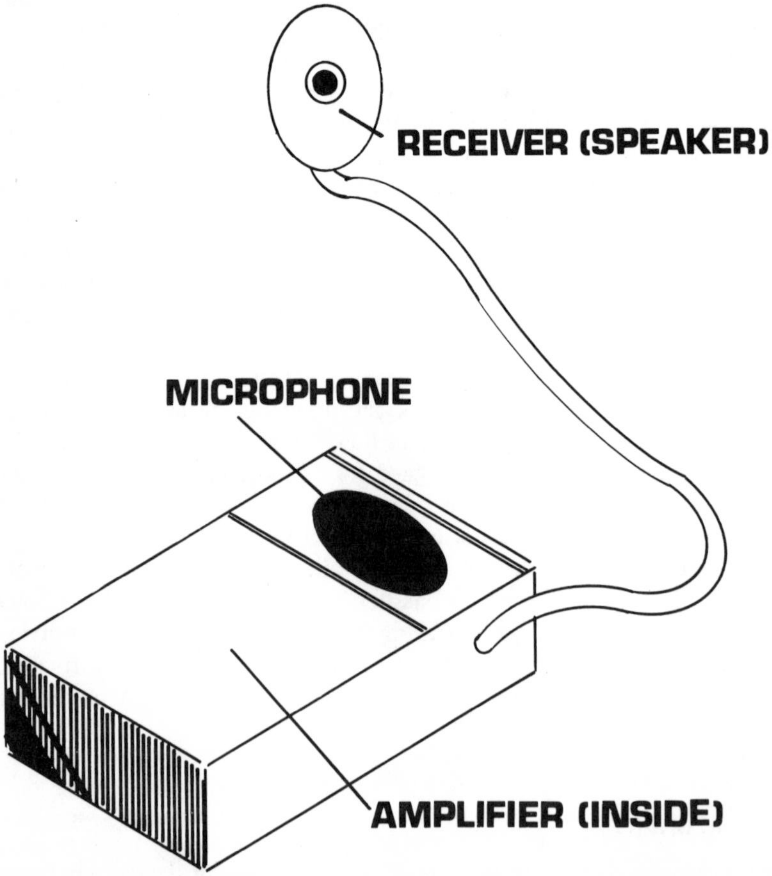

Figure 19-1. Components of a hearing aid.

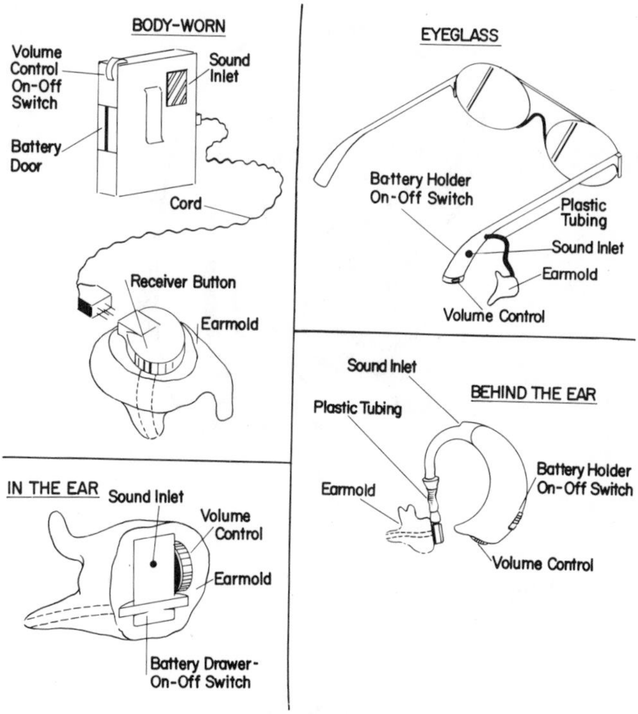

Figure 19-2. Styles of hearing aids. (Source: Belt-ne, Inc., Chicago, Ill.)

styles that are used at ear level: the *behind-the-ear aid,* which looks like a shrimp and fits around and behind the ear (Figure 19-3); the *eyeglass aid,* in which the hearing aid components are located in eyeglass temples; and the *in-the-ear aid,* which is the smallest of the three and fits in the concha of the ear (Figure 19-4). Ear level aids are sometimes modified in a CROS (contralateral routing of signals) arrangement for use with persons who have a severe loss or unusable hearing in one ear. This arrangement can be found in behind-the-ear or eyeglass aids and involves a microphone that picks up sound on the bad side and transfers it across the head to the good ear. Other unusual but seldom used styles are described in Hodgson (1977). The components of these aids are all within the hearing aid case except for the receiver of the body aid, which is at the end of a long cord extending from the case of the hearing aid. The receivers of the ear level aids are concealed, and their sound is funneled through (plastic) tubing.

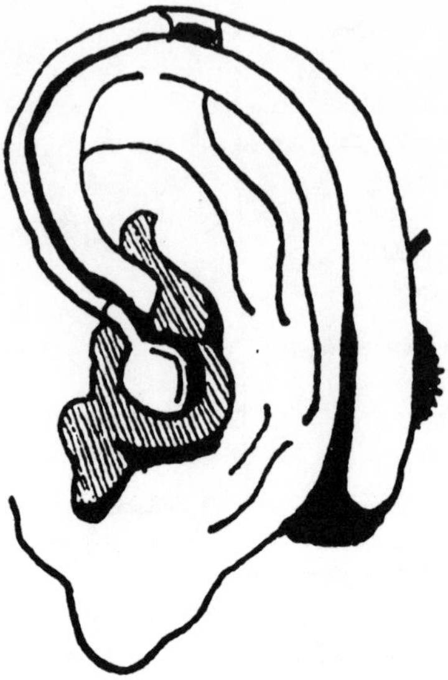

Figure 19-3. Behind-the-ear hearing aid positioned on the ear. (Source: ASHA, 1977.)

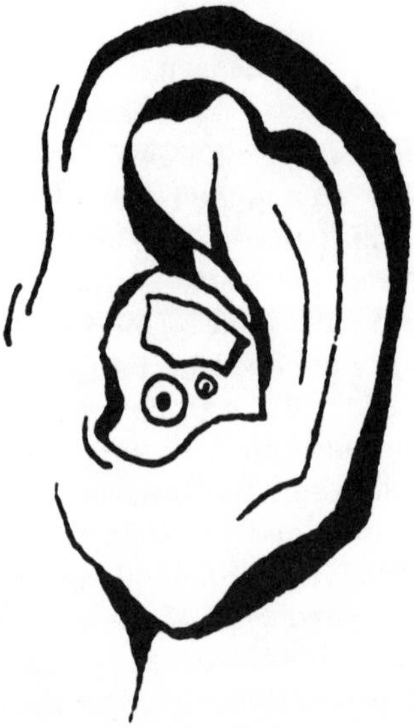

Figure 19-4. In-the-ear hearing aid positioned in the ear. (Source: ASHA, 1977.)

Sales and Popularity

Body aids are more powerful than the ear level models, even though they are cosmetically less appealing. They also tend to have larger controls, which makes them easier to manipulate for an elderly person. They have been found to be quite popular in the institutionalized elderly (see Chapter 18). In-the-ear aids have lately enjoyed a tremendous surge in popularity. Up until now, however, the behind-the-ear aid has been the most popular. In 1974, for example, it comprised 67% of total sales. Eyeglass aids were next most popular at 23%; in-the-ear aids, 3%; and body aids, 7%. The CROS eyeglass and CROS behind-the-ear aids comprised about 5% of the total sales (Pollack, 1975b). In-the-ear aids are very compact, and the controls and batteries are rather tiny, making them difficult for the elderly to manipulate. However, these aids are contained in one unit which slips in the ear, and they may, therefore, be easier to put on than other aids. Some elderly persons known to the authors are quite happy with them.

EARMOLDS

With most aids, the sound is eventually introduced into the ear canal. This is accomplished by attaching a custom-fitted earmold on the tip of the receiver or tubing (Figure 19-2). These molds are made by taking an impression of the concha and ear canal area and then sending such an impression to a laboratory to have a smooth, finished product produced. Some molds are also made directly from the impression in an "instamold" procedure. The purpose of the earmold is to prevent sound from escaping once it is sent into the canal. Amplified sound that escapes from the ear may enter into the microphone once more and be even further amplified. If this happens, there will be a whistling sound produced by the hearing aid. This sound is called *feedback* and is an indication that the earmold is either not properly seated or that it does not fit.

Feedback can be stopped by turning the hearing amplification down, but, of course, this is not a final solution, since the person may not be able to hear as loudly as necessary. Occasionally when feedback occurs, the tubing is cracked or the receiver is damaged. So if re-adjustment of the earmold in the person's ear canal will not stop the whistling noise, then the temporary solution is to turn the hearing aid down or to cover the mold with a little petroleum jelly, which will provide a seal around the mold. The next step is to call for specialized help to see if the earmold or other parts need replacement. Sometimes a mold will make the ear sore. If this occurs, the dealer or audiologist can be asked to adjust it for a better fit.

The earmold can be detached from the aid and cleaned when its channel becomes clogged with earwax or other debris. The mold can be removed from a body aid by simply snapping it off. On ear level aids except in-the-ear, the plastic tubing is disconnected from the aid. Tubing that eventually becomes stretched where it attaches to the aid can be replaced so that feedback will not occur. Warm, soapy water and a pipe cleaner can be used to clean the mold if it is detachable, but only dry pipe cleaners should be used for in-the-ear aids. The molds should be dried off completely afterwards. Alcohol or other cleaning solvents should not be used to clean the mold.

A few hearing aids use a vibrator that is strapped over the head and placed on the mastoid. It introduces a bone conduction signal, and in these cases an earmold is not needed.

CONTROLS

The major controls of the hearing aid include the volume control, the battery compartment, the telephone switch, the output control, and the tone control (Figure 19-5).

Volume Control

The volume control adjusts the level or the gain of the amplified sound. It is usually visible as a half-moon shaped object with ridges and protrudes from some part of the instrument. Often this control doubles as an on–off switch, which will click when turned completely off. In other cases, the battery must be pulled out to turn off the aid. When the aid is not in use, the battery should be removed to conserve its power. Sometimes, there are numbers on this control to guide a person in using it, but often there are none, so that checking for feedback is one method to determine where the maximum setting is located and if the aid is working. If the hearing aid is off the user's ear, the volume control can be moved to the two extreme settings. If the aid is functioning, the maximum setting will generally produce feedback, since the amplified sound will be able to re-enter the microphone. The volume control is usually set at a comfort level for the patient after the hearing aid and earmold are in place.

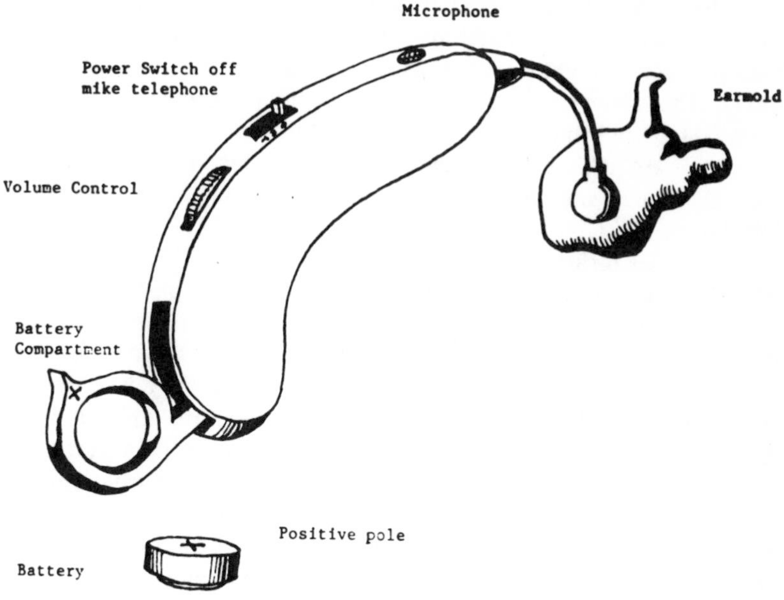

Figure 19-5. Behind-the-ear hearing aid showing various components and controls. (Source: ASHA, 1977.)

Battery Compartment

The battery supplies the energy to operate the aid. It has a positive and negative side and must be put into its compartment in the right position to be effective. The compartment usually has a plus (+) or minus (−) sign to indicate the position of the battery. The small batteries for ear level aids have a flattened and a rounded side, and there are corresponding surfaces in the compartment that serve as a guide for insertion of the battery. If the hearing aid does not work after putting in a battery, it is possible that the battery is in backwards or that the battery is dead. It is an easy matter to reverse the position of the battery to see if that will help, and a battery tester may be used to check the power of the battery. These testers can be obtained from the same source where the batteries are purchased. Most batteries are 1.3–1.5 volts, but this depends on battery size and will be marked on the battery package. When the power gets below about 1.0–1.2 volts, the battery should be replaced. Old batteries should be thrown away or they may be turned in for credit on new batteries.

Most hearing aid batteries are made of silver oxide, nickel cadmium, or mercury materials. Silver oxide and nickel cadmium batteries are thought to be superior to the mercury type (Smith, 1977). The silver oxide batteries provide more power and consistency, though a somewhat shorter life, than the mercury. The nickel cadmium are rechargeable and thus more economical. However, more than one rechargeable battery of this type may be needed for a full day of use. Unfortunately, they are more popular in Europe and are sometimes difficult to buy in this country.

Hearing aids should be stored in a cool, dry place, but one misconception common among hearing aid users is the idea that batteries ought to be stored in the refrigerator for longer life. Actually this causes water condensation when the battery is removed from the cool refrigerator to a normal temperature. This in turn leads to corrosion and shortens battery life. Some manufacturers discourage their retail sales representatives and users from refrigerating batteries (Kelley, 1976). They find that the batteries last just as long without refrigeration. If the battery is kept in the refrigerator, at least it should be kept in a plastic bag and left there for a while after removal from the refrigerator. Smith (1977) cites two studies on battery performance which indicate that batteries purchased from a discount store with an undefined stock rotation policy performed just as well as those from stores that rotate their stock every 3 months. The consumer-conscious elderly person may wish to attempt such an experiment in his own surroundings, since the generality of these findings is not known. It is known that batteries of the same type may vary drastically in the hours of service life, so a number of batteries should be tried before conclusions are drawn (Smith, 1972).

Telephone Switch

Many hearing aids have a telephone switch, which allows a different method for hearing through the aid when talking on the telephone. The telephone receiver must be placed as close as possible to the aid. For an ear level aid, the listening part of the telephone goes just behind the ear, and for a body aid the phone should be inverted from its usual position. Telephones built recently will not accommodate the telephone switch of the hearing aid. In the Bell System, a special small adapter can be obtained which will fit over the telephone receiver and make the system functional. These can be carried in a pocket or purse. In the General Telephone System these adapters will not work, but the company will install phones that are compatible with this hearing aid feature (Pollack, 1975b). However, if the switch is left in the telephone (T) position, regular use will be hampered. Care should be taken to make sure this knob is in the microphone (M) position except when using the telephone. Actually, many users prefer the regular microphone position even when talking on the phone.

Maximum Power Output Control

Most aids have a maximum power point to prevent them from amplifying any extremely loud sounds. Refined forms of this control called automatic volume control (AVC) or automatic gain control (AGC) are also available and are used to provide more comfort for the user who cannot tolerate the loud sounds heard through the aid.

Pitch Control

Hearing aids may have a control for altering the frequency response or the pitch emphasis of the amplified sound. This control will be set by the audiologist or the dealer and should not be altered. If the user is not satisfied with the way the aid sounds, some adjustment can often be made by altering this control or by having the dispenser change the earmold or receiver.

ELECTROACOUSTIC ANALYSIS

The tone emphasis and other control characteristics, like gain control, telephone control, maximum power, as well as hearing aid harmonic distortion, can be measured by electroacoustic analysis of the aid. This requires a special test box and equipment to carefully measure sounds introduced to and amplified by the aid. To standardize methods of reporting these and other hearing aid characteristics, the Hearing Aid Industry Conference in 1961 adopted a uniform set of procedures. Recently, a new modified standard has been adopted by the American National Standards Institute, which is designated ANSI S3.22-1976 (Pollack, 1975b; Kasten, 1977). These test procedures will often be helpful to the audiologist in the hearing aid evaluation or in orientation for the new hearing aid user.

HEARING AID EVALUATION

In obtaining a hearing aid, the safest course is to obtain advice from a physician (preferably an ear specialist) on the medical status of the ear and to consult with an audiologist for a hearing aid evaluation. A recent federal regulation makes medical clearance mandatory before a hearing aid purchase except for persons over 18, who may sign a waiver if none of the following conditions apply (Federal Register, 1977, p. 9295):

1. Visible congenital or traumatic deformity of the ear
2. History of active drainage from the ear within the previous 90 days
3. History of sudden or rapidly progressive hearing loss within the previous 90 days
4. Acute or chronic dizziness
5. Unilateral hearing loss of sudden or recent onset within the previous 90 days
6. Audiometric air-bone gap equal to or greater than 15 dB at 500 Hz, 1000 Hz, and 2000 Hz
7. Visible evidence of significant cerumen accumulation or a foreign body in the ear canal
8. Pain or discomfort in the ear

Persons under 18 are required to obtain a hearing aid evaluation from an audiologist in all circumstances.

Audiology work settings are enumerated in Chapter 17, and the procedures used for hearing aid evaluation with elderly subjects, including institutionalized patients, are explained in Chapter 18. After these selection procedures are carefully followed, the aid is usually obtained from a hearing aid dealer or dispenser. Aids should generally be obtained on a trial basis with 30-day return privileges.

USE OF A HEARING AID

New hearing aid users will find that the first few days and weeks after the aid is obtained present several challenging experiences. Learning to put the aid on can be a major hurdle, requiring practice and patience. The dealer or audiologist should help the new user go through this once or twice. Generally, one should turn the aid off while inserting it and rotate the mold back and forth until it goes in and feels snug. Some elderly patients cannot adjust the gain control after it is on, and thus they may need to set the volume and either turn the aid off or put up with a little feedback while they insert the aid. Navarro (1977) has reported on the use of a special mold which has a small handle the elderly patient can use to grasp the mold while putting it in the ear. This can be of real benefit to the aged person with inadequate dexterity.

Another new experience for the hearing aid owner is clothing noise for the body aid user and wind noise for those with ear level aids. These are picked up by the microphone of the aid and can at times be quite irritating. When possible, the aid should be used in a carrier or soft material should be used near the aid to reduce clothing noise. The user should avoid getting the aid in the direct blast of the wind. The internal hum of the aid may be heard by the person along with many more environmental noises than he is used to hearing. The new aid user, however, can learn to ignore some of these unpleasant noises the same way people with normal hearing learn to "turn off" unpleasant noisy sounds in the environment. It is a good idea for the new user to wear the aid for just a few hours at a time at first, and to do so in quiet listening situations. If sounds continue to be unpleasant after a reasonable trial period, the audiologist or dispenser should be consulted.

Some new hearing aid users will make an easy adjustment and wear the aid all waking hours from the time they receive it. Others, especially those who have very mild or quite severe losses, may require a long time to adjust. It is recommended that all elderly subjects receiving a hearing aid for the first time have a recheck from their dispenser and a hearing aid orientation from an audiologist. These procedures will help immensely in the adjustment period and will generally give the person a chance to compare experiences with others who are also new users.

The following are a summary of suggestions to help the newly aided person:

1. Begin with a comfortable volume level.
2. Begin with easy listening challenges.
3. Don't overtire yourself.
4. Relearn the trick of concentration.
5. Don't be afraid to ask for help.
6. When in church or group meetings, sit up close.
7. Experiment with difficult listening environments or situations (noisy places, TV or stereo listening, telephone use). Try different volume settings on the aid or tone controls on the stereo. Use the telephone with and without the aid. Parttime hearing aid use may be a solution.

8. Listen with your eyes. Be visually observant.
9. Be patient and keep trying.

CARE AND MAINTENANCE OF THE AID

The care and maintenance of the aid may be the responsibility of the elderly person. If so, the person needs thorough exposure to this information when the aid is issued. For some elderly persons or for residents of extended care facilities, others such as a spouse or staff member may need to help in maintaining the aid. In these cases, a listening check should be made on the aid each day before placing it on the person. In this way, batteries can be replaced regularly (about once a week depending on use), and other malfunctions can be detected.

Kasten and Warren (1977, pp. 196–197) have listed a series of do's and don'ts which should help to prolong hearing aid life:

1. Excessive heat and cold may very well damage a hearing aid. Never leave it on a radiator, near a stove, in a sunny window, or in any other hot place. Do not wear the aid when using a hair dryer, or near a sun lamp, heat lamp, or diathermy instrument. In extremely cold or wet weather, do not wear the aid outside unless absolutely necessary.
2. Do not drop the hearing aid on a hard surface. As a precautionary measure, hold the aid over a table or bed, rather than over the floor, when changing batteries or performing maintenance.
3. Moisture damages a hearing aid. Never wear it in the rain or while taking a bath. If you perspire excessively and you have a behind-the-ear eyeglass aid, avoid wearing it during strenuous activity in hot weather. If the climate is humid or if you perspire, store the hearing aid overnight in a tightly closed container with a silica gel packet to absorb the moisture.
4. Don't apply hair spray when wearing the aid. It may damage the microphone.
5. Clean the battery contacts occasionally to remove corrosion, by scraping very gently with a sharpened pencil eraser. Battery contacts may be dried with a cotton swab in cases of humid weather or heavy perspiration.
6. Never attempt to open the case of the hearing aid. You may cause more damage and will likely void the manufacturer's warranty.

When an aid is nonfunctional or weak or is not performing well in other ways, there are a few simple remedies which may be tried. If the aid is giving a weak signal or none at all:

1. Place a new battery in the aid, taking care to put it in properly and completely. Check the battery contacts and clean them with a sharpened pencil eraser if they show corrosion.
2. Check the telephone switch to make sure it is in the (M) position.
3. Turn the volume control of the aid up and down, listening for scratchiness or "cutting on and off."
4. Check the cord of a body aid to see if it is intact and firmly connected to its sockets. Roll it in the fingers to see if this causes intermittency.

If the aid is producing inappropriate feedback:

1. Try reseating or adjusting the earmold.
2. Check the tubing to see if there are any cracks or leaks.
3. See if the earmold is clogged, cracked, or loose from the tubing or receiver.
4. If the feedback persists when the sound outlet is plugged, the mold, tubing or receiver is probably faulty and will need replacement or repair.

If all else fails, call the local dispenser and arrange for repair. If the aid gives continual trouble and/or the dispenser is not providing satisfactory service, most states have "hot lines" sponsored by the National Hearing Aid Society to deal with these complaints. Periodically, the hearing aid user should see an audiologist for an evaluation of his hearing and hearing aid. This should be done even when the aid is performing satisfactorily and especially in cases when the aid has been malfunctioning.

OTHER COMMUNICATION DEVICES

A number of other devices besides the hearing aid can assist the hard-of-hearing person (ASHA, 1975). These include special alarm clocks which shake the bed or produce a flashing light, doorbell attachments which activate a flashing light or air fan, and a variety of telephone and TV amplifiers. One device, called a sound lamp, will turn on in response to any number of auditory sounds including a doorbell, a baby crying, a telephone, or any alarm which might sound. These devices can be purchased from local hearing aid dealers, telephone companies, electronic and appliance shops or by mail order from companies such as Hal-Hen (36-14 Eleventh St., Long Island City, N.Y. 11106).

SUGGESTED READINGS

Coreliss, E. Facts about Hearing and Hearing Aids. Washington, D.C.: U.S. Government Printing Office, 1971.

Cutler, W. H. Dispensing systems. In M. C. Pollack (ed.), Amplification for the Hearing-Impaired. New York: Grune & Stratton, 1975.

Kasten, R. N., and Warren, M. P. Learning to use the hearing aid. In W. R. Hodgson and P. H. Skinner (eds.), Hearing Aid Assessment and Use in Audiologic Habilitation. Baltimore: Williams & Wilkins, 1977.

Miller, M. H. Hearing Aids. Indianapolis: Bobbs-Merrill, 1972.

RPAG, Retired Professional Action Group. Paying Through the Ear: A Report on Hearing Health Care Problems. Philadelphia: Public Citizen, Inc., 1973.

Smith, K. E. Earmolds and hearing aid accessories. In W. R. Hodgson and P. H. Skinner (eds.), Hearing Aid Assessment and Use in Audiologic Habilitation. Baltimore: Williams & Wilkins, 1977.

Teter, D. L. Clinical considerations of hearing aids. In J. L. Northern (ed.), Hearing Disorders. Boston: Little, Brown, 1976.

REFERENCES

ASHA Committee on Communication Problems of the Aging. Resource Materials for Communicative Problems of Older Persons. Washington, D.C.: U.S. Department of Commerce, 1975.

ASHA. Breaking the Silence Barrier. In-Service Training Program. Washington, D.C.: American Speech and Hearing Association, 1977.

Berger, K. W. The Hearing Aid: Its Operation and Development. Detroit, Michigan: National Hearing Aid Society, 1970.

Donnelly, K. Interpretating Hearing Aid Technology. Springfield, Ill: Charles C Thomas, 1974.

Federal Register. Rules of the Food and Drug Administration for the hearing aid industry. Federal Register, February 15, 9286–9296, 1977.

Hodgson, W. R. Special cases of hearing aid assessment: CROS Aids. In W. R. Hodgson and P. H. Skinner (eds.), Hearing Aid Assessment and Use in Audiologic Habilitation. Baltimore: Williams & Wilkins, 1977.

Hodgson, W. R., and Skinner, P. H. (eds.). Hearing Aid Assessment and Use in Audiologic Habilitation. Baltimore: Williams & Wilkins, 1977.

Kasten, R. N. Electroacoustic characteristics. In W. R. Hodgson and P. H. Skinner (eds.), Hearing Aid Assessment and Use in Audiologic Habilitation. Baltimore: Williams & Wilkins, 1977.

Kasten, R. N., and Warren, M. P. Learning to use the hearing aid. In W. R.

Hodgson and P. H. Skinner (eds.), Hearing Aid Assessment and Use in Audiologic Habilitation. Baltimore: William & Wilkins, 1977.

Kelley, K. J. Quality control in battery manufacture. Hearing Aid Journal, February, 7 (1976).

Miller, M. H. Hearing Aids. Indianapolis: Bobbs-Merrill, 1972.

Navarro, M. R. An earmold for the geriatric patient. Journal of Speech and Hearing Disorders, 42, 44–46 (1977).

Pollack, M. C. (ed.). Amplification for the Hearing-Impaired. New York: Grune & Stratton, 1975a.

Pollack, M. C. Electroacoustic characteristics. In M. C. Pollack (ed.), Amplification for The Hearing-Impaired, New York: Grune & Stratton, 1975b.

Rubin, M. (ed.). Hearing Aids: Current Developments and Concepts. Baltimore: University Park Press, 1976.

Smith, K. E. Variability of battery life in children's hearing aids. Audecibel 21, 148–152 (1972).

Smith, K. E. Earmolds and hearing aid accessories. In W. R. Hodgson and P. H. Skinner (eds.), Hearing Aid Assessment and Use in Audiologic Habilitation. Baltimore: Williams & Wilkins, 1977.

Chapter 20
Role of the Speech/Language Pathologist

This chapter explores the profession of speech/language pathology with respect to historical development, training, services offered, and approaches to helping the elderly. A strong position is taken that speech and language pathologists must increase their efforts in the area of geriatrics. Of particular attention is increased service to the demented patient, a new dimension of therapy.

BEGINNINGS

Disorders of speech and language have been recognized and treated since the dawn of history. Evidence of this is reflected in Biblical records of Moses' alleged speech problem (Exodus 4:11), references to stuttering in ancient Chinese scripts (Van Riper, 1971), and the writings of classical Greek scholars who mentioned stuttering, aphasia, articulation, and voice problems (Paden, 1970). In general, the history of the treatment of speech disorders has mirrored the treatment of other problems subsumed under the generic term "behavior disorders." In primitive times and societies, speech problems were often considered the result of demons, and treatment was undertaken through witchcraft by shamen.. In classical Greek and Roman times, a much more naturalistic and humanistic view of such problems prevailed, and dramatists or rhetoricians and physicians provided rehabilitative assistance. Religious animism prevailed in the Middle Ages, and priests assumed responsibility for treatment, largely through exorcism. With the onset of the Renaissance, the thinking of ancient Greeks and Romans was rekindled, bringing with it the re-emergence of medical treatment of speech disorders by physicians. For the most part, that attitude persisted until the mid-

1800s when educators joined with physicians to try to bring relief to those with communicative handicaps.

As Paden (1970) has noted, significant contributions by Americans were not apparent until the early 1900s. Three major developments occurred in the first two decades of this century to highlight the presence of speech pathology as a profession in the United States. First, the public schools in several larger cities began to employ speech correctionists. For example, the Chicago public schools employed 10 speech correctionists by 1910; Detroit, two by 1910; and the State of Wisconsin, eight by 1916 (Paden, 1970). Second, there was a growing list of scientific publications regarding speech problems in the professional literature by the end of the 1920s. Third, universities were beginning to offer courses in speech problems and rehabilitative procedures. A physician by the name of "Smiley" Blanton, who received training at Cornell Medical College, began the first university speech clinic at the University of Wisconsin. This university sprinted beyond any others in the United States, granting the first Ph.D. in speech pathology to Sara Stinchfield in 1921. Later, other university programs at Columbia, the University of Pennsylvania, the University of Iowa, the University of Illinois, Pennsylvania State College, and Temple University were begun.

In 1925, a tiny but dedicated group of professionals split away from the National Association of Teachers to Speech (NATS) and formed the American Academy of Speech Correction (AASC). The AASC remained affiliated with the NATS for many years, and the latter organization offered support as a strong parent organization. In 1947, the organization name was changed to the American Speech and Hearing Association (ASHA), which has grown in strength and stature from 11 members in 1925 to over 25,000 in 1977. The organization now sponsors four highly respected professional journals: *Journal of Speech and Hearing Disorders, Journal of Speech and Hearing Research, Asha,* and *Language, Speech, and Hearing Services in the Schools.* In addition, ASHA holds a national convention and a rotating regional convention each year. All states have an affiliated state association for speech and hearing professionals, and most of these state programs are strong, viable organizations.

TRAINING

The American Speech and Hearing Association will now issue its Certificate of Clinical Competence in Speech Pathology (CCC-SP) only to those who have attained a master's degree or its equivalent for an accepted program of study. Because of the tremendous breadth of speech/language pathology, students are obligated to receive education in many ancillary areas including psychology, education, physics, general biology, statistics, and child development. Within the professional coursework, speech/language pathology students receive training in the nature, diagnosis, and treatment of most disorders of communication as well as anatomy, physiology, speech and hearing science, audiology, counseling, and many others depending upon the orientation of the training institution and interest of the student.

In addition, to be eligible for the CCC-SP, a student must complete at least 300 hours of supervised clinical practicum for a variety of disorders specified by ASHA. Following completion of the master's degree or its equivalent, the candidate for CCC-SP must satisfactorily complete 9 months of full-time professional work (Clinical Fellowship Year) under the supervision of a certified speech/language pathologist. All candidates are also required to pass a national examination before certification is granted.

The American Speech and Hearing Association maintains an agency known as the American Board of Examiners in Speech Pathology and Audiology (ABESPA), which serves as the parent organization for the Education and Training Board (ETB). This latter board maintains responsibility for granting accreditation to university training programs which meet certain academic, professional, and service standards for the preparation of speech/language pathologists.

Finally, all certified members of ASHA are bound by the Association's Code of Ethics. This code specifies standards of professional conduct, treatment, public relations, and interprofessional communication. A Board of Ethics is designated by ASHA to review cases where violations of the Code of Ethics might have occurred. Violators may lose ASHA membership and certification.

SERVICES AND WORK SETTINGS

Speech/language pathologists offer a rather wide variety of services depending upon professional setting and the population served. Most clinicians provide diagnostic and therapeutic services, with fewer members of the profession offering consultation, training, and administration of clinical, academic, or governmental agencies. Still others are primarily engaged in research activities. Most speech/language pathologists are employed in public schools, community clinics, and hospitals. The remaining professionals are found in universities; local, state, and federal agencies; private practice; the armed forces; and private industry.

Because of the higher incidence of medical problems observed among the elderly, hospitalization is certainly more probable in this group. Therefore, a special review of speech pathology services in the hospital setting would seem warranted. The data to be presented are taken from a rather comprehensive survey completed by Strandberg (1977a, b). From the 717 responding hospitals, it was determined that patients ranging from 45 to 64 years were the most frequently treated, and those over age 64 ranked second in frequency of treatment. Furthermore, the rank order of disorders treated beginning with the most common appears as follows:

Aphasia
Apraxia/dysarthria
Language disorders
Articulation disorders
Voice disorders
Neurologic disorders
Cancer-related disorders
Cleft palate
Cerebral palsy

Neurologists constituted the most common referral source followed in order by pediatricians, otolaryngologists, physiatrists, internists, general practitioners, psychiatrists, and orthopaedic surgeons.

APPROACHES TO SERVING THE ELDERLY

As may be discerned from earlier chapters and those that follow, the speech/language pathologist has a service of considerable importance and professional credibility to offer to the older population. Unfortunately, for a variety of reasons, those in the profession of communication disorders are not providing adequate service for the aged. The thesis of the final section of this chapter is that much needs to be done on the part of all professionals to ensure that speech and language therapy is available to an increasingly larger number of older people. This thesis is presented from two points of view. In the first, a case is made for increased service to those patients with communication problems traditionally handled by the speech/language pathologist. The second proposes a new dimension of service to the elderly not currently offered in most settings.

Increased Service for Traditional Cases

Undeniably, there is a large and unknown number of elderly people for whom speech and language services are desperately needed and not offered or not available. Those of us in the profession of speech/language pathology who serve predominantly rural areas are acutely aware of the typical small, isolated town with its many elderly residents with serious communication impairments. Often our professional services are not available and, if available, unknown and/or unappreciated. Similarly, those of us working in urban locations are fully cognizant of the many patients in institutions or underpriviledged sections who, for many reasons, may not be receiving care for speech and/or language problems. Why does this deplorable situation exist? Certainly some of the blame lies with the profession of speech and language pathology, but the response of other health professionals and agencies must also be implicated.

With respect to the profession of speech and language pathology, two critical issues must be raised. First, the importance of gerontology is often minimized in training programs to the point that graduating students have a limited appreciation of the broad range of communicative problems observed among the elderly. As mentioned in Chapter 1, very few graduate programs in communication disorders offer specific coursework in geriatrics. As a result, many graduates unwittingly consider this information to be of secondary importance and unfortunately this attitude extends to clinical management. Weiss (1971) echoed this point when he stated:

> Since the major concern of the speech pathologist is communication, it is ironical but not surprising that a large segment of our aged population receives virtually no communicative assistance. Several reasons can be offered to explain the comparative lack of interest in working with the aged. Some speech pathologists feel that aged persons are challenging, but not necessarily stimulating. Other possible drawbacks such as poor prognostic implications and the brevity of remaining life period (whether productive or nonproductive) are also stressed. (p. 640)

The solution is obvious, though perhaps not simple. Training programs in speech/language pathology must begin to offer specific coursework in gerontology beyond the courses concerned with individual disorders (e.g., aphasia, voice disorders, neuromotor disorders, etc.). Such additional training will provide a better understanding of geriatric patients and a revised appreciation of their rehabilitative potential and right to services.

The second point to be raised with respect to the profession of speech and language pathology relates to outreach and advocacy. Historically, it has been axiomatic within our profession that active case seeking and public education is inappropriate and perhaps unprofessional. Rather, until recently a passive role has been assumed and the tragic result has been unneeded patient suffering. A great many things can be done to reverse this passive role and to permit systematic advocacy on behalf of the profession and the patients whom it serves. Speech/language pathologists in hospitals, community rehabilitation centers, and university clinics must undertake a massive public education program both for the layman and health professional. Certainly, this may require substantive increases in federal and state funding, but it must be recognized that large sums of money are already available and should be properly tapped. For example, the Department of Health, Education, and Welfare recently awarded a substantial grant to the American Speech and Hearing Association to establish regional workshops that would provide for dissemination of information regarding professional responsibilities with geriatric individuals. As another example, Program IMPACT of the Higher Education Act of 1965, Title I, and the Idaho State Commission for Higher Education Facilities awarded the College of Health Related Professions at Idaho State University a grant to provide continuing education workshops for nursing home personnel. For the speech pathology and audiology component, statewide workshops were conducted that involved patient screening, consultation, and classroom presentations in selected nursing homes.

By way of summary, Howell (1971) highlighted the need for public advocacy by stating:

> I am convinced, as a geropsychologist, that the services that your profession (speech/language pathology) does have to offer the elderly are vastly more important than many of the services that psychologists offer to elderly individuals with hearing and speech problems. Your services are crucial to the total well-being of the patient, but your profession must make this publicly known so that your services will be publicly demanded. (p. 9)

As mentioned earlier, however, implicating the profession of speech and language pathology is only one side of the coin. Certainly, we must extend ourselves, but it is a two-way street. Perhaps one of the most deplorable failures of the American health profession in general is an overwhelming lack of teamwork and cooperation. Nearly everyone can cite several personal examples of patients for whom proper referral was not made or, when referrals did occur, inadequate cooperation and coordination ensued. It is quite safe to say that most training programs in medicine, nursing, psychology, social work, physical therapy, etc., have very limited involvement with speech and language pathology. This undoubtedly creates a glaring ignorance among professionals as to the scope of our profession and the services it may provide. Howell (1971) illustrated this point when she noted:

> It became evident to me that this field [speech/language pathology] was badly misunderstood in terms of its functions and capabilities by otherwise well-trained professionals in the health field. The response to presentations by speech pathologists ranged from that of considering such a service a "frill" to an almost layman's belief that anybody (with some training in any health profession) could teach all that was necessary to an aphasic patient and his family with regard to communication problems. (p. 8)

A case in point is the statement in Chapter 12 concerning the potential assistance offered by a speech pathologist to the neurologist in early assessment and evaluation of neurologic disease. Most neurologists simply do not take advantage of such a service.

A New Dimension of Treatment

Beyond the amplification of existing services for cases traditionally treated by the speech/language pathologist there may be additional client populations which would benefit from remediation. Specifically, those with intellectual and memory deteriorations have occasioned growing interest among other health professionals as possible candidates for treatment. As Miller (1977) has observed:

> In the all too recent past the general approach to management has been one of therapeutic nihilism. The assumption, either explicit or implicit, has been that dementia is incurable and its effects irreversible. All that can be done is to look after the patient's basic needs as humanly as possible until nature takes its inevitable course. (p. 120)

Certainly, this attitude has also prevailed among speech and language pathologists.

However, there is a growing awareness that this viewpoint is not totally accurate and that for many of these patients there are means of arresting, mitigating, and reversing the effects of dementia. From a medical standpoint, there are certain pharmacologic agents that have shown promise. For example, cerebral vasodilators, such as cyclandelate, have appeared to arrest intellectual and memory deteriorations in arteriosclerotic dementia (Miller, 1977). It is quite reasonable to assume that future medical developments will evidence just as promising outcomes.

Perhaps more important, however, is the growing evidence that psychological and social intervention strategies are producing positive behavior changes among demented patients. One rather promising approach has been reality orientation, where demented patients have been given rather continuous opportunity for rehearsal of information related to orientation of time, place, and person. For example, Brook, Degun, and Mather (1975) engaged 18 demented subjects in a reality orientation program for 16 weeks. According to rating scale values by the nursing staff, the more mildly involved patients evidenced noticeable improvement. One of the critical variables affecting improvement appeared to be active participation by the therapist. Other promising avenues of intervention have included normalization (Wolfsenberger, 1970) and behavior modification (Libb and Clements, 1969; Mueller and Atlas, 1972). In short, changes, albeit modest ones, are possible with such subjects, and increased effort would seem warranted to improve the quality of life for many older demented patients.

As noted earlier, there has been limited involvement of speech and language pathologists with demented subjects even though clinical observations would confirm the potential for communicative intervention. For example, Bloomer (1971) noted:

> I have seen older patients respond to therapy after long months or even years of virtual neglect. The progress may be slow, but progress is made. (p. 14)

Similarly, Weiss (1971) reported:

> Some generalizations made about the aged would seem to indicate that: 1) they need fewer communicative skills because they typically live in restricted and sheltered environments, 2) they are not nearly so interested in communication as when they were younger, 3) they have a negative attitude toward rehabilitation and toward life, and 4) their "world" has diminished so drastically that it provides little opportunity and incentive for communication. I doubt that these assumptions foster objective and enthusiastic interest in communication of the aged, or that they are entirely justified. The writer's experiences while working in a geriatric environment generally do not concur with these impres-

> sions. The aged usually are quite interested in communication, and many of them who have speech and language problems want to improve their communicative skills. Heretofore, however, remedial speech programs for the aged have been comparatively meager. Many times have aged persons expressed in vain the desire to talk with someone, or to improve their communicative skills. (p. 641)

It is clear to the present authors that systematic research efforts are critically needed to delineate the role of speech and language pathologists in the treatment of patients with intellectual impairments. This endeavor should begin with a careful documentation of the speech and language characteristics of normal elderly people—this research endeavor is well under way. Furthermore, there should be careful delineation of the typical changes in communicative function observed among demented patients—little experimental work has been undertaken in this area. Given this substrate of knowledge, the speech and language pathologist should develop experimental therapy programs and, through carefully controlled outcome research, determine if speech/language pathology can help these patients to live with a richer quality of existence. Butler and Lewis (1977) summarized this message well when they said:

> Any evidence pointing toward older people as untreatable is usually found in the minds of therapists rather than in empirical studies. Powerful forces of countertransference and cultural prejudice are at work, including personal fear and despair over death. Therapeutic pessimism and nihilism are inappropriate, invalid, and inhumane. The elderly, like the young, can gain from insight and understanding, from objectivity and empathy. Biology is not destiny in old age any more than in youth. (p. 264)

SUGGESTED READINGS

Butler, R. N., and Lewis, N. I. Aging and Mental Health. St. Louis: C. V. Mosby, 1977.

Miller, E. Abnormal Ageing. London: John Wiley & Sons, 1977.

Paden, E. P. A History of the American Speech and Hearing Association 1925–1958. Washington, D.C.: American Speech and Hearing Association, 1970.

Weiss, A. E. Communicative needs of the geriatric population. Journal of the American Geriatrics Society, 19, 640–645 (1971).

REFERENCES

Bloomer, H. H. Speech and language disorders as a function of aging. Hearing and Speech News, 39, 14–15 (1971).

Brook, P., Degun, G., and Mather, M. Reality orientation, a therapy for psychogeriatric patients: A controlled study. British Journal of Psychiatry, 127, 42–45 (1975).

Butler, R. N., and Lewis, M. I. Aging and Mental Health. St. Louis: C. V. Mosby, 1977.

Howell, S. C. Advocates for the elderly: A contribution to the reshaping of the professional image. Hearing and Speech News, 39, 7–9 (1971).

Libb, J. W., and Clements, C. B. Token reinforcement in an exercise program for hospitalized geriatric patients. Perceptual and Motor Skills, 28, 957–968 (1969).

Miller, E. Abnormal Ageing. London: John Wiley & Sons, 1977.

Mueller, D. J., and Atlas, L. Resocialization of regressed elderly patients: A behavioral management approach. Journal of Gerontology, 27, 390–392 (1972).

Paden, E. P. A History of the American Speech and Hearing Association 1925–1958. Washington D.C.: American Speech and Hearing Association, 1970.

Strandberg, T. E. A national study of United States hospital speech pathology services, report number one. Asha, 19, 69–76 (1977a).

Strandberg, T. E. A national study of United States hospital speech pathology services, report number two. Asha, 19, 160–163 (1977b).

Van Riper, C. The Nature of Stuttering. Englewood Cliffs, N.J.: Prentice-Hall, 1971.

Weiss, A. E. Communicative needs of the geriatric population. Journal of the American Geriatrics Society, 19, 640–645 (1971).

Wolfensberger, W. The principle of normalization and its implications for psychiatric services. American Journal of Psychiatry, 127, 291–297 (1970).

Chapter 21
Speech and Language Therapy

The intent of this chapter is to discuss such issues as: which patients should be referred to a speech pathologist for help, when therapy should begin, and the effectiveness of speech and language therapy. These issues are discussed relative to the speech and language disorders presented in Section III.

As pointed out in the preceding chapter, apparently a great deal of misapprehension still exists among health professionals about the rehabilitative potential of the aged. In this regard, Rusk (1971) stated that "... the realistic potential of the older patients for making significant functional gains from therapy is widely underestimated. Age alone should not be a reason to exclude, a priori, an older patient from the benefits of therapy" (p. 659). Clinical experience and research have shown that encouraging results can be obtained with elderly patients even though therapeutic progress may be slow (McCoy and Rusk, 1953; Wallace, 1964; Bloomer, 1971).

Philosophically, the major objective for speech/language therapy for the aged is maximizing and maintaining communication skills for independent living, emotional adjustment, and effective environmental contact (Hefferin, 1968; Kaplan and Ford, 1975). The therapeutic emphasis should be on the highest possible degree of communication skills obtainable that will enable the elderly person to function in the environment. The communicatively impaired aged are capable of achieving improved speech and language skills, and once these improvements have been maximized they should be maintained for as long as feasible. Ignoring a disability is far more costly to the individual and to society than an early aggressive program of rehabilitation (Rusk, 1971). The theme of this chapter, then, is to advocate early therapeutic intervention with the communicatively handicapped and to instill in the reader the notion that age is not a sufficient reason for excluding the elderly from rehabilitative services.

WHO SHOULD BE REFERRED FOR SPEECH AND LANGUAGE THERAPY?

Given that age should not be a limiting factor in referring a patient for rehabilitative services, the question still remains as to who ought to be seen by the speech pathologist. In general, anyone who is unable to communicate or who is not easily understood should at least be evaluated. It is the contention of these authors that a speech and language evaluation should be a part of any admission routine in a nursing home or long-term care facility. Where this practice has not been in effect, its implementation should be preceded by an initial screening of all residents. In addition to identifying the elderly who need therapy services, such a plan is also beneficial for the nursing home staff. Knowing which residents have communication problems and the nature of the disorder will help the house staff work with these individuals in more appropriate and effective ways. This same principle also applies for hospitalized elderly patients. Patients who have neurologic problems, vascular disorders, cancer of the speech mechanism, and articulation or voice disorders all need help and should receive therapy.

Based on an 11-year study by Kaplan and Ford (1975) one might reasonably expect about 15% or more of nursing home residents to require speech therapy services. Other evidence suggests that Kaplan and Ford's data are somewhat conservative. For example, Bloomer (1960) found that 45% of the residents in a county hospital facility had speech and language impairments. Page (1967) reported that 56% of the geriatric patients studied in an institution had handicapping speech and language disorders. Data collected by these authors from 10 nursing homes around the State of Idaho are similar to those of Bloomer and Page. In the average Idaho nursing home, about 40% of the residents had speech and language disorders, 17% had aphasia, and 23% had some form of dysarthria. A number of voice and intellectual degeneration cases were found as well. These data varied depending on the type of facility being screened. Where the nursing care facility had a selective admission policy, fewer patients were identified who needed speech and language services than might be expected in a county-operated home. The point to be made here is that a significant number of geriatric patients in health care facilities need speech and language therapy. Only those patients whose medical condition precludes participation in therapy should be excluded. This latter decision must remain with the physician.

INITIATION OF THERAPY

The question as to when speech/language therapy should begin has not posed a problem with respect to most communication disorders. Generally, once the problem has been noted and diagnosed, therapy is typically initiated soon thereafter. However, this has not been the case with laryngectomees and patients suffering from neurologic insults. In each instance, factors related to the particular nature of these two disorders must be taken into account. For example, the laryngectomee must have time to heal and the neurologic patient passes through a spontaneous recovery phase, both of which have important relationships to the initiation of therapy.

DYSARTHRIA

Therapy for the dysarthric is aimed primarily at maximixing the level of available speech functioning in the elderly patient. The philosophy and techniques used to rehabilitate older dysarthrics are essentially the same as those used with younger patients but modified to account for the physiology of the aging patient (Rusk, 1971). The essence of the therapy techniques applied to dysarthria is neuromuscular facilitation (Farber, 1973; Mysak, 1975).

Even though some authors maintain that speech therapy for the dysarthrias is largely of psychological value to the patient (Stein, 1942; Minnigh, 1971), others hold that these "negative" opinions seem to be premature (Canter, 1965; Samra, Riklan, Levita, Zimmerman, Waltz, Berymann, and Cooper, 1969). Samra et al. reported that several of their patients who received intensive speech therapy showed signs of improvement. Canter (1965) also affirmed that speech therapy may be extremely beneficial for dysarthric patients who remain neurologically stable for periods of time. The use of neurologic and pharmacologic treatment programs for these patients increases the likelihood of having a neurologically stable patient to work with in therapy.

APHASIA THERAPY

When and for Whom?

A recurring question about aphasia is whether or not speech and language therapy accomplishes worthwhile results for the aphasic person beyond what could be expected from spontaneous recovery.

A second question concerns the issue of when to start therapy with the neurologically impaired patient. The comments in this section also apply to the disorders of agnosia and apraxia of speech.

Although there have been various opinions expressed in the literature, perhaps four studies answer these questions best. The first study was by Butfield and Zangwill (1946). These authors studied two groups of aphasics, one which began therapy less than 6 months post trauma and the other which began therapy more than 6 months post insult. Their data suggested that there was a spontaneous recovery period and that earlier therapy made a significantly greater difference in language recovery. A second study by Wepman (1951) verified Butfield and Zangwill's findings. Like these earlier authors, Wepman also used early and late therapy groups with 1 year pre and post trauma being the differentiating factor. Unlike either of these two earlier studies, a third study by Vignolo (1964) compared a control group of aphasics with a therapeutic experimental group. From this study Vignolo concluded that the majority of spontaneous recovery took place during the first 2 months and that early, intensive aphasia therapy has a specific positive effect if such therapy lasts for at least 6 months. The fourth study by Kertesz and McCabe (1977) reported that recovery rates from aphasia were clearly related to the time of examination after onset. These authors also used a control group (spontaneous recovery) and an experimental (treatment) group for comparisons.

Taken together, the findings from these studies indicate that: 1) time elapsed from injury before therapy was begun is an important and significant factor in aphasia recovery, 2) the effects of speech/language therapy have the greatest positive effect when coincidental with the spontaneous recovery process, and 3) intensive therapy has a decidedly positive effect on recovery from aphasia, even for patients in whom spontaneous recovery has run its course. As to when actual aphasia rehabilitation can begin, Policoff (1970) suggested that therapy could start "...as soon as the patient is in physiological balance and his life is no longer at risk" (p. 99). In most instances this would be 2 to 3 days post insult.

Age as a Rehabilitation Factor

The literature indicates that prognosis for speech rehabilitation is less favorable for elderly aphasic patients. Vignolo (1964) found that improvement appears to be much less frequent in people over age

60 than those who are younger. Similarly, Sands, Sarno and Shankweiler (1969) concluded that age appeared to be the most potent variable influencing recovery and that older aged patients do not do as well. Two recent studies by Smith (1971) and Kertesz and McCabe (1977) verified these earlier findings. Smith found overall language impairment from aphasia was greater with advanced age. Kertesz and McCabe investigated recovery patterns in aphasia and found that age was correlated with recovery rates in the first 3 months post insult. The younger patients had higher initial recovery rates. An early study by Mitchell (1958) summarizes these points. As shown in Table 21-1, a greater percentage of younger aphasics (less than age 60) made substantial improvement as a result of speech and language therapy than the older aphasic group did. However, by inspecting Table 21-1, one may also note that the older group's therapeutic progress was almost equally divided between the slow improvement and substantial improvement categories. The older patient can improve from therapy, but the gains are not as dramatic as for younger aphasic patients.

ALARYNGEAL SPEECH THERAPY

Initiation

Gardner (1971) suggested that therapy should begin for a laryngectomee as soon as possible after the physician has given approval. This approval is usually given a few days after the nasogastric tube has been removed and the integrity of the pharyngoesophageal segment has been established. However, other factors may further delay initiation of therapy such as poor health and weakness, radiation therapy, plastic surgery, extensive scarring which prevents dilation or relaxation of the pharyngoesophageal sphincter (Diedrich

Table 21-1. Age and percentage improvement from aphasia therapy

		Improvement			
Age group	Deterioration	None	Slow	Substantial	Adjustment
45–49 (N = 13)	8	23	8	46	15
60 + (N = 42)	7	29	29	24	12

Source: Adapted from Mitchell (1958).

and Youngstrom, 1966), and dysphagia or an inability to swallow. Clinical experience has shown that those laryngectomees who must overcome these problems are not likely to develop good esophageal speech. In addition, patients who wait a long time (more than 2 years according to Gardner, 1971) will probably not develop very good esophageal speech either. In the latter instance, motivation seems to be the prime factor, as suggested in Chapter 15.

Efficacy

The factor of age as related to successful acquisition of esophageal speech has been the subject of several studies. While some investigators reported no significant difference between ages of good and poor esophageal speakers (Diedrich and Youngstrom, 1966; Snidecor, 1969), other studies maintained that age is a negative factor in learning to use esophageal speech well (Svane-Knudson, 1960; Smith, Rise and Gralnek, 1966). Svane-Knudson's data indicated that the older a patient is, the less likely he will attain adequate esophageal speech. Smith et al. also maintained that advanced age is a failure factor, and Table 21-2 presents a synopsis of their data.

The conflicts between these viewpoints are probably best resolved by Berlin's (1964) position, which holds that age alone is not necessarily the prime cause of failure. Rather, other factors associated with aging such as incentive, attitude, needs, and social role are far more important. In other words, age, in and of itself, does not determine levels of aspiration or motivation.

DYSPHAGIA

Both the laryngectomee and the neurologically impaired patient may have difficulty swallowing (dysphagia), but for different reasons. The laryngectomee may sustain injury to the cranial nerves (IX, X, XII) subserving the swallowing mechanism. Radiation therapy in-

Table 21-2. Comparison of age with speech proficiency

Age groups	Good speech (%)	Poor speech (%)
30–50 (N = 17)	88	12
50–70 (N = 97)	68	32
70+ (N = 14)	29	71

Source: Adapted from Smith et al. (1966).

volving the mouth region may also impair the laryngectomee's ability to initiate swallowing (Larson, 1972). Neurologically involved patients may be unable to swallow properly because of central lesions involving the medulla oblongata or as the result of peripheral disturbances affecting the nerves or muscles subserving swallowing.

Dysphagia can be managed therapeutically in most cases by teaching the patient how to swallow volitionally rather than reflexively. However, the neurologically impaired patient, particularly nonfluent aphasics and those with apraxia of speech, may have an oral apraxia component that will make voluntary swallowing actions difficult to achieve.

According to Larson (1972), successful dysphagia rehabilitation requires a team effort. He suggested that the speech pathologist should evaluate the swallowing mechanism, indicate how the problem should be managed, and, if necessary, train a person to feed the patient. This feeder can be a family member, a volunteer, or an aide. The nurse should coordinate through her nursing care plans the recommendations of the speech pathologist, the dietitian, and the physician. The physician determines the patient's ability to tolerate dysphagia rehabilitation.

SUGGESTED READINGS

Dickson, S. (ed.). Communication Disorders: Remedial Principles and Practices. Glenview, Ill: Scott, Foresman, 1974.

Perkins, W. H. Speech Pathology: An Applied Behavioral Science (2nd Ed.). St. Louis: C. V. Mosby, 1977.

REFERENCES

Berlin, C. I. Hearing loss, palatal function, and other factors in post-laryngectomy rehabilitation. Journal of Chronic Disorders, 17, 677–684 (1964).

Bloomer, H. H. Communication problems among aged county hospital patients. Geriatrics, 18, 291–295 (1960).

Bloomer, H. H. Speech and language disorders as a function of aging. Hearing and Speech News, 39, 14–15 (1971).

Butfield, E., and Zangwill, O. L. Re-education in aphasia: A review of 70 cases. Journal of Neurology, Neurosurgery and Psychiatry, 9, 75–79 (1946).

Canter, G. J. Speech characteristics of patients with Parkinson's disease, III: Articulation, diadochokinesis, and over-all speech adequacy. Journal of Speech and Hearing Disorders, 30, 217–224 (1965).

Diedrich, W. M., and Youngstrom, K. A. Alaryngeal Speech. Springfield, Ill: Charles C Thomas, 1966.

Farber, S. D. Sensorimotor Evaluation and Treatment Procedures for Allied Health Personnel (1st Ed.). Indiana University Occupational Therapy Program, Bloomington, 1973.

Gardner, W. H. Laryngectomee Speech and Rehabilitation. Springfield, Ill: Charles C Thomas, 1971.

Hefferin, E. A. Rehabilitation in nursing home situations: A survey of the literature. Journal of the American Geriatrics Society, 16, 293–313 (1968).

Kaplan, J., and Ford, C. S. Rehabilitation for the elderly: An eleven-year assessment. The Gerontologist, 15, 393–397 (1975).

Kertesz, A., and McCabe, P. Recovery patterns and prognosis in aphasia. Brain, 100, 1–18 (1977).

Larson, G. L. Rehabilitation for dysphagia paralytica. Journal of Speech and Hearing Disorders, 37, 187–194 (1972).

McCoy, G., and Rusk, H. An evaluation of rehabilitation. Rehabilitation Monograph 1. New York: University-Bellevue Medical Center, 1953.

Minnigh, E. C. The changing picture of parkinsonism, Part II: The Northwestern University concept of rehabilitation through group physical therapy. Rehabilitation Literature, 32, 38–39, 50 (1971).

Mitchell, J. Speech and language impairment in the older patient. Geriatrics, 13, 467–476 (1958).

Mysak, E. Dysarthria and oropharyngeal development and evaluation. Physical Therapy Review, 55, 235–241 (1975).

Page, E. R. Speech and language characteristics of institutionalized and geriatric patients. In Proceedings 7th International Congress of Gerontology (Vol. 4). Vienna: Viennese Medical Academy, 1967.

Policoff, L. D. The philosophy of stroke rehabilitation. Geriatrics, 25, 99–107 (1970).

Rusk, H. A. Rehabilitation Medicine. St. Louis: C. V. Mosby, 1971.

Samra, K., Riklan, M., Levita, E., Zimmerman, J., Waltz, J. M., Berymann, L., and Cooper, I. S. Language and speech correlates of anatomically verified lesions in thalamic surgery for parkinsonism. Journal of Speech and Hearing Research, 12, 510–540 (1969).

Sands, E., Sarno, M. T., and Shankweiler, D. Long-term assessment of language function in aphasia due to stroke. Archives of Physical Medicine and Rehabilitation, 50, 202–206, 222 (1969).

Smith, A. Objective indices of severity of chronic aphasia in stroke patients. Journal of Speech and Hearing Disorders, 36, 167–207 (1971).

Smith, J. K., Rise, E. N., and Gralnek, D. E. Speech recovery in laryngectomized patients. Laryngoscope, 76, 1540–1546 (1966).

Snidecor, J. C. Speech Rehabilitation of the Laryngectomized. Springfield, Ill.: Charles C Thomas, 1969.

Stein, L. Speech and Voice. London: Methuen, 1942.

Svane-Knudson, V. The substitute voice of the laryngectomized patient. Acta Otolaryngologica, 52, 85–93 (1960).

Vignolo, L. A. Evolution of aphasia and language rehabilitation: A retrospective exploratory study. Cortex, 1, 344–367 (1964).

Wallace, M. Speech therapy with geriatric aphasia patients. In R. Kaslenbaum (ed.), New Thought on Old Age. New York: Springer, 1964.

Wepman, J. M. Recovery From Aphasia. New York: Ronald Press, 1951.

Chapter 22
Role of the Health Professional

Health professionals can combine their expertise to provide effective total treatment for communicatively impaired older people. In this chapter, the possibilities and difficulties of achieving a multiprofessional approach are discussed. Also summarized are specific actions which health care providers may take in caring for the patient's physical disorder, dealing with emotional aspects, and in communication. Finally, the role of the professional in coordinating and arranging for other help through community and professional resources is discussed.

In this chapter, as in this book as a whole, the focus is on giving guidance to the health professional who would like to improve his or her relationship with the elderly communicatively-impaired patient. It is hoped that a case has been made demonstrating the very great needs of the elderly in communication areas. Presumably the professional, having read earlier chapters, has an understanding of common hearing, speech, and language disorders. He or she knows about the role of the key communication disorder specialists, the audiologist, and the speech/language pathologist. Yet little has been said to direct the health professional in specific, active efforts. Thus, the aim of this chapter is to fill that gap.

In the ever expanding health care field, it is a considerable challenge to make a complete list of the various professionals and their associates. Certainly such a list will include physicians, dentists, dental hygienists, nurses (RNs and LPNs) and their aides, occupational therapists and their assistants, physical therapists plus their aides, nutritionists, optometrists, psychologists, social workers, rehabilitation counselors, laboratory or x-ray technicians, pharmacists, activity directors, health care administrators, and perhaps even ministers. Of course, such a list is not exhaustive, but at least it indicates some direction to the suggestions being proposed herein.

AWARENESS OF COMMUNICATION DISORDERS IN DELIVERY OF HEALTH CARE

Knowledge and awareness of common communication disorders is, of itself, a large step in the right direction. It helps, for example, to know that presbycusic hearing loss develops gradually and tends to be worse in the high pitches. Consequently, hearing and understanding women's and children's voices often creates a great challenge for some elderly persons. Similarly, awareness of the different types of aphasia assists in understanding the various symptoms and communication patterns of these patients.

This type of knowledge is needed, since far too little thought may occur in connection with the communication aspects of care. For instance, when the patient with hearing loss presents himself for a physical examination, it is possible that he cannot understand some of the physician's questions. If he tries to bluff, he may appear to be senile, and, if, in turn, the elderly person is treated as if he were senile, the establishment of a good relationship between patient and professional may be jeopardized.

In typical health care, a great deal of information is usually communicated to the patient via hearing. As Bettinghaus and Bettinghaus (1976) pointed out, in the hospital:

> . . . the patient is told about medication, is told when to awaken, when to eat, how to bathe and many other commonplaces. For the average patient the system works well. For the hearing-impaired patient the system may not work well. Yet few health care facilities have made formal provisions for alternative ways of passing along information . . . (p. 131)

The informed professional should recognize that up to 40% of the aged may have hearing loss, and, in long-term care units, on the average 80% will have a loss (see Chapter 4). Thus, health personnel can always be on the alert to compensate for this difficulty. This is probably most important in acute care, since the professional may have only a short time to make appropriate adjustments for effective communication. Bettinghaus and Bettinghaus (1976) illustrate the implications in this situation:

> The physician, the nurse, the dietician, x-ray technician, the orderly, and the laboratory technician may all need to communicate with any given patient. In a large facility, not only one physician but many different physicians may need to communicate with the patient.
>
> When the patient is aged and has a hearing impairment, a strain may well be placed on the relationship . . . . The patient who has de-

> veloped a long-term relationship with a personal physician benefits from the physician's knowledge of and adjustment to the disability .... The same patient, when placed in a complex health care facility, will lose that benefit. Some of the personnel on the hospital ward may not realize the patient has a hearing disability. Other staff who realize the impairment may not accommodate for it in a manner that is comfortable for the patient, and the patient-provider relationship will deteriorate. (pp. 130–131)

The importance of communication can be demonstrated also with respect to speech disorders. As a case in point, Skelly (1975) has interviewed a number of aphasic patients who reported their feelings about communication with the health professionals during the course of their illness. She found a number of commonly reported complaints, including the following:

1. Their feelings of fear and anguish would have been reduced in the immediate post-trauma period if they had received reassurance and some explanation of what had happened to them.
2. They could understand what was being said fairly soon after the onset of the aphasia and long before they could respond to what was heard.
3. They were insulted by professionals because they were talked about as if they were not there or treated like little children.
4. Because people assumed they could not understand much, few if any, explanations were given them about procedures or decisions.
5. They were aware of and sensitive to nonverbal cues given by hospital workers which indicated annoyance or impatience.
6. Too many strangers, who did not seem to be related to the patient's illness, would come unexpectedly to observe them like some animal in a zoo and were a source of irritation.
7. People asked too many questions at one time or repeated the same question too quickly, which made answering all the more difficult.
8. They needed more time to respond to questions, but few people waited long enough for an answer.
9. Because of their illness they "heard slower" and people talked too fast.
10. Noise was especially irritating in health care facilities because people talked too loudly, TV sets were always blaring, doors were slammed, equipment rattled or squeaked, and loudspeaker announcements were too loud and frequent.

The evidence suggests that health care professionals who are aware of these common feelings can provide much more in the way of understanding and support than they otherwise could.

The informed health care professional is cognizant that, besides the common sensory disabilities like hearing and vision, there are also changes in health, physical mobility, and environment for the typical older person. These have been discussed in this text (see Chapter 3) because they can influence effective communication. In fact, emotional reactions which accompany new fears, new surroundings, new family life styles, and new associations with different people increase the need for open channels of communication. An awareness of and an understanding approach to these circumstances can do much to smooth the health care relationship. Novick (1967) reported on the relocation of 125 institutionalized elderly patients. In moving from one facility to another, special communication efforts were made to counteract the fear of the unknown and to assure the patients that familiar people would still be present in the new setting. Under these circumstances the death rate in the new building was lower than it had been before. Better research of this sort needs to be done, but it does suggest that health care is improved through good communication even in the face of environmental change.

THERAPEUTIC ROLE OF THE HEALTH PROFESSIONAL: PROMOTING A TEAM APPROACH

Though a particular health professional may not be qualified to deliver the needed specialized therapy, he may contribute valuable care if his expertise can be combined with that of other professionals attending the patient. Leutenegger (1975) pointed out that:

> . . . none of us, as rehabilitation specialists, can function effectively autonomously. The greatest values accrue to the patient who is approached by a staff completely imbued with the team approach . . . . Not only must the staff discuss the patient's needs and attitudes, but they need also to talk with the patient about what and how he is doing.
>
> Other members of the staff, as well as family members, need to see the full array of the patient's problems. Each professional person has the responsibility to help all other members of the staff to see the problem as they see it. (pp. 121–122)

Federal law has recently mandated programs like the Professional Standards Review Organization (PSRO) and Utilization

Review (UR) to ensure the necessity, quality, and appropriate use of health services for various recipients of federal monies (Federal Register, 1974). Another program sponsored in part by federal funds brought speech and hearing professionals together with various nursing home health professionals (ASHA, 1977). The thrust of programs like this is to bring health professionals together to thoughtfully evaluate the care the patient is receiving as compared with the care he ought to be receiving. It is recognized that one professional, acting independently, cannot fully anticipate the best rehabilitation for the patient. Of course, such review occurs in facilities not associated with federal funding, and there is recognition by many professionals of the value of such a process.

One excellent example of a professional team approach is provided by the Geriatric Center of Mansfield Memorial Homes (Mansfield, Ohio). Professionals from this facility have reported on their program, which has been in existence for over 11 years (Kaplan and Ford, 1975). This nursing home is a 99-bed private, nonprofit, skilled nursing unit. The professional team includes persons trained in dietetics, social work, medicine, nursing, pharmacy, recreation, sociology, psychology, and occupational, physical, and speech therapy. Adjunctive professionals are drawn from the fields of dentistry, optometry, and podiatry.

One goal of this team is to achieve restoration of the elderly patient's physical and social capabilities so that he can return to independent living, if possible. Bettinghaus and Bettinghaus (1976) have emphasized the desirability of independent living arrangements for the elderly whenever possible because of the traumatic effect of a permanent move compared to the change of pace when a brief visit to a health care facility is involved. In the 11-year period reported on by Kaplan and Ford (1975), 1864 patients were admitted to the facility. For this group, there were staff conferences for coordinative purposes about 50 times per year. The strength of this team rehabilitative effort is indicated by the fact that 1135 persons, age 62–99, were discharged, 693 of whom to independent living arrangements.

Despite such happy successes with team approach therapy, there is often tremendous inertia in getting health professionals to work together routinely. A major deterrent to cooperative action is education. Even with an exposure to the information contained in this text or others like it from other fields, it is not reasonable to expect any one professional to have much more than a general knowledge of other professions. For example, evidence has been cited in this book which indicates a lack of attention by some health professionals to the communication problems of their patients (see Chapters 18 and 20). But neglect in understanding other professions is evident among the communication disorder specialists as well. Leutenegger and Stovall (1971) were aware of this situation in the training of students in the speech and hearing field, and so they organized a course to improve interdisciplinary exposure. To their seminar, entitled "The Role of the Speech Pathologist in a Multiprofessional Approach to the Chronically Ill and Aged," they invited various lecturers. These included a physiatrist, a neuropathologist, a health care administrator, a public health nurse, a physical therapist, an occupational therapist, a dentist, a social worker, a physician, and a clergyman. As part of the course, students were allowed to observe in action a consultative team from the Public Health Section of Chronic Disease and Aging. Leutenegger and Stovall reported that this observation experience effectively demonstrated the value of mutual problem solving rather than serial referral among specialists. Many of the students at the beginning of the course tended to prescribe therapy for sample cases they evaluated without consideration of the roles of other professionals. Students did not tend to envision their roles in terms of using or consulting with other professional people who were also caring for the patient. Fortunately, by the end of the course, many of these attitudes had changed to a multiprofessional problem-solving approach.

Such attitudes as those initially shown by these students are probably quite representative of feelings found in students being trained in many health professions. Without exposure to such a multidisciplinary course, these attitudes may persist well into a person's professional years. It is urgent that more health care students receive training of this sort, for, while some work settings provide an introduction to a team approach, many do not.

SUGGESTIONS FOR DEALING WITH THE ELDERLY

In this section, a number of general suggestions are offered for providing acute and long-term health care when working with the elderly patient having communication disorders. Also included in appendices are specific suggestions for communicating with the gerontologic patient. These pointers may apply to any person talking to the elderly, whether that person is a professional, family member or friend.

General Suggestions for the Hearing Impaired

Sometimes it is difficult to tell whether the elderly patient is hard of hearing or is confused from neurologic impairment or has both conditions. This may cause some ambiguity in terms of how to manage the case. In acute care, when there is any doubt about hearing ability, an evaluation of hearing (see Chapter 6) should be arranged. In long-term care, some type of abbreviated hearing measurement should be arranged for all patients when they are admitted to the facility or soon thereafter. In the case of outpatients, health professionals may wish to employ the Hearing Handicap Scale (HHS) as a paper and pencil screening device in order to identify those who should be referred for audiological or otological evaluation. The use of HHS in this fashion is described in Chapter 6, and a copy of both forms of this scale is contained in Appendix A of that chapter. Such a self-evaluation scale is certainly not a foolproof method for identifying those with hearing impairment, but it does have the advantage that it can be easily administered, perhaps while patients are waiting for their appointments in health professionals' offices. Furthermore, a simple 30% cut-off has been shown to identify a substantial proportion of elderly subjects with serious hearing loss, without excessive over-referral of those who do not have hearing impairment (Shenoy, Tannahill, and Schow, 1975). The value of using HHS this way is in alerting patients to the availability of help for hearing problems they may be ignoring. It should not be a basis for discouraging formal evaluation of those who suspect they have a loss.

Once the hearing status is known, appropriate care can be initiated for those patients who have definite hearing disability. After medical referral, or aural rehabilitation, or both, it will probably still be necessary for the health care provider to make adjustments to compensate for the loss or to assist the patient. Some will need help with a hearing aid. Suggestions for providing this assistance are contained in Chapter 19. Others may not be able to use amplification, and, in these cases, when loss is still present, the professional should be alert to the hearing problems of this patient in order to facilitate good care. Whether or not a hearing aid is used it is important to have regular otoscopic examinations to keep the ear canals clear. This is a simple matter which may improve hearing, but it is often neglected (McCartney and Alexander, 1976; Nerbonne, Schow, and Goset, 1976). The older hard-of-hearing person has a tendency to withdraw or to feel paranoid when left out of conversations. He should therefore be encouraged to participate in group activities, and a fellow patient with good hearing can be asked to go with him on various occasions and give helpful clues. TV and radio listening can occasionally be a problem, since the person may play these at a loud level and disturb other patients. Special amplifiers can be provided or purchased to rectify this problem (see Chapter 19). Specific suggestions for communicating with the hard-of-hearing patient are contained in Appendix A.

General Suggestions for the Aphasic or Agnosic Patient

The care for brain-injured patients with aphasia or agnosia should follow a predictable daily routine whenever possible. Since the person may be quite disoriented and confused, this will give some stability and be quite reassuring to him. In connection with these routine activities, the care provider should make efforts to communicate with the patient, giving him an opportunity to hear simple speech in connection with familiar events.

The health professional should be careful not to discuss the condition of the patient in his presence, since, while he may not understand completely, he may sense the mood or other visual clues, and it is possible that parts of the message which he does understand would alarm him. In terms of prognosis, it is better not to give a patient false hope by saying things like, "Your speech will soon come back," but rather encourage him to do his best, since this will improve his chances for recovery.

It will often be beneficial for the patient to listen to TV or radio, since this provides verbal stimulation. This can be encouraged if he seems to enjoy it. Also, the aphasic person should be invited to participate in group activities, since this will provide language stimulation and have social value. It should be remembered, however, that aphasic patients sometimes have difficulty regulating their emotions and sometimes will laugh or cry uncontrollably. Therefore, members of the health team should be alert to change an activity or a discussion which is emotionally stressful or to remove the person from the situation. It is important to avoid being overly solicitous, but it is also good to express to the patient an understanding of this unusual behavior. Appendix B lists suggestions for communicating with the aphasic or agnosic.

General Suggestions for the Apraxic Patient

Inasmuch as apraxia is the result of brain damage as is aphasia and is often seen in conjunction with aphasia, the care for these individuals should be identical to that described earlier for aphasics. With respect to communicating with an apraxic person, one must understand that in the absence of more generalized brain damage, understanding will not be impaired. Furthermore, the apraxic will often exhibit considerable difficulty articulating certain words which may be quite frustrating to the listener as well as the speaker. Specific suggestions for communicating with the apraxic patient are in Appendix C.

General Suggestions for the Dysarthric Patient

It must be understood that the person with dysarthria may exhibit a speech problem as the result of many precipitating factors. Furthermore, the degree of severity may range from complete incapacitation with respect to oral communication to only a mild articulatory deficit. As a result of this considerable variability in communicative skill, it is difficult to prescribe an exact set of communicative care procedures. Certainly, as with all other elderly individuals with communication problems, it is wise to keep dysarthrics in the social and communicative world. As with apraxic patients, the dysarthric may evidence considerable frustration in his efforts to communicate but usually will not exhibit any impairments in understanding. Appendix D lists tips for communicating with the dysarthric patient.

General Suggestions for the Laryngectomee

In these cases the patient, unless he is hearing impaired, will generally have no difficulty in understanding what is said to him. Nevertheless, the care provider will need to exhibit understanding when the patient is trying to communicate at various times. When the health care provider has difficulty communicating with a laryngectomee, he must exercise considerable patience and as tactfully as possible ask the patient to repeat. One might say, for example, "I missed that one. I'm sorry. Could you give it to me again." Most laryngectomy patients can increase articulatory precision and with such a reminder will be able to make the message intelligible. In addition, the subject may have difficulty swallowing, and all health professionals should be cognizant of this fact. This condition puts tremendous emotional burdens on the patient (see Chapter 15 and 23), and understanding and sympathy are important. Appendix E contains suggestions for communicating with these patients.

General Suggestions for the Confused or Intellectually Impaired Patient

As discussed in Chapter 14, confused or intellectually impaired often tend to be disoriented in terms of time and place. There will particularly be a loss in short-term memory, frequent difficulty in comprehension, and occasionally rambling or incoherent speech. These patients may also have intervals of delirium or hallucination and periods of depression or paranoia (Bollinger, Waugh, and Zatz, 1977).

As with other brain-injured patients, it is important to provide a calm, relaxed atmosphere and follow a regular routine in daily care. The room arrangement can also be examined and adjusted to avoid shadows at night in order to promote calm and reduce hallucinations. Health professionals can help these patients become oriented to time and physical facilities through a number of approaches, such as calling the person by name regularly and including references to the time of day in normal conversation with the patient. For example, say "It is 2 p.m., Mrs. Jones, and nearly time for your nap." Large calendars on which important dates are marked and large clocks can be helpful. Signs or photos can be used to label the patient's own room and bed. Personal items should be in obvious view when possible. Patients can be shown where various rooms or objects are located and then asked to lead the way to these places.

The patient at first may need help with simple activities like hanging up clothes or turning on the radio at a level where it is not too loud. It may help to go through simple procedures in self-care with the patient by dividing these into several different steps which the patient should follow one at a time. Then the patient should be watched while he does these on his own. Confused persons can be encouraged to attend group activities, watch TV, or listen to music on the radio. Visitors are usually good for these people also, especially when they are familiar persons and when there are not too many present at once. Suggestions for communicating with these patients are contained in Appendix F.

REFERRALS—COMMUNITY RESOURCES

One valuable service which health professionals can render when they are familiar with communication disorders is to refer persons who may need assessment or rehabilitation. Many hospitals have departments of speech pathology and audiology, and progressive nursing homes will have consultant services available in these specialties. Other settings for these services are listed in Chapters 17 and 20. However, such resources are of no value to those who need them unless client and service somehow get together. Physicians and nurses, particularly, are charged with assessing needs of their patients, starting basic health care programs, making appropriate referrals, and arranging consultations (Leutenegger, 1975). In this context, three of the standards for geriatric nursing read as follows (Moses, Grant, Brown, Knowles, and Lane, 1970, pp. 1894–1897);

> Standard 1: The nurse observes and interprets minimal as well as gross signs and symptoms associated with both normal aging and pathologic changes and institutes appropriate nursing measures.
>
> Standard 6: The nurse employs a variety of methods to promote effective communication and social interaction of aged persons with individuals, family, and other groups.
>
> Standard 8: The nurse assists older persons to obtain and utilize devices which help them attain a higher level of function and ensures that these devices are kept in good working order by the appropriate persons or agencies.

All of these standards imply the involvement of communication disorder specialists. So, the nurse who is familiar with communication disorders and their symptoms can assist the patient in getting the help he needs.

Even though the nurse and physician have prime responsibility in the area of referral, any professional health care provider may coordinate and arrange for specialized help. Health professionals should be aware of community resources as listed in Chapter 23 and help patients to take advantage of these services. The health care worker can also work with the family to obtain services, or additionally they can arrange for finances or provide moral support for these efforts. In short, the role of the health professional in the area of communication disorders is a very broad and very important one. It entails knowledge, awareness, interdisciplinary cooperation, specific communication efforts, and being alert to referral possibilities.

SUGGESTED READINGS

ASHA. Upgrading services to nursing home patients with communicative

disorders. Breaking the Silence Barrier Participant Manual. Washington, D.C.: American Speech and Hearing Association, 1977.
Bettinghaus, C. O., and Bettinghaus, E. P. Communication considerations in the health care of the aging. In H. J. Oyer and E. J. Oyer (eds.), Aging and Communication. Baltimore: University Park Press, 1976.
Bollinger, R. L., Waugh, P. F., and Zatz, A. F. Communication Management of the Geriatric Patient. Danville, Ill.: Interstate, 1977.
Christensen, J., Hutchinson, J., Nerbonne, M., and Schow, R. Speech and Hearing Problems: A Guide for Nursing Home Personnel. Pocatello, Idaho: Department of Speech Pathology and Audiology, Idaho State University, 1976.
Jodais, J. If your patient doesn't understand. In J. Jodais (ed.), Personal Care of Patient. Philadelphia: W. B. Saunders, 1970.
Leutenegger, R. R. Patient Care and Rehabilitation in Communication-Impaired Adults. Chapter 9. Springfield, Ill.: Charles C Thomas, 1975.
Maloney, C. C. The occupational therapist on a geriatric rehabilitation team. The American Journal of Occupational Therapy, special issue: Programs for the Elderly, 30, 300–304 (1976).

REFERENCES

ASHA. Breaking the Silence Barrier. In-Service Training Program. Washington, D.C.: American Speech and Hearing Association, 1977.
Bettinghaus, C. O., and Bettinghaus, E. P. Communication considerations in the health care of the aging. In H. J. Oyer and E. J. Oyer (eds.), Aging and Communication. Baltimore: University Park Press, 1976.
Bollinger, R. L., Waugh, P. F., and Zatz, A. F. Communication Management of the Geriatric Patient. Danville, Ill.: Interstate, 1977.
Federal Register. Current utilization review requirements for long-term care facilities, (November 29, 1974).
Kaplan, J., and Ford, C. S. Rehabilitation for the elderly: An eleven-year assessment. The Gerontologist, 15, 393–397 (1975).
Leutenegger, R. R. Patient Care and Rehabilitation of Communication-Impaired Adults. Springfield, Ill.: Charles C Thomas, 1975.
Leutenegger, R. R., and Stovall, J. D. A pilot graduate seminar concerning speech and hearing problems of the chronically ill and the aged. Asha, 13, 61–66 (1971).
McCartney, J., and Alexander, D. Geriatric audiology nursing home project: First year evaluation. Presented at the Annual Convention of the American Speech and Hearing Association, Houston, 1976.
Moses, D. V., Grant, M. D., Brown, M. I., Knowles, L. N., and Lane, H. C. Standards for geriatric nursing practice. American Journal of Nursing, 70, 1894–1897 (1970).
Nerbonne, M., Schow, R., and Goset, F. Prevalence of conductive pathology in nursing home population. Research Laboratory Report. Department of Speech Pathology and Audiology, Idaho State University, Pocatello, 1976.
Novick, L. J. Easing the stress of moving day. Hospital, 41, 64–74 (1967).

Shenoy, M., Tannahill, C., and Schow, R. Self assessment of hearing in a geriatric population. Paper presented at Annual Meeting of the Illinois Speech and Hearing Association, Chicago, 1975.

Skelly, M. Aphasic patients talk back. American Journal of Nursing, 75, 1104–1142 (1975).

APPENDIX A: COMMUNICATION TIPS WITH THE HARD-OF-HEARING OR DEAF

1. Whenever possible, communication with hearing-impaired persons should occur in a quiet environment. Radios, TVs, and stereos should be turned down and other background noises should be eliminated by closing doors or windows if feasible. Visual distractions can also interfere and should be reduced so that the listener can concentrate fully on the message.
2. Since considerable information is available by watching the lips, facial expressions, and gestures, the environment should be arranged for optimal lighting on the faces of those speaking to the hearing-impaired person. Turn on lights, rearrange positions to avoid glare, and achieve good lighting when possible. Also, distortions produced by eating, chewing gum, or covering the mouth with hands or fingers should be avoided.
3. Before speaking, get the attention of the hearing-impaired person by touching the shoulder, clearing the throat, or otherwise attracting attention.
4. Speak distinctly and somewhat more slowly than normal without elaborately mouthing or exaggerating the words. Don't shout, but speak at a good, loud level.
5. Give the person a clue as to the topic of conversation. "We're discussing politics, Dave," can politely be interjected when someone joins the group or if the person with a hearing loss seems confused. Also, avoid sudden shifts in the topic, and when there are topic changes this can be emphasized.
6. Avoid long involved sentences. Use appropriate gestures. When necessary to repeat, rephrase the sentence making it shorter and simpler if possible.
7. When telling a long or involved story or giving important instructions, wait to make sure the person understands before going on. The listener can be asked to repeat or be questioned on key aspects of the message. "Did you understand why you need to be there?" "Did you get the address?"

Additional Tips for Talking to Hearing Aid Users

1. When a person is using an aid, speak slowly and distinctly as to any hearing-impaired person. Don't talk too loudly or shout.

2. Encourage the hearing aid owner to wear the aid when you talk to him.
3. Be knowledgable about hearing aid function so that you can help the user having difficulty with amplification.
4. If he reports the aid is not working, check its function (see Chapter 19), and then, if there is nothing you can do, encourage him to seek professional help from the dispenser or audiologist.
5. Encourage the hearing aid user to have a hearing aid evaluation on a regular 1–2 year basis, at which time his hearing can be tested and his aid can be checked. With heavy use, some hearing aids will perform optimally for only 3–5 years. Also, hearing changes with time, and a different aid may be needed. Furthermore, hearing aids need to be analyzed electroacoustically to detect and correct subtle distortions of sound (see Chapter 19).

APPENDIX B: COMMUNICATION TIPS WITH THE APHASIC OR AGNOSIC PERSON

1. Communicate in a quiet, relaxed atmosphere free of competing conversations or background noises.
2. Tell the aphasic person what you are doing or are about to do. Be sure you have his attention before giving any instructions.
3. The agnosic or aphasic person usually has a preferential sensory modality (vision or hearing) through which he communicates best.
4. Keep instructions or questions short, simple, and direct. Use gestures to help communicate your intent. Questions that can be answered with "yes" or "no" are usually preferable.
5. Talk to the aphasic person at a slower rate, distinctly, and at an adult level. Avoid speaking loudly or with overexaggeration. Raising your voice or shouting will not necessarily help the person understand you.
6. Don't overreact or be surprised if an aphasic person swears even though they usually cannot speak. Remember, these people have difficulty in selecting their words and monitoring what they say.
7. Avoid discussions about abstract, emotional, or controversial topics. An aphasic person can comprehend what you say much better if you talk about specific events, objects, or people. In any event, let the aphasic person set the conversational tone and pace.
8. Encourage all attempts these people make at communicating, including social expressions, gestures, or pointing. Don't interrupt by offering all kinds of words or phrases or by doing their talking for them. Be patient, listen, and be aware of situational cues.
9. An aphasic patient often has visual field defects or blind spots in his sight. Present written materials and other items where they can be easily seen. If the person wears glasses be sure they are clean and properly positioned.
10. Since many elderly people have a hearing loss, be sure that hearing aids are being worn and in working order before attempting to communicate with them.

APPENDIX C: COMMUNICATION TIPS WITH THE APRAXIC PERSON

1. Patience and tolerance are the major attributes of a good listener for an apraxic patient. If the listener displays frustration and mild intolerance, it will often exacerbate the frustration of the apraxic, who is frequently fully cognizant of the errors being made.
2. An occasional phrase of support or understanding during moments of struggle is often helpful. For example, the listener might say, "I understand that you know what you want to say but are having difficulty getting it out. I'm in no hurry."
3. If the listener has difficulty understanding the patient, he may honestly say so and ask the patient if he wouldn't mind trying it again. Often, repeating back that segment of the message that was understood is helpful. For example, the listener might say, "I understand that you would like me to get you something, but I didn't quite understand what it was. Would you mind helping me out by trying it again?"
4. Often, it may be clear to the listener what a person with apraxia is attempting to say. It is perhaps better to nod encouragement rather than "filling in" the troublesome word. Otherwise, the person with apraxia may ultimately experience frustration and a reduced motivation to communicate.
5. Since understanding may not be impaired with this disability, it is unnecessary to reduce message complexity, raise the intensity of the voice, or alter articulatory patterns when communicating with the apraxic person.
6. It is unwise for the health care professional or family member to attempt any form of corrective exercise for the apraxic patient without specific training by a speech pathologist.

APPENDIX D: COMMUNICATION TIPS WITH THE DYSARTHRIC PERSON

1. It must be recognized that most persons with dysarthria, as is true for all normal talkers, do not typically speak with maximum precision. This is perhaps more true of the milder cases. Therefore, such subjects have a relatively wide range of precision and, when required, can articulate more precisely thereby increasing intelligibility. Accordingly, if the listener does not fully understand what is being said, some form of positive indication (verbal or nonverbal) will probably result in clearer speech.
2. In the more severely involved cases, the speech may be quite slow and marked by considerable effort. The listener must be patient and tolerant of the rate. In addition, he must not demand responses from the person that are lengthy and complex, since such utterances may lead to rapid fatigue. When fatigued, the dysarthric talker may have even greater problems with his intelligibility. When this occurs, of course, a rest is in order.
3. Since intensity of speech may be reduced and precision impaired, with dysarthrics the listeners and speaker should do whatever possible to make the environment conducive to good communication. It should be quiet, there should be no competing utterances while the dysarthric is speaking, and the speaker and listeners should face one another while talking.
4. In the extremely severe cases, paper-and-pencil or a communication board may be necessary to permit the patient an opportunity to make his basic desires and needs known.
5. In most cases of dysarthria, hearing and understanding are not likely to be abnormally impaired. Therefore, raising the voice, exaggerating articulatory precision, and slowing rate is unnecessary.
6. It is unwise for the health care professional or family member to attempt any form of corrective exercise for the dysarthric patient without specific training by a speech pathologist.

APPENDIX E: COMMUNICATION TIPS WITH THE LARYNGECTOMEE

Communicating with the Hospitalized Laryngectomee

1. Ask questions that require only a "yes" or "no" answer. The laryngectomee can use head gestures to indicate his response.
2. Where more information is required, provide either paper and pencil or a "magic" slate for the laryngectomee to use.
3. Be sure that the call button is within easy reach for the laryngectomee. Remember, he cannot call out for help.
4. Obtain a "loaner" artificial larynx for the patient to use while he is in the hospital. Artificial larynges that must be placed against the neck are unsatisfactory since vibration of the healing tissues is painful. Intraoral devices like the Cooper-Rand artificial larynx are much better.

Communicating with the Laryngectomee Who Can Talk

1. Avoid talking in noisy places. Alaryngeal speech tends to be somewhat quieter and less intelligible.
2. Watch the person's lips as he talks in order to obtain additional cues about what is being said.
3. If you are unsure what was said, try rephrasing what it was that you thought was spoken. The laryngectomee will then have some feedback to see if you are "getting the message."
4. Be patient; it usually takes a laryngectomee a little more time to say what he wants and if he feels pressured he cannot speak as well.

APPENDIX F: COMMUNICATION TIPS WITH A PERSON HAVING INTELLECTUAL AND MEMORY IMPAIRMENTS

1. Often these individuals are not well oriented with respect to time and place. Furthermore, they may not be aware of who is addressing them. This lack of orientation and recognition is often very difficult for family members to understand and appreciate. Nevertheless, when speaking with these patients, frequent reminders of time, place, and person are often necessary to maintain the conversation.
2. Patients with intellectual and memory impairments will frequently exhibit rambling, poorly integrated discourse with occasional jargon behavior. In such instances, the listener must attempt tactfully to "bring the patient back" to the immediate conversation either by a question or reminder.
3. On some occasions, the discourse may be so disoriented that the probability of meaningful conversation is negligible. On such occasions, the disabled person should not be prodded to interact, and attempts to resume the conversation should be attempted later.
4. The intellectually impaired individual is often very susceptible to treatment as a child by either health professionals or family members. Talking as to a child should be avoided. Because intellectual processing is impaired, however, reducing the complexity of utterances and permitting ample time to respond is most helpful.
5. In initiating conversations, the confused person may need to have his attention aroused. Bollinger, Waugh, and Katz (1977) recommend touching the person or prefacing remarks by calling his name.
6. It is unwise for the health care professional or family member to attempt any form of corrective exercise for the patient with intellectual or memory impairments without specific training by a speech pathologist.

Chapter 23
Role of the Family

The family has a very important role in helping the communicatively handicapped patient cope with his disorder. This chapter discusses what the family can do in the areas of socialization, acceptance of the patient's limitations, and understanding the need of the elderly patient to communicate. Additional information is also given about some community resources that can be called on by the family for help.

As a person gets older his family assumes an ever increasing amount of importance. The family is the older person's main source of emotional strength, companionship, and, more importantly, a prime source of help in an emergency or in the case of illness (Riley and Foner, 1968). As mentioned in Chapter 3, one of the phenomena of aging seems to be that as a person gets older there is a progressive trend toward fewer formal group relationships and closer ties with specific individuals. These last social ties to which the elderly cling are often those of their immediate family. During the later years of life, frequent interaction with one's relatives appears to be the rule rather than the exception in the United States (Sweetser, 1975). For example, Riley and Foner (1968) indicated that 84% of elderly people age 65 and older live within an hour's distance from at least one of their children. Furthermore, elderly people who are sick or whose activity or mobility is limited by chronic ailments are more likely to live with one of their children (Duffy, 1975).

Because of the changes which have taken place in our society, families generally no longer live in close proximity to each other. This does not mean, though, that there is little or no communication between family members or that families do not help each other when problems arise. Since the elderly person's family is an important socioeconomic element, this final chapter is directed toward the family and its role.

DELIVERING HEALTH CARE

With the high cost of centralized health care services many families find that home care is their only viable alternative. Research has shown that if a family is available and if it can get the needed direction and encouragement from a health care team, the communicatively handicapped patient can often live at home and receive better care as well (Lehmann, DeLateur, Fowler, Warren, Arnhold, Schertzer, Hurka, Whitmore, Masock, and Chambers, 1975). For this reason, delivery of health care services should not be directed solely to the aged person with a communication disorder but should be a family-oriented activity. It is recognized that quite frequently the family needs help as much as the patient does. Most families want to do something to help in time of need, but in some cases their efforts are unguided, nonproductive, or even counterproductive. Unfortunately, the geriatric patient with a communication problem is not always understood, even by family members, as to his limitations and reduced abilities. For these reasons, the rehabilitative challenge presented by the older communicatively impaired patient will also require the family to seek and expect help from the health care professionals. When a family has some understanding of the nature of an elderly patient's disorder, what can be reasonably expected, and how to effectively help, then adjustments are easier to make, misunderstandings are avoided, and worthwhile patient care results.

THERAPEUTIC ROLE

The family of an aged handicapped person is often required to assume the role of a nurse, occupational therapist, physical therapist, psychologist, rehabilitation audiologist, and speech therapist for months or years without any warning or training. In the case of the aged person who has a hearing loss, both the family and the patient need to know how to communicate with each other effectively and need to know the importance of monitoring residual hearing. Both the spouse and laryngectomee need to know about stoma protection and care, the limitations of alaryngeal speech, and the special health care problems this type of operation presents in the elderly. Similarly, family members should seek information about the physical and emotional problems of the aphasic, hearing impaired, apraxic, dysarthric, or intellectually impaired patient and how to cope with them. Essentially, the elderly patient with a communication disorder needs a lot of personal support, and the family is frequently best equipped to provide this type of daily, long-term help. In fact, Youmans and Yarrow (1971) pointed out that an intact, supportive, and intimate social environment is an important sociopsychological factor in resisting disorders in old age and is a significant factor in survival.

HELPING THE HARD-OF-HEARING OR DEAF FAMILY MEMBER

Sometimes it would seem that members of the family of someone with hearing impairment suffer as much and perhaps even more than the impaired person himself. The elderly person with hearing loss may appear serene and calm, basking in the peace and quiet which the impairment provides, while all around him everyone else tries in vain to communicate. Of course, it is not generally pleasant to be cut off from daily communication, and having such a disability is worse than it may seem. Nevertheless, the family suffers as well.

Common complaints about the hearing impaired by the family include:

1. He hears what he wants to.
2. He blames everyone else for his hearing problem.
3. He won't use his aid or, when he uses it, he still acts like he can't hear.

The family member should realize that it is possible to hear some parts of conversation or some voices more easily than others. Thus, the hearing impaired are usually innocent of the thing they are so often accused of, namely, hearing only what they want to hear. When a person has a hearing loss, it often requires great concentration and use of visual and other clues to fill in parts of the message which are not heard. If full effort is not put forth, the conversational meaning can easily be missed. With normal hearing, by contrast, one can hear and understand with very little effort. When the hearing impaired are tired or not watching carefully, it may require more concentration than they can muster to participate in communication.

It is not an easy thing sometimes to accept the fact that one has a disability. Considering the gradual way in which presbycusic losses develop, it is not surprising that many elderly persons who have a loss deny it and blame others "who don't enunciate". With gentle comments, the family member may be able to help the impaired person recognize that he possibly has a problem and encourage him to seek proper help. When a hard-of-hearing elderly person is seen by a physician or an audiologist, it is helpful for a member of the family to go with him. It is also important to attend aural rehabilitation classes with the new hearing aid user (see Chapters 6 and 18).

Finally, it should be recognized that hearing aids are only "aids" to hearing, and they do not generally restore auditory skills to normal performance. In addition, it is often difficult to become adjusted to hearing aid use. This difficulty is sometimes compared to the adjustment for contact lenses, which is generally much harder than learning to use conventional glasses. Berest (1977) reported that the median hearing aid adjustment time is about 6 months, and some persons are never able to use a hearing aid in all situations. Therefore, it behooves the family member to generate as much patience and understanding as possible in interactions with the hearing impaired. Adjustment can be facilitated when the hearing-impaired person attends hearing aid orientation sessions as recommended in Chapter 18. New hearing aid users should be encouraged to attend such sessions and family members should go with them since they will learn ways to help in the adjustment process. Chapter 19 also contains information which family members should study in order to help in the management of the hearing aid. Specific suggestions for communicating with the hard-of-hearing and deaf are contained in Chapter 22, Appendix A.

SUGGESTIONS FOR COPING WITH APHASIA, AGNOSIA, AND APRAXIA OF SPEECH

The family of an elderly individual suffering from aphasia, agnosia, or apraxia of speech is usually confronted with a number of problems. Family members reading this book should know that other families in the same situation have had similar problems and reactions. For example, Malone (1969) conducted a study where he interviewed the families of 20 aphasic patients. From this study he found that the most frequently mentioned problems were: 1) the spouse was forced to assume a different role—for example, if the disabled person were a husband, the wife found herself having to assume a more independent, dominant role to making family decisions; 2) the family's income was reduced, forcing the wife or other family members to go to work; 3) the family's social life was dramatically reduced; and 4) health problems were much more prevalent. Malone also found that the most frequent reactions to these problems were: 1) irritability, hostility, or frustration; 2) guilt feelings; 3) oversolicitiousness or an overprotective attitude; and 4) rejection.

Hildred Schuell (1964) emphasized three factors in counseling families of aphasic patients. These suggestions, based on her long clinical experience, were (pp. 328–331):

1. Accept the fact that dramatic changes toward improvement are not likely. Find out what a reasonable therapeutic goal will be and do not fruitlessly expend time, energy, and money on the unattainable.
2. It is important to understand the nature of the family member's disorder and that the elderly aphasic patient is not necessarily feeble minded or mentally deranged.
3. Learn to make the best possible adjustment to an altered life style, focusing on the importance of living as normally as possible within daily routine that gives meaning to life.

In adopting the role of a speech therapist in the home or in other settings, family members, in some respects, can do far more than any professional. Family members know each other better than any therapist ever will. Hence, the family will know what will motivate the elderly aphasic family member, what his interests are, and how to recognize fatigue and depression much quicker.

Family members can help the elderly aphasic understand what it is that is being said to them by using gestures, facial expressions, speaking a bit slower, and by using shorter phrases. Some important things family members can do to help the aphasic communicate with them are: 1) help him learn to use "yes" and "no" appropriately with gestures; 2) give him time to say what he has in mind: 3) provide word cues when needed; 4) do not ask several questions at one time; and 5) reduce or eliminate competing noises when talking to him. Additional suggestions for communicating with these persons are contained in Chapter 22, Appendices B and C.

HELPING THE DYSARTHRIC FAMILY MEMBER

The family member who has a dysarthric speech problem characteristically has an impaired ability to speak clearly or precisely, and in most instances this is his major communication problem. That is, these individuals can usually write, read, and understand what is said to them. Other members of the family should exercise patience and understanding when communicating with a dysarthric person.

If the speech of the dysarthric family member is difficult to understand, asking him to repeat, speak more carefully, or use gestures may prove helpful. Additional suggestions for communicating with the dysarthric family member may be found in Appendix D of Chapter 22.

HELPING THE LARYNGECTOMEE

The elderly person who has lost his larynx because of cancer has some fears or concerns which family members usually share as well. The major fear is in connection with the word "cancer" and its extremely negative connotations (Stoll, 1958). In this regard, the fear of death and losing a loved one is probably the greatest worry. The first 5 years following a cancer operation are of most concern because any residual cancer will usually make its presence known during that time. Until a "clean bill of health" is given, the fear of dying from cancer remains as a nagging specter. Secondary to this major fear are worries of the laryngectomee's ability to function normally, the aggravation expressed by the laryngectomee of being old and feeling even more useless, and concerns about being able to speak again.

Families of elderly persons should face their prime fear, death from cancer, with more optimism than people in the past have. As was pointed out in Chapter 15, the 5-year survival rate for laryngectomees is getting better. In any case, regular physical check-ups constitute the best insurance. The secondary worries can be compensated for or managed with some help and training. Of major importance is an optimistic attitude and the desire to try and overcome the problems of concern. Family members, in particular, can aid a great deal with their encouragement and positive attitude. Finally, a number of options are available to reestablish the ability to communicate, and the material in Chapter 15 indicates what they are.

Beyond being sure that the laryngectomee is given positive support and receives therapy there is one other thing that families of these patients should know about: giving artificial respiration to a laryngectomee. Individuals wishing further information and training in this matter should contact the American Cancer Society in their area. Suggestions for communicating with the laryngectomee are contained in Chapter 22, Appendix E.

HELPING THE INTELLECTUALLY DEGENERATED

The problem of intellectual degeneration in the elderly should not simply be ignored with the attitude that there is nothing the family can do to help. As suggested in Chapter 20, prescribable medications are available which may help reduce the effects of intellectual decline. The family might well take the lead in getting appropriate medical help if it is not suggested by its physician.

A key word which should guide the family in effectively helping the aged, intellectually impaired family member is "normalization." The intent here is to keep the surroundings and daily routines as familiar as possible. Institutionalization may complicate efforts at maintaining a familiar environment or activities. Even so, the family should try to keep the surroundings as familiar as possible in the nursing home by providing a favorite chair to sit in, the chest of drawers customarily used, favorite paintings or pictures of the family to look at, and other items which were normally used and enjoyed in previous years. It is further suggested that abrupt changes in dietary habits should be avoided. The family can help by informing the necessary health care personnel in what the person normally eats. Additionally, nursing homes may have reality therapy programs which can be supplemented by the family. Family members can help maintain the elderly person's contact with reality by taking them out for short walks, auto rides, or home visits if the health of the aged individual permits.

Family members can also help the elderly person remember who is visiting them by stating their name and telling some earlier incident or fact about themselves which will facilitate recall. Families also need to appreciate the fact that even with relatively good health the elderly person with an intellectual degeneration problem will probably continue to decline. Hence, family members should not over react if "Grandpa" does not remember them even with prompting. At all times family members should try to interact on an adult level. Communication tips for the person with intellectual degeneration are contained in Chapter 22, Appendix F.

COMMUNITY RESOURCES

To preserve some feeling of dignity and usefulness, the communicatively impaired older patient needs to be functionally independent in all of his daily activities. This goal can be facilitated if family members obtain proper counseling and know how and where to get help. As Lowey (1975) points out, availability and accessibility of existing services alone does not guarantee that they will be utilized. Obstacles such as difficulty in communicating, the effort required to manage bureaucratic forms, standing in time-consuming lines, an inability to get to the agency, and not really knowing who to see or where to go may prohibit the communicatively handicapped elderly person from obtaining the help needed. Many of these problems can be best solved by younger family members who have both the energy and ability to get the required help.

A number of community resources are available to help the family care for their impaired elderly. Church groups can provide emotional and spiritual support and, in most instances, home help with meals, housekeeping, and socialization. Self-help organizations, such as Lost Chord clubs sponsored by the American Cancer Society and stroke clubs, promote therapy, socialization, and disseminate helpful information in the communities where they serve. Other community agencies, such as the American Heart Association, the American Cancer Society, the Easter Seal Society for Crippled Children and Adults, and the American Red Cross also provide educational information and assistance in locating help, and in some instances therapeutic services are also made available. These agencies are supplemented in their efforts by senior citizens volunteer organizations which promote such services as Meals-onWheels, Handi-cabs, or transportation in private cars to obtain medical help. Government agencies which offer help are the Federal Social Security Administration, the Veterans Administration hospital centers and outpatient clinics, state public health services, and state mental health services. In addition to all of these resources for health care services many universities and colleges have speech and hearing training programs which can provide therapeutic services for communication disorders. Speech and hearing services are also available through community rehabilitation centers, speech and hearing clinics, and private speech therapists and audiologists, all of which are usually listed in the yellow pages of the phone book under such listings as "rehabilitation services" or "clinics," "speech pathologists," and "audiologists."

SUGGESTED READINGS

Buck, M. Dysphasia: Professional Guidance for Family and Patient. Englewood Cliffs, N.J.: Prentice-Hall, 1968.

Taylor, M. L. Understanding Aphasia: A Guide for Family and Friends. Patient publication 2, The Institute of Physical Medicine and Rehabilitation, New York University Medical Center, 1958.

REFERENCES

Berest, S. Family involvement in aural rehabilitation. Hearing Instruments, 28, 10, 22 (1977).

Duffy, B. J., Jr. Medical care of the elderly. In M. G. Spencer and C. J. Dorr (eds.), Understanding Aging: A Multidisciplinary Approach. New York: Appleton-Century-Crofts, 1975.

Lehmann, J. F., DeLateur, B. J., Fowler, R. S., Jr., Warren, C. G., Arnhold, R., Schertzer, G., Hurka, R., Whitmore, J. J., Masock, A. J., and Chambers, K. H. Stroke rehabilitation: Outcome and prediction. Archives of Physical Medical and Rehabilitation, 56, 383–389 (1975).

Lowey, L. Social welfare and aging. In M. G. Spencer and C. J. Dorr (eds.), Understanding Aging: A Multidisciplinary Approach. New York: Appleton-Century-Crofts, 1975.

Malone, L. Expressed attitudes of families of aphasics. Journal of Speech and Hearing Disorders, 34, 146–150 (1969).

Riley, M. W., and Foner, A. Aging and Society (Vol. 1: An Inventory of Research Findings). New York: Russell Sage Foundation, 1968.

Schuell, H., Jenkins, J. J., and Jimenez-Pabon, E. Aphasia in Adults. New York: Harper and Row, 1964.

Stoll, B. Psychological factors determining the success or failure of the rehabilitation program of laryngectomized patients. Annals of Otology, Rhinology, and Laryngology, 67, 550–557 (1958).

Sweetser, D. A. Sociologic perspectives on aging. In M. G. Spencer and C. J. Dorr (eds.), Understanding Aging: A Multidisciplinary Approach. New York: Appleton-Century-Crofts, 1975.

Youmans, E. G., and Yarrow, M. Aging and social adaptation: A longitudal study of health old men. In S. Granick and R. D. Patterson (eds.), Human Aging 2, U.S. Department of Health, Education, and Welfare, DHEW Pub. No. (HSM) 71-9037, pp. 95–103, 1971.

Index